D1472115

Second Edition

Elder Care
in Occupational Therapy

Second Edition

Elder Care

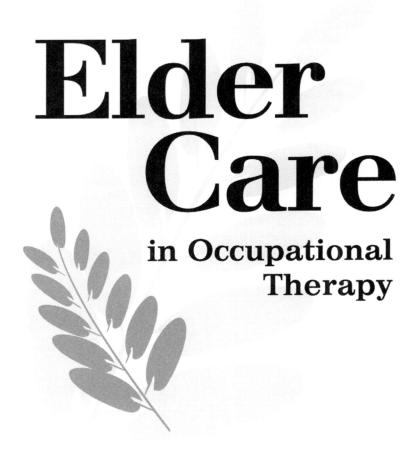

in Occupational Therapy

Sandra Cutler Lewis, MFA, OTR/L
Wyndmoor, Pennsylvania

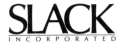

An innovative information, education, and management company
6900 Grove Road • Thorofare, NJ 08086

www.slackbooks.com

ISBN: 978-1-55642-527-1

Copyright © 2003 by SLACK Incorporated
Illustrations by Jon Di Venti
Cartoon image concepts by Sandra Cutler Lewis MFA, OTR/L (pp. 397-410)

The procedures and practices described in this book should be implemented in a manner consistent with the professional standards set for the circumstances that apply in each specific situation. Every effort has been made to confirm the accuracy of the information presented and to correctly relate generally accepted practices. The authors, editor, and publisher cannot accept responsibility for errors or exclusions or for the outcome of the material presented herein. There is no expressed or implied warranty of this book or information imparted by it. Care has been taken to ensure that drug selection and dosages are in accordance with currently accepted/recommended practice. Off-label uses of drugs may be discussed. Due to continuing research, changes in government policy and regulations, and various effects of drug reactions and interactions, it is recommended that the reader carefully review all materials and literature provided for each drug, especially those that are new or not frequently used. Any review or mention of specific companies or products is not intended as an endorsement by the author or publisher.

SLACK Incorporated uses a review process to evaluate submitted material. Prior to publication, educators or clinicians provide important feedback on the content that we publish. We welcome feedback on this work.

Published by: SLACK Incorporated
                       6900 Grove Road
                       Thorofare, NJ 08086 USA
                       Telephone: 856-848-1000
                       Fax: 856-853-5991
                       www.slackbooks.com

Library of Congress Cataloging-in-Publication Data

Elder care in occupational therapy / Sandra Cutler Lewis.-- 2nd ed.
   p. ; cm.
Includes bibliographical references and index.
 ISBN 1-55642-527-9 (alk. paper)
 1. Occupational therapy for the aged.
 [DNLM: 1. Occupational Therapy--Aged. 2. Chronic
Disease--rehabilitation--Aged. 3. Terminal Care--Aged. WB 555 L676e
2002] I. Title.
RC953.8.O22 L49 2002
615.8'5--dc21
                                                                        2002013516

Printed in the United States of America.
    Contact SLACK Incorporated for more information about other books in this field or about the availability of our books from distributors outside the United States.
    For permission to reprint material in another publication, contact SLACK Incorporated. Authorization to photocopy items for internal, personal, or academic use is granted by SLACK Incorporated provided that the appropriate fee is paid directly to Copyright Clearance Center. Prior to photocopying items, please contact the Copyright Clearance Center at 222 Rosewood Drive, Danvers, MA 01923 USA; phone: 978-750-8400; website: www.copyright.com; email: info@copyright.com.

Last digit is print number: 10   9   8   7   6   5   4   3

To life.

CONTENTS

Acknowledgments

My Early Years

My building blocks for developing a zest for "wanting to know and understand" came from my parents, Jack Cutler and Ethyle Reisman Cutler. They inspired me, at an early age, to always look at the world in a new light; life and study were part of the discovery process. My maternal grandmother, Bertha G. Reisman, taught me that history and wisdom were intertwined with people who were older. She provided me with songs and stories from the past. I cherished them then, and I cherish them today. Harriet Cutler Treatman, my older sister, brought laughter, adventure, and the ability to enjoy the moment into my life (even going to the supermarket to pick up a can of soup could be exciting).

My Professional Years

For more than 30 years, I have been an occupational therapist. Along the way, many individuals have played a part in my professional development. One person, in particular, stands out as having prompted me into writing, and that individual is Doris Kaplan (former director of occupational therapy at Norristown State Hospital for more than 20 years). It was she who taught me specifics of professional writing, and it was she who encouraged me to pursue this area of work. I can rightfully say that through these 30 years my association with occupational therapists, certified occupational therapy assistants, aides, physicians, nurses, recreational therapists, psychologists, physical therapists, and speech therapists (in a variety of work settings) has been one of great satisfaction and professional growth.

At this time, I would also like to express my gratitude to Alicia Kuenning for her highly professional and expert services in making this manuscript accessible for publication.

My Immediate Family Involvement

Last, but certainly in no way least, is my wonderful and loving family. To my son, Ethan Lawrence Lewis, I would like to thank him for continually involving me in new ways of thinking and helping me to develop my own inquisitiveness. To my oldest daughter, Judy B. Hoffman, I would like to thank her for her vivacious and poetic spirit as well as her undaunted determination in pursuing answers to an ongoing recent illness. She has taught me to value courage and perseverance. To my youngest daughter, Sharon Deborah Bloomgarden, I would like to acknowledge that her inquiring mind, creativity, and supportive nature have inspired me to want to achieve my fullest potential. It is her example of being able to analyze a situation and work through to a desired outcome (despite an encounter with a severe automobile accident) that has taught me to understand and appreciate insightfulness and bravery. To my dearest husband, Paul Lewis, I would like to thank him for his companionship and friendship of more than 40 years of marriage. His dedication and devotion to me with this project (and, indeed, many previous projects) have made it possible for me to complete this new edition.

Concluding Remarks

Meaningful interactions with individuals such as family members, friends, teachers, other professionals, and clients can serve to enrich our lives. It is these very experiences that help us to become more in touch with the "human" condition as we provide service to others.

About the Author

Sandra Cutler Lewis, MFA, OTR/L received her bachelor's and master's degrees from the University of Pennsylvania, Philadelphia. She has published articles pertaining to geriatrics in the following periodicals: *The Gerontologist, The American Journal of Occupational Therapy, Hospital and Community Psychiatry, Osteopathic Annals, The Activity Director's Guide, The Gerontology Special Interest Section Newsletter, The Occupational Therapy Forum,* and *The Journal of the American Geriatrics Society*. She has authored three books, *The Mature Years: A Geriatric Occupational Therapy Text, Providing for the Older Adult: A Gerontological Handbook,* and *Elder Care in Occupational Therapy*. Ms. Lewis has been a reviewer for a number of the American Occupational Therapy Association's (AOTA) position papers concerning gerontic occupational therapy; a professional publishing house; a paraprofessional, commercial publishing house; and a professional multi-disciplinary journal. She has served as a contributing author to AOTA's *Role of Occupational Therapy with the Elderly, First Edition* and as a member of the Editorial Review Board for Module III of the second edition of AOTA's *Role of Occupational Therapy With the Elderly*. Ms. Lewis has been listed in *Who's Who of American Women* and is a lifetime member of Sigma Phi Omega, the National Gerontology Academic Honor and Professional Society.

Work experience in adult care has included a community evening arts program in a settlement house, psychiatric occupational therapy in a private mental hospital, occupational therapy in a rehabilitation center, and acute care occupational therapy in a general hospital. For 19 years, Ms. Lewis served as the supervisor of geriatric and restorative services for the department of occupational therapy at a large state mental hospital. While in this capacity, she was a member of a multi-disciplinary, community-based program that focused upon preventing institutionalization as well as serving clients within the institution. She was also responsible for developing a field-work Level II curriculum for occupational therapy students wishing to specialize in geriatrics.

Ms. Lewis has been a consultant to nursing homes, an environmental consultant in planning a new activities wing at an acute private psychiatric unit (which was part of a general hospital), and a consultant to a university-based home-care training center where she was part of a multi-disciplinary team and shared in the responsibility for the development and presentation of an intensive 15-week curriculum for home health aides.

Ms. Lewis has spent 7 years working directly with residents in subacute skilled nursing facility settings for rehabilitation companies as a full-time employee. One of these nursing homes was affiliated with an assisted living facility. She has also served as a private contractor for rehabilitation agencies and is well acquainted with the Prospective Payment System (PPS) in these settings.

For more than 10 years, Ms. Lewis has worked as a private contractor for two home health agencies (one religiously affiliated and the other hospital based). In both of these agencies Ms. Lewis has served mostly elderly clients from a variety of racial, cultural, and economic backgrounds (e.g., the inner city, the suburbs, small boroughs and villages, assisted living facilities, private one-room apartments, large estates, boarding homes, college professors, barely literate clients, and individuals who spoke no English). While working in these settings Ms. Lewis has become familiar with the PPS requirements for home health.

Ms. Lewis has lectured on topics pertaining to gerontology at a number of universities and colleges. She has also coordinated and presented at a variety of workshops and seminars to employees at institutions and community centers. Her audience has included physicians, psychologists, physical therapists, recreational therapists, social workers, occupational therapists, nurses, gerontologists, student nurses, residents, architects, lawyers, nursing home administrators, nurse's aides, and activities workers. She has spoken at a number of multi-disciplinary conferences and has initiated several educationally oriented community projects related to the elderly.

Sandra Cutler Lewis, MFA, OTR/L is currently working as a private contractor and a consultant devoted solely to the concerns of the late life adult.

INTRODUCTION

A major focus of this book is to provide a pragmatic and comprehensive text for occupational therapy and certified occupational therapy assistant students. Another purpose of this revised edition is to serve as a resource for practitioners already in the field or for those clinicians who are interested in entering geriatrics. Over time, the care of older adults has become a significant avenue of interest for therapists and assistants. Indeed, many of our institutions of higher learning that support occupational therapy and assistant programs are now devoting whole specialty areas dedicated to intervention and wellness programs that affect late life adults. So, too, this book has come to reflect the enormous growth and development of occupational therapy programs that are currently available to older adults.

The remainder of the introduction is concerned with topics that relate to information, organization, and structure of this second edition of *Elder Care in Occupational Therapy*.

I would like to address the issue of changing terminology and thought. As we go to press, the American Occupational Therapy Association (AOTA) is beginning to use a new framework for practice. Familiar terms such as treatment, performance components, occupational performance, and performance context are being replaced by intervention, areas of occupation, context, client factors, and occupational engagement and participation. Intervention (formerly known to many as "treatment") is composed of three parts: (1) a plan, (2) implementation of the plan, and (3) review. At various work settings, a plan may be termed by a number of titles such as "the care plan," "the plan of care," "the treatment plan," or "the intervention plan." For the purpose of illustration and information, it is important to briefly review some of the specifics that are a part of this newly formed occupational therapy framework. In an article by Jessica Alley (2002, April 8). Rebuilding OT. *Advance for Occupational Therapy Practitioners, 18*(7), 13-14, the *New Occupational Therapy Practice Framework: Domain and Process* was discussed. This is a written revision of *Uniform Terminology* (UT) that has taken approximately 4 years, with 18 rewrites. This proposal was approved on May 1-3 (in Miami Beach, FL to the 2002 Representative Assembly). Mary Jane Youngstrom, MS, OTR, FAOTA, chair of the AOTA's Commission on Practice, has been crafting the framework (with input from the association's membership). The commission itself spent 2.5 years writing the framework. It became essential to clarify the fact that occupational therapy is grounded in occupation. The document is composed of two sections—domain and process. According to Youngstrom, "[the domain] is the area of human experience that we care about [and] that we offer assistance to others in... and the process [is] where we try to explain our area of interest [and] what the process looks like when we do it." Some of the most apparent changes in this new document will be in the area of language.

Specifically, "performance areas," as termed in UT, are now labeled as "areas of occupation" and what were known as "performance components" have been separated into "performance skills." The framework, a much broader document than UT, reflects the evolution of occupational therapy. As Youngstrom states, "we want to give practitioners a way to think about, talk about, and apply occupation across the OT process." Members of the AOTA can download the complete text of this new document at AOTA's website, www.aota.org (under Practice and Ethics).

Throughout this second edition, evaluations, energy conservation techniques, and environmental adaptations are described in a variety of ways for a variety of conditions. One "size" does not fit all. For instance, energy conservation techniques for a client with chronic pulmonary disease is not exactly the same for a client with osteoarthritis (even though a number of techniques may be similar). Each diagnosis or condition has special needs that should be addressed separately. Similarly, environmental adaptations and evaluations are specifically described for each disease entity (even though some overlap may occur from time to time). The idea, here, is for the reader to become empowered so that he or she is able to immediately extract the information that is needed.

Although the Health Care Financing Administration (HCFA) is now titled the Centers for Medicare and Medicaid Services (CMS), some forms such as the HCFA 485 or the HCFA 855 are referred to in this text using the HCFA abbreviation, as these forms are currently being used.

The following comments relate directly to the rationale for this text's organization and structure. The concept of wellness (and programs relating to it) deals with healthy community living. These approaches are concerned with a healthy lifestyle and supportive environmental changes that can be used to help the older adult remain independently living in the community for as long as possible. Wellness is not a remedial program. Instead, it presents a change in the lifestyle to promote and maintain health. Wellness programs are detailed and documented in Unit 1. In Unit 3, a number of community programs (such as home health, home modification, and driver training [or retraining]) are presented. While these programs take place in the community, they are definitely remedial. Therefore, they have been separated from the wellness concept and are placed within the world of modalities that involve "remedial intervention." In these instances, where an illness and loss of function have occurred, occupational therapy expertise is needed to improve the client's condition. While all the programs in Unit 3 are relevant, it is driver training/retraining that I consider to be one of the most important ways in which an individual can remain independent in his or her community. It is presented last so that its impact will be remembered. It is probably one of the most essential life skills (unless one lives in a city with excellent public transportation or a town that is a small, self-contained community where all essentials are within a short walking distance) that permits one to perform everyday needed activities (e.g., physician visits, the beauty or barber shop, shopping, religious services, cultural events, the pharmacy) without having to depend upon others.

Finally, appendices are included to describe a variety of programs, resources, and concepts. These are not intended to be "add-ons." Rather, their purpose is to serve as "quick and ready" references for significant issues and information.

In closing, I would like to emphasize that never have there been more options and opportunities for clinicians and practitioners to serve late life adults than the present. This is a time for innovative programming and thoughtful intervention. With more people living longer, the need is great to ensure that these individuals will be able to lead independent lives within their communities for as long as possible. Never before has our profession had so much to offer to so many.

—Sandra Cutler Lewis, MFA, OTR/L
OT Consultant and Independent Contractor

Unit 1

Older Adults and Gerontic Occupational Therapy

A HISTORICAL OUTLOOK

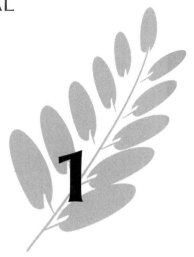

GERONTIC OCCUPATIONAL THERAPY—A DEFINITION

According to Neistadt and Crepeau, *occupational therapy* can be defined as the science and art of helping individuals to perform daily activities that are important to them despite disability, impairment, or handicap. The term *occupation* in occupational therapy refers to all of the activities that occupy a person's time that are meaningful to him or her.[1] These activities were known in occupational therapy as occupational performance areas and as such were divided into three major areas: *activities of daily living, work and productive activities*, and *play and leisure activities*.[2] However, the New Occupational Therapy Framework utilizes the term "areas of occupations" and categorizes these occupations into seven areas (please refer to Appendix T).

Another term of recent conception that is vital to occupational therapy is *occupational science*. This is an academic discipline that centers upon the critical role of daily activities in promoting a sense of well-being and health in our lives. The focus rests upon the nature of occupation and its effects upon human beings.[3]

In any discussion dealing with the elderly, it is helpful to define and distinguish the difference between the following terms: gerontology, geriatrics, and gerontic. *Gerontology* refers to a multi-disciplinary science that is the study of aging. *Geriatrics* is the medical practice that deals with diseases that are associated with older people and aging. *Gerontic* is used to describe occupational therapists who specialize in elderly care and development.[4]

HISTORICAL PERSPECTIVES

The Formative Years

The profession of occupational therapy was founded on March 15, 1917, in Clifton Springs, NY, and was known as the National Society for the Promotion of Occupational Therapy. This was later renamed the American Occupational Therapy Association. The founding persons were individuals who represented a variety of professions, skills, interests, and backgrounds. The host of the meeting, George Barton, was an architect who had tuberculosis. He had also become a strong advocate for occupational therapy (after a long convalescence during which he experienced the benefits of occupational intervention).[5] It was Barton who coined the term "occupational therapy."[6] Other members of this meeting included Thomas B. Kidner, the vocational secretary of the Military Hospital Commission of Canada, who was also a former architect, and Eleanor Clarke Slagle, the Director of the Henry B. Favill School of Occupations. She had formerly been associated with Hull House and was interested in habit training and balanced daily routines. These founders' views asserted that moral intervention, scientific medicine ideology, the arts and crafts movement, social reform, and the women's professions be the high point of the creed of the fledgling profession.[5]

Another early advocate of occupational therapy was Dr. Adolph Meyer. He was a psychiatrist working in the late 19th and early 20th centuries who believed that the rhythms of life (work, play, rest, and sleep) must be kept balanced to promote health and well-being. Intervention, in his view, became a blending of work and pleasure that included recreation and productive activity. Further, Meyer affirmed that it was important that instructors respect the native capabilities and interests of their clients.[7] Thus, Meyer's concepts were helpful in developing a basis for establishing occupational therapy as a profession.

Two other individuals, Susan E. Tracy and Herbert J. Hall, were also involved in occupational therapy's formative years. Susan E. Tracy was a nurse who believed that self-help instruction involving wholesome interests and activities was important. She conducted a number of courses in "occupation" while training nurses. Herbert J. Hall, a physician, prescribed occupation, which he termed the "work cure" for his clients as a type of intervention to direct one's interests and regulate one's life. He developed a training program (primarily for nurses and social workers) that focused upon work as a form of intervention.[8]

However, it is Dr. William Rush Dunton, Jr. who is considered by many to be the father of occupational therapy. He was involved in the utilization of occupational therapy as an intervention for clients with mental illness. In 1919, Dr. Dunton, Jr. published *Reconstruction Therapy*. This book established guiding principles for occupational therapy that are still meaningful to the profession today. These quotes from his book serve as our professional credo:[9, p.10]

◇ "That occupation is as necessary to life as food and drink.

◇ That every human being should have both physical and mental occupation.

◇ That sick minds, sick bodies, and sick souls may be healed through occupation."

The Reconstruction Aides

During World War I, reconstruction aides, mostly civilian women, were trained by lectures that included psychology of the handicapped, fatigue and work cure, personal hygiene, anatomy, kinesiology, ethics and hospital administration, and classes that provided instruction in cord work, wood work, weaving, bead work, ceramics, and basketry. These women worked with clients who had surgical and orthopedic problems as well as emotional and nervous disorders.

This was also the period when a scientific approach to treating the physically disabled evolved. Some examples include: devices that were developed to measure strength and range of motion (ROM), adaptation of pieces of equipment designed to help promote specific motions for increasing strength and ROM, and the kinesiological analysis of activities that were initiated to allow activities to be chosen as the basis for remediation of specific physical limitations.[7]

As gerontic practitioners look forward to treating our clients in the 21st century, it is wise to remember that we have a unique and rich heritage that remains the cornerstone of our profession's future. Some of these concepts include:[8]

◇ The utilization of the client's needs, values, and interests in stimulating constructive activity.

◇ The use of existing skills and the development of new skills to remediate pathology:

▲ A respect for manual and creative labor as a restorative modality.

▲ The importance of interpersonal relationships and interaction in establishing and maintaining a therapeutic process.

▲ The development of adaptive techniques and devices to decrease disability.

▲ The basic concept that occupation (purposeful and meaningful activity) can be a positive force in influencing an individual's state of health.

Over the past 50 years, the field of gerontic occupational therapy has gradually developed. The inception period for those therapists specializing in working with older adults can be placed in the 1940s. At that time, occupational therapists had already treated older Americans who had disabilities or diseases of old age (e.g., cerebrovascular accident, arthritis).[4]

Intervention modalities had begun to expand, and homemaker activities and activities of daily living were added to craft and work modalities. Neurodevelopmental and biomechanical intervention modalities were also used with elderly clients.[4]

The contemporary arena has further expanded to areas such as poetry, computers, reminiscences, energy conservation, pet therapy, reality orientation, adaptive equipment, work simplification, dysphagia intervention, and environmental adaptations.

As early as 1947, Hildenbrand had discussed the goals of gerontic occupational therapy as follows: prolong the life span and enable aging persons to enjoy better vitality and health, adjust to the changes involved in aging, and continue to be useful to society.[10] Hildenbrand was also very concerned about forced retirement (prevalent at that time) and its effect on the aging individual. She was interested in establishing job analysis of the physical and mental abilities of each job. This, she felt, would help to eliminate age as a criterion for acquiring a job.[4]

The 1950s and 1960s continued to see expanded growth in gerontic occupational therapy. By 1963, Willard and Spackman's third edition of *Occupational Therapy* included a chapter on occupational therapy in geriatrics.[11] By the late 1970s, the Gerontology Special Interest Section (which serves as a resource on research, literature, and practice issues) was formed. In 1986, the first edition of *The Role of Occupational Therapy With the Elderly* was developed.[12]

The expansion of therapists seeking specialization with older adults has consistently grown through the decades following the late 1940s until the present.

CONCEPTUAL MODELS, DEMOGRAPHICS, LIFE DEVELOPMENT, AND OCCUPATIONAL ACTIVITIES

2

CONCEPTUAL MODELS USEFUL IN GERONTIC OCCUPATIONAL THERAPY

As occupational therapy began to expand in service delivery, theoretical practitioners, educators, and researchers began to look for new avenues to organize the theoretical concepts that were developing. These concepts and frames of reference will be briefly discussed to serve as a springboard from which a practicing therapist may derive methodology and intervention approaches. Only models and theories that are likely to be useful in gerontic occupational therapy will be discussed.

The Biomedical Model

In this model, the focus is upon musculoskeletal pathology and activity that may be interfering with movement when an individual is performing occupations. Diagnosis and symptom reduction are the primary forums with the postulation that the disease state has remitted and symptoms are reduced so that the individual may be able to resume former occupations and tasks. This approach is most common with therapists who work in medical institutions and settings. Examples of diagnoses under this model include cardiopulmonary disease, tendon and ligament damage, connective tissue disease, autoimmune diseases, and orthopedic injuries and disease.[13]

Claudia Allen: The Cognitive Disability Model

Allen uses a neuroscientific perspective and presents us with six cognitive levels that are related to information processing.

LEVEL 6—PLANNED ACTIONS

This level is theoretically characterized by the absence of disability. Deductive reasoning may be used, and attention may be directed toward anticipating errors and in making plans to prevent mistakes. The sensory cues are rich and varied (e.g., able to comprehend and use written instructions, diagrams, speed, time) and well understood. Persons are able to imagine the effect that their actions will have.

LEVEL 5—EXPLORATORY ACTIONS

At this level, attention is held by variations in motor actions that are of an exploratory nature. Inductive reasoning is used from specific to general. The learning environment needs to be adapted to concrete, visible, and meaningful stimuli.

LEVEL 4—GOAL-DIRECTED ACTION

Individuals in this category may not be able to consider the consequences of their actions before they begin to act. Persons at this level can involve themselves in a number of familiar concrete manual activities. Sensory cues such as touching and seeing are the most important cues at this level. Individuals can imitate a demonstrated direction one step at a time (directions must be clearly visible). Persons in this category experience a great deal of difficulty correcting mistakes.

LEVEL 3—MANUAL ACTIONS

At this level individuals are not able to correct many errors (even when they are demonstrated to them). Thought processes are restricted to compliance with a typical procedure. Motor actions may be either very slow or at times hyperactive. Time awareness is restricted to the here and now. Individuals are not able to connect their manual actions to a purposeful goal unless another person directs them.

LEVEL 2—POSTURAL ACTIONS

This level involves spontaneous actions that involve proprioceptive responses (e.g., bending, pacing). Persons with dementia may have difficulty initiating a movement. Exercise that moves body parts is recommended. However, the therapist may be needed to help move body parts when initiating movement during exercise. Attention may be sustained for 5 to 10 minutes.

LEVEL 1—AUTOMATIC ACTIONS

Individuals at this level have an impaired awareness level. They appear to respond to internal cues and often have a glazed look. These people are able to perform automatic actions involving drinking, walking, and eating. The attention span is momentary, and the therapist may need to stimulate these individuals to take food and drink.[14]

Allen affirms that task analysis plays a vital function in its relationship to the client's cognitive level. The *Allen Cognitive Level Test* (ACL) is helpful in determining an individual's cognitive level. Allen asserts that environmental compensation is a successful strategy that can be used with persons suffering from dementia and depression.[14]

In general, when utilizing this model, intervention and comprehension for a cognitive disability calls for the suppression of the symptoms and the support of successful task behavior.[8,14]

Ann Cronin Mosey: Three Frames of Reference

From a historical point of view, the work of Mosey needs to be explored as she, early on, was a major contributor in developing the concept of an occupational therapy frame of reference. Although her book may no longer be in print (and many therapists might rank her work as outdated), it still has value and deserves to be considered as a part of our profession's historical development.

Mosey developed a biopsychosocial model that focuses upon the client's mind, body, and environment. Her basic tenet rests upon recapitulation of ontogenesis that concerns the development of adaptive skills (perceptual-motor, cognitive, drive object, dyadic interaction skills, primary group interaction skill, self-identity skills, and sexual identity interaction skill). Generally, this model focuses upon knowledge, skills, abilities, and values that individuals need to learn in order to function productively. Dysfunction results when there is a lack of development in a necessary skill component.

Mosey uses five different sequential developmental groups (parallel, project, egocentric, cooperative, and mature). The three frames of reference (developmental, analytical, and acquisitional) are based upon seven philosophical assumptions concerning individuals and their relationships toward the human and the nonhuman environment.[15]

In examining these three frames of reference, Larson further demonstrates practical application. For instance, analytical frames relate to psychology (e.g., loss of skills and adapting to loss). Developmental frames relate to the personal, physical, and social maturation of the individual. The acquisitional frame of reference is useful in acute care, rehabilitation, and the community setting (wherever there is a concern for learning new skills or relearning and adapting to old skills).[13]

Mosey affirms that occupational therapy is focused upon promoting functional independence by means of strategies that are directed toward enhancing the client's participation in occupational performances (now termed areas of occupation) and the development of performance components (now termed performance skills). Changes occur through delineating learning needs and teaching the learning process. Mosey asserts that therapy is an action-oriented experience that involves learning by doing. The therapist's and assistant's primary focus is to help individuals gain greater insight into the self and to develop their specifically needed skills.[15]

Mary Reilly: The Occupational Behavior Perspective

This model has been useful with clients in a neuropsychiatric setting. Reilly views the health of individuals in terms of their level of adaptation to their environment. In this model, the objective of occupational therapy is to assess the developmental level of the client's occupational roles so that appropriate remediation and growth can be fostered.

Being able to practice a healthy balance of rest, work, and play is paramount. Some basic tenets for Reilly's model include the following:[16]

- ✧ Occupational behavior is acquired developmentally.
- ✧ Client programming needs to be graded.
- ✧ Occupational therapy needs to provide decision-making environments for clients.
- ✧ Intervention should foster the aesthetic, cognitive, and self-realization needs of clients.

✧ Occupational therapists should tailor programs to meet the individual client's abilities, occupational roles, interests, and age, as well as provide a learning environment where normal daily patterns of play, work, and rest can be practiced.

The Group Work Model (Generalized)

Individuals who perform occupations in a social relationship may benefit from the generalized concept of group process. Besides psychiatry there is a host of other settings that involve groups. Clients in acute care hospitals, rehabilitation centers, and subacute rehabilitation units may perform occupations in a parallel group setting. Clients seen in the home setting may be part of a family group, and, therefore, are influenced by the family members' expectations and interactions. Members of adult day care intervention programs, assisted living situations, or congregate housing programs may work on tasks together and, therefore, are affected by the other group members.[13] Some therapists do not believe this to be a true frame of reference. Furthermore, it might be considered to be an approach or method.

The Motor Control Model

This model is composed of four intervention approaches that have been developed and designed to remediate movement deficits after brain trauma. The researchers and therapists associated with this model include the Rood approach, Bobath's neurodevelopmental treatment, Brunnström's movement therapy, and proprioceptive neuromuscular facilitation (PNF) (Voss, Ionta, and Meyers). The PNF treatment approach is usually used with clients who have experienced a CVA.[13]

The Cognitive-Perceptual Model

This model is concerned with the process of cognition and perception that relates to the way an individual responds to the environment when performing occupations. This approach derives information from neuropsychology, neuroscience, and fields that focus upon the development of motor control. *Cognitive-perceptual dysfunction* occurs when the brain becomes damaged (such as in a cerebral vascular accident). Therapists working with this model might provide remedial training (tasks that assist in reorganizing the impaired central nervous system's functions). For example, dressing and bathing training will enable the client to don/doff clothes and wash himself or herself as well as provide sensory stimuli that can activate new neural pathways to improve motor function. Therapists working with the *adaptive approach* would assist the individual to compensate for dysfunction and adapt the environment (using grab bars and a bath bench in the tub to assist with bathing and a long-handled zipper pull to assist with dressing). With the adaptive approach, the therapist accepts that the cognitive-perceptual defect as permanent, and intervention consists of assisting the older adult to compensate for dysfunction by adapting the environment.[13]

Gary Kielhofner: The Model of Human Occupation

The *model of human occupation* utilizes and applies general systems theory. This includes the concept that the systems are self-maintaining and open in a dynamic interaction with the environment. The evolution and change in the system are guided by a feedback loop.[8,17]

The *human occupation system* is made up of three subsystems—volitional, habituation, and performance. The *volitional* subsystem (which is motivated by personal causation, interests, values, and a belief in efficiency of skill) is considered the highest. The *habituation* subsystem arranges behavior into roles and patterns. This subsystem is influenced by: internalized expectations, perceived incumbency (a person's awareness of his or her role), and role balance. The habituation subsystem is governed by the volitional system. The *performance* subsystem is governed by both the habituation subsystem and the volitional subsystem. It is comprised of motor, process, and communication skills.[8,17]

Occupational dysfunction is seen as the interface of the individual with the environment, and is a cessation, decrease, inappropriateness, ineffectiveness, or imbalance of output. Environmental factors become paramount and are essential when evaluating for occupational dysfunction.[17]

When considering the older adult, this model can be applied broadly. It can be applied to gradual declines in strength, to traumatic injury or illness, or to how an individual responds to retirement. For example, for an individual experiencing physical changes, the therapist might provide information about adaptive equipment or environmental changes (e.g., reduced glare for lighting). For the older adult facing retirement, the therapist might guide that individual to review his or her life roles and interests so that an appropriate selection of alternative tasks can replace work tasks.[13]

There are a variety of models from which the therapist and assistant may choose. Models may be adapted or intertwined to meet the needs and values of each client. No two individuals are alike. Problem solving and finding the most effective method, model, and approach are essential to the rehabilitation process and well-being of each client.

DEMOGRAPHICS OF THE CURRENT AND THE PROJECTED ELDERLY POPULATION

Statistics demonstrate that Americans, as a population, are getting older. In 1960, approximately 12.7 million Americans were over 65. By 1991, the number was 31.5 million. The figure is projected to be 52.1 million by 2020. At that time, the age group over 85 will include about 6.7 million people.[18]

Furthermore, it is now predicted that in 50 years one in four Americans will be 60 or older. Worldwide predictions forecast that one person in five will be 60 or older. That translates to 2 billion people over 60 in 50 years. In 50 years, there will be more people, worldwide, over 60 than under 18.[19] By 2050, according to the U.S. Bureau of the Census, women in the United States will outnumber men by about 7 million.[20]

The older population in the United States is becoming more diverse. Current projections by the U.S. Bureau of the Census estimate that in 1990 one in 10 elderly persons were of a race other than white. This population is projected to double by 2050. The Hispanic population is expected to grow from 4% to 16%.[21]

The special needs of the elderly will become a momentous force in the future. Caregivers of all professions will be called upon to harness their skills and energy so that they can act with humanity, proficiency, and efficiency. In the past 20 years, more professionals have sought an interest in serving the elderly, and the need for caring and well-trained personnel has continued to grow.

In the United States, the federal government has expanded numerous social programs. These include: the inception of Social Security during the 1930s, the establishment of Medicare (1965), the establishment of the Older Americans Act (1965), the passage of the Age Discrimination in Employment Act—first initiated in 1967 and later amended in 1986 to abolish mandatory retirement, the establishment of Supplemental Security Income (1974), the passage of the Employees Retirement Income Security Act (1974), and the establishment of the National Institute of Aging (1975).[21]

As the elderly population continues to grow, so too have the number of health professionals, and the gerontic therapist and assistant are no exception. According to a membership survey, the American Occupational Therapy Association reported that in 1991 approximately 30% of OTRs and almost 40% of COTAs worked with older adults.[22]

LIFE DEVELOPMENT IN THE LATER YEARS: THEORIES OF AGING AND DEVELOPMENT

From the moment of conception to the moment of death, all living organisms are aging. Human development involves changes that occur during the lifetime of an individual. Schuster, who utilizes a holistic approach to aging, has defined the five major areas in which human development occurs as: spiritual, biophysical, cognitive, social, and affective.[23] The following information will be concerned with those theories that relate mostly to aging and the aging process.

Moral/Spiritual

Kohlberg believed that moral developmental theory consisted of seven stages:[24]

✧ *Stage 1* (punishment and obedience) involves physical consequences to determine the value of an action.

✧ *Stage 2* (instrumental relativism) consists of reciprocity (e.g., if you do this for me, then I'll do that for you).

✧ *Stage 3* (interpersonal concordance) involves behavior that is judged by intent.

✧ *Stage 4* (law and order) consists of behavior that is based upon a person's willingness to respond to and respect authority and duty.

✧ *Stage 5* (social contract legalistic approach) advocates action that is based upon individual rights, with standards agreed upon by society (e.g., free agreement and contract with flexibility).

✧ *Stage 6* (universal ethical principle) consists of behavior that is determined by individual decisions of conscience as related to universal ethical principles (e.g., the Golden Rule).

✧ *Stage 7* (ontological religious approach) involves the cosmic and contemplative experience.

Biophysical Theories

These theories are concerned with an explanation of the physical process of aging up to the moment of death. Questions such as what triggers the process of aging, how do cells age, and what the mechanisms may be for the processes of aging (whether the process occurs independently or pathologically or if it is due to other externally related influences) concern theoreticians who work in this arena.[25]

Altered Functional Forms of the Immune System

These theories postulate that as age advances, the immune system begins to form antibodies against its own proteins and incorrectly identifies them as antigens. There is an increase of immature T lymphocytes in the blood and a decrease in the primary immune response of B cells.[8]

FREE RADICAL THEORY

This theory contends that unstable free radical chemical molecules produce alterations of chromosomes and collagens and are also responsible for pigment accumulation agents.[8]

PROGRAMMED AGING THEORY

In the programmed theory of aging, Leonard Hayflick gives much credence to the concept that an organism is capable of a constant and specific number of cell divisions. Cell death occurs when these divisions are fully completed.[8]

CROSS-LINKAGE THEORY

In this theory, it is proposed that as aging occurs the molecular strands of selected cellular proteins such as DNA and collagen enzymes connect cross-wise. The formation of these new cross-links, over time, produces proteins that are altered both functionally and structurally. These changes can cause failures in related tissues, cells, and organs.[25]

DNA-RNA THEORY

In this theory, defective enzymes produce substrates within the cell. This can seriously impair the normal metabolic process.[8]

INTENTIONAL BIOLOGICAL PROGRAMMING THEORY

This theory affirms that senescence occurs by means of programmed changes that occur within an organism's life cycle. There is an aging chronometer (i.e., biological clock) that controls the speed of the metabolic process.[8, 25]

GENE THEORY

This theory holds that one or more genes are programmed to stop or initiate functioning of specific processes throughout a person's life and is used to explain longevity over generations within a given family.[25]

COGNITIVE-INTELLECTUAL DEVELOPMENTAL THEORY

A major theory in this realm is based on the work of Jean Piaget. Piaget's general theory of cognitive development is based upon two biological attributions. The first, organization, is the tendency of the living organism to integrate progress into cohesive systems. The second, adaptations, is the instinctive tendency of organisms to interact with their environment through accommodation and assimilation.[8] Piaget postulates that there are five major stages of intellectual development:[8]

 ❖ *Phase 1 (sensorimotor—birth to 2 years)*. Learning occurs through manipulation of the senses. Deductive reasoning may be used by the end of this phase.

 ❖ *Phase 2 (preconceptual—2 to 4 years)*. Simple language, repetition, and symbolic play are utilized. Individuals begin to make use of comparison and classification of items by simple characteristics (e.g., color or size).

 ❖ *Phase 3 (intuitive—4 to 7 years)*. Words are used to express ideas. The generalization of symbols becomes paramount.

 ❖ *Phase 4 (concrete operations—7 to 11 years)*. Logical thought is now fully utilized. Objects can be organized into a series and then be reversed (e.g., multiplication and division, addition and subtraction).

 ❖ *Phase 5 (formal operations—11 years and ongoing)*. Abstract thought is now understood and utilized.

Practical application of Piaget's theories can be useful when working with older adults. For instance, if a practitioner is treating a cognitively disabled older person, it is helpful to know where this individual's cognitive development is in terms of capabilities so appropriate intervention can be planned and initiated.

Social and Affective Related Theories

ERICKSON'S EIGHT STAGES OF EGO DEVELOPMENT

Erickson identified eight stages of development that utilize a psychodynamic perspective. Each stage centers on a psychosocial conflict that the individual must resolve in order to progress into the next developmental stage. In old age, known as the *maturity stage*, the individual has the opportunity to accept and respect his or her life as one of fulfillment and cohesiveness. The conflict arena in this stage is one of ego integrity vs. despair. The virtue that can be developed at this time is wisdom.[8,25]

PECK'S DEVELOPMENTAL THEORY

R.C. Peck believed that Erickson's stages of development could be expanded. According to Peck, there are three old age stages (rather than just one stage). It is during this time that one's life experiences can be used to arrive at new approaches for accomplishing tasks. The three old age stages are:[8,25]

 ❖ *Ego differentiation vs. work/role preoccupation*: Developing alternative activities upon retirement

 ❖ *Body transcendence vs. body preoccupation*: Harnessing intellectual or creative activity to combat the tendency to dwell on bodily ills and dysfunction

 ❖ *Ego transcendence vs. ego preoccupation*: Overcoming withdrawal by developing an awareness of the significance of one's achievements as contributions to the future

Occupational therapy, with its interventional focus upon balanced occupational performance areas, now termed areas of occupation, can complement Peck's references to the multiple dimensions of worth and self-identity.[25]

HAVIGNURT'S SOCIAL TASK DEVELOPMENT THEORY

This theory affirms that adulthood is divided into three periods (early adulthood, middle age, and old age). In old age, the developmental tasks for an individual to master include: adjusting to retirement (which is often accompanied with a reduced income), the loss of a partner or spouse, fulfilling civic and social responsibilities, establishing relationships with others of similar age, and adjusting to the deficits of declining strength and health.[8,25]

MASLOW'S HUMANISTIC VIEW OF DEVELOPMENT: THE PYRAMID OF NEEDS THEORY

Abraham Maslow believed that development is based upon *need gratification* (also known as *growth maturation*). He asserted that there exists a hierarchy, or pyramid, of seven basic needs. The bottom of the pyramid is supported by the fulfillment of physiological needs and includes in ascending order: safety, belonging and love, esteem, the need for self-actualization, the need to know and understand, and aesthetic needs.[8,25]

DISENGAGEMENT THEORY

The Disengagement Theory of Cumming and Henry proposes that older adults disengage through general reduction in energy levels, increased preoccupation with self-needs, and less societal involvement. These two theorists contend that withdrawal or disengagement can help individuals prepare for their eventual death.[8,25] This is a controversial theory.

THE ACTIVITY THEORY

The activity theory, the opposite of disengagement, holds that successful aging occurs among those persons who maintain the highest possible involvement in activity. Old age, then, even with its increasing limitations, can still be regarded as a time of fulfillment in activity and as a time when the wisdom of the years may be utilized and harvested by society.[8]

THE CONTINUITY THEORY

This theory affirms that as people become adults, they develop specific preferences and habits that become a part of their personalities that last throughout their life span. As individuals grow older, if their personalities remain integrated, there is an increasing consistency of that personality.[8] Fidler's Life-Style Performance Model reflects an emphasis upon the continuity of lifestyle performance over time. This model can be very helpful to practicing therapists and assistants in its use across all levels of the life span and across a variety of cultures.[8,26]

PERSON-ENVIRONMENT TRANSACTION PERSPECTIVE

A.N. Schwartz postulates that there is a mutual interaction and influence of individuals with their environment. Positive self-esteem provides the basis of an individual's competence. Successful aging, then, depends on the ability of individuals to structure their social and physical environment so that they can compensate for the losses that occur in old age, and so that they may continue to function effectively. This viewpoint, which involves a continuous developmental adaptation process, fits well with the occupational behavior approach to gerontic occupational therapy.[27, 28]

There is a multitude of theories on the development of the human being over a life span. We have discussed those that mainly pertain to the older adult and those that most affect gerontic occupational therapists and assistants. No one client actually fits 100% into a specialized theory. However, these theories can be intertwined and adapted to meet specific needs and situations. It is wise to have a knowledge base of human development so that appropriate and meaningful intervention can be provided to older persons.

WORK, RETIREMENT, RECREATIONAL, AND LEISURE ACTIVITIES

Work

Webster's Dictionary defines *work* as "an activity in which one exerts strength or faculties to do or perform something... the labor, task, or duty that is one's accustomed means of livelihood."[29] Work represents a very important life activity that often defines "who" a person is.

Barron postulates that work assumes five universal functions: it regulates life activity, it offers status and identification, it provides income, it makes available opportunities for meaningful life experiences, and it provides opportunities to associate with others.[30]

These are major attributes as to how individuals spend their time in the work force. If one leaves the work force, it is imperative that replacement activities be found that may act as substitutes and that may provide similar satisfactions.

It should be noted that many older adults are choosing to work longer (some on a part-time basis) due to economic need and/or the desire to perform meaningful activity. In the United States, Congress has just passed legislation allowing workers between the ages of 65 to 70 to collect Social Security benefits regardless of how much income they may earn. Due to the aging of the "baby boom" generation, it is expected (if the majority of this group leaves the work place) that there will be fewer younger workers to support the retirees. If this occurs, more employers are expected to court older workers.

In the United States, it has been reported that Social Security will face insolvency in 2034 (if there are no corrective measures initiated).[31] This gives even more impetus for longer working years for future generations. Occupational therapists have the opportunity to act as advocates for aging workers—to promote their well-being through wellness programs and by developing compensatory and adaptive techniques. Practitioners can also contribute by ensuring the rights of older adults to continue working and the "means" by which to pursue work activities throughout their lives.[32,33] Some of these "means," as stated above, may include: designing work stations, adaptive seating, injury prevention, and the use of ergoeconomic principles.

Historically, individuals have made enormous contributions in their old age. Benjamin Franklin, Leonardo da Vinci, Michaelangelo, Isaac Bashevis Singer, Georgia O'Keefe, Gian Carlo Menotti, Agnes de Mille, Imogen Cunningham, Alan Greenspan, John Huston, Martha Graham, Grandma Moses, and Frank Lloyd Wright are some examples of talented older men and women, through the ages and in the present, who have generously contributed to society as artists, dancers, architects, screen directors, political leaders, economic advisors, writers, actors, poets, and choreographers.

Creativity and productivity can be a lifelong process that knows no age limit. To these individuals, withdrawing from their occupation or work was not even considered to be a part of their plans. For them, work was an all-absorbing and ongoing experience. Competent and willing workers of any occupation and age should not be limited by age alone for continuing to be employed.

Retirement

Retirement can be described as a "withdrawal from one's position or occupation or from active working life."[34] It is the opposite of work.

Although the previous discussion on work dealt with the concept of extending the working years, there is evidence that some older people are retiring early through buy-out packages, down-sizing, saturation, or dissatisfaction of the work being performed.

If one is not to have an abrupt awakening, planning for retirement is essential. Financial investments and reinvestments, dealing with losses (friend, spouse, significant other), development of meaningful leisure-time activities, alternate housing, and understanding biological or nutritional needs associated with aging are some of the many areas to be considered in the planning process. A person who is contemplating retirement needs something to which he or she can "retire to."

Social activities become increasingly important after retirement. Volunteer work in the community or unpaid work for the family is one avenue in which older adults can find productive and meaningful occupations. Advisory roles to businesses, institutions, persons, or organizations is another way to stay involved in activity that provides a sense of worth.[33] Retired senior volunteer services, literacy counseling, foster grand-parent programs, Service Corps of Retired Executives, and Volunteers in Service to America are some examples of specific advisory groups available to the older adult. Many other older people also choose to serve as volunteers for religious organizations.

Continuing education programs at colleges and universities as well as Elder Hostel programs are ways in which older adults can involve themselves in rewarding and fulfilling learning experiences.[33]

Ludwig and Kornblau affirm that occupational therapists should consider promoting reasonable accommodations whenever possible that would enable older persons to participate in volunteer or educational programs (e.g., a volume-controlled telephone might be helpful if an elderly volunteer experiencing some hearing loss desires to work at the information desk of a hospital).[33]

It is common today for individuals to spend 30 to 40 years in retirement. For some people that may be the same amount of time they spent working.[35]

Retirement has become a period of the life cycle that could readily use the skills of the occupational therapist—whether it be in recommending physical adjustments in the home, exploring ways of making activities of daily living more efficient and less tiring, or maintaining the well-being of an individual.

Leisure

Leisure can be defined as "freely selected activity pursued simply for the pleasure of it."[36] Activities in which older individuals may choose to participate are varied and depend upon the meaning and relevance that each individual associates with the activities. Trips/travel; exercise; cooking clubs; volunteer activities; religious activities; card and checker playing groups; planned visits to a park, tavern, or restaurant; gatherings; cinema activities; visits with friends and family; puzzles; computer activities (e-mailing grandchildren is a favorite); bowling; photography and arts groups; theater clubs; grandparenting activities; crafts and sewing groups; spectator sports; home embellishments; entertainment; and television are some of the ways that older adults can spend their leisure time. Avocational/hobby interests held in younger days can continue to be pursued in later years as lifelong interests. They can often serve as transitional activities that help bridge the gap from the work world to the world of retirement.

The therapist and the assistant can play an important role in assisting older adults to participate in meaningful pursuits. Activity analysis, supportive techniques, and assistive devices often aid in ensuring the older person's ability to enhance or facilitate performance of a purposeful activity.[37]

PROBLEMS ARISING IN CARING FOR THE ELDERLY

3

ABUSE AND ABANDONMENT

Elder abuse or maltreatment of older persons occurs in about 4% of the elderly population in the United States.[38] Abuse of the older person may occur in several areas—emotional or psychological, sexual, physical, financial or material, and neglect. The abuse may be in the home or in an institutional setting. *Psychological or emotional abuse* refers to treatment of an older adult that decreases the self-esteem of that individual; *physical abuse* involves physically hurting the older adult. *Sexual abuse* refers to sexual activity without the person's given consent (including the person who is unable to give consent). *Financial or material abuse* involves theft or misuse of the older person's property or funds. It may also involve financial schemes and asking the older adult to sign papers that they don't understand. *Neglect* may be active (lack of caregiver's intervention when the caregiver has adequate knowledge of appropriate care) or passive (neglect occurs by the caregiver's lack of knowledge or inability to render appropriate care).[8,39]

In the family, abuse may arise for a number of reasons. One major factor is due to the constant strain of caring for a chronically ill and dependent parent who may also be incontinent and confused. Also, some caregivers (because the average life span has become extended) are elderly themselves and are not able to physically and emotionally render service. At times, these caregivers reach a breaking point in being able to provide appropriate care.[8,39]

If a therapist or an assistant suspects abuse (e.g., signs of physical abuse, malnutrition, fear of being touched, or the older adult mentioning that he or she has been abused in some way), the practitioner should discuss these concerns with the caregiver. It should be noted that the therapist should look for patterns of neglect over time rather than unrelated incidents. If true abuse is suspected, the therapist is legally obligated to report suspected abuse to appropriate aging agencies.[39]

Abandonment occurs when the older dependent adult is left alone without any arrangements for another caregiver to provide service. Some frail elderly are left at the doorsteps of hospitals with no one to claim them.[39]

CAREGIVER NEEDS

Respite care and the mobilization of social networks may aid the caregiver.

Occupational therapists working in home health have the perfect opportunity to improve the older client's abilities and decrease some of the caregiver's responsibilities. For instance, practitioners can help elders reduce their dependency on family members by teaching the older adult self-care techniques to improve the older person's self-esteem. Meanwhile, the amount of energy the caregiver needs to provide to the older adult is reduced. Specific areas could involve: informing the client how to use energy conservation techniques, recommending assistive devices, encouraging the older person to assist with household tasks (e.g., plant care, mending, folding laundry), teaching of adaptive self-care skills as needed, and recommending support services.[40]

WELLNESS

NEW IMPLICATIONS FOR OCCUPATIONAL THERAPY IN DEVELOPING WELL ELDERLY PROGRAMS

The concept of wellness is predicated in the belief that there are identifiable lifestyle factors that can prevent, or at the least delay, the onset of serious illness or disability.[41]

Occupational therapy is beginning to add wellness programming as another modality to the practitioner's bag of interventions. Since populations are growing "greyer," it becomes of the utmost importance to design meaningful programs that will enable older adults to remain in the community and lead productive lives as long as possible.

The University of Southern California Well Elderly Study

The University of Southern California (USC) Well Elderly Study is a prime example of occupational therapy engaging in the community with a wellness emphasis.

In an address to the American Medical Association's 16th Annual Science Reporters Conference on October 21, 1997, Dr. Florence Clark discussed some of the outcomes of the USC Well Elderly Study. Primarily, she commented that this study indicated that preventative occupational therapy could have a major impact on the outlook and well being of the elderly by improving their mental and physical health, slowing declines in bodily pain, decreasing emotion-based limitations, and increasing vitality.[3]

The findings of the USC Well Elderly Study demonstrated that occupational therapy is an effective way to promote health and increase the quality of life of America's rapidly growing older adults. The results of the research show promise for helping elders to maintain their independence in the community. This is critical because it is the loss of independence that most senior citizens fear, and it is the high cost of dependent care that is threatening the financial security of the United States as well as the health care system in general.[3]

A brief discussion of the clinical trial is helpful because its results demonstrate its effectiveness to promote "wellness" among elderly persons. The USC Well Elderly Study was a randomized clinical trial. Participants were assigned randomly to one of three groups. After they completed a battery of questions, they were screened by a geriatrician. The three groups consisted of (1) occupational therapy (lifestyle redesign), (2) social activity control (each member received 2.5 hours per week at which time non-professional coordinators conducted activities such as crafts, movies, dances, and outings), and (3) no intervention control. The participants consisted of 361 seniors ranging in ages from 60 to 89. Basically, these older persons were low income, urban, lived independently, and were culturally diverse (Caucasians, African-Americans, Hispanics, and Asians). Twenty-seven percent had disabilities (as defined by the participant).[3]

All participants were evaluated both at the initiation of the study and 9 months later with tests that measured physical health, social functioning, mental health, and life satisfaction.[3]

The four core concepts that framed the design of the Lifestyle Redesign Program were:[3]

1. Occupation is life.
2. Occupation is able to create new visions of the possible self.
3. Occupation has a curative effect on mental and physical health and on a sense of routine and life order.
4. Occupation has a definite place in preventative care.

In this study, a qualitative approach to needs evaluations became an important way to comprehend and address the unique needs of a given group of clients. Questions such as: What types of things do you find meaningful? What types of things do you believe act as barriers to prevent you from doing what you want to do? What types of activities/things do you do each day? are useful and serve as excellent springboards for understanding clients' needs. Once the needs evaluation is conducted, the findings can be used to modify the Lifestyle Redesign Program so that it has meaning in a local setting.[3]

The goal of the Lifestyle Redesign Program was to maintain or increase the independence, well-being, and health of older persons who were already living independently. Elderly persons met in their own small groups (approximately 10 members and the occupational therapy leader) for 2 hours each week for a period of 9 months. The occupational therapist also met for a period of 9 hours of individual interaction with each participant (usually in his or her apartment/dwelling) during the program. Group sessions were held at the same place, day, and time of the week, and each session lasted for the same time. Group sessions permitted spontaneity, improvisation, and variety. Guest speakers provided specialized materials and skills, snacks would change from one session to another, and materials were presented in various formats. Each participant was recognized as an expert; because these older persons had lived to their present ages indicated that they had, in some way, been successful in solving life's many challenges. Selecting and reproducing feedback phrases in a printed format was yet another method that was helpful in promoting the therapeutic process, and in providing handouts of the participants' responses during the discussion periods.[3]

Typical theme and topical content areas included an introduction to the power of occupations; aging, health, and occupation; transportation and occupation; finances and occupation; social relationships; home and community safety; cultural awareness (can also include areas such as outings, exploration of special events); dining as an occupation; time and occupation and as a conclusion—an integrative summary and ending of the group. The methods of program delivery consisted of didactic presentations (such as material the occupational therapist brought to the group—e.g, joint conservation), peer exchange (participants story-telling to the group—e.g., how challenges among group members were met), direct experience (someone actively doing something), and exploration (reflecting on meaningfulness of the didactic content to each person's life).[3]

There were four major elements that enabled the participants to possess long-term strategies for promoting well-being and health by means of involvement in occupation. *Occupational self-analysis* became an important factor. Participants were challenged to reflect about who they were as occupational persons and to think about the occupations that they had always found or were presently finding most rewarding. They were then asked to evaluate the extent to which they were experiencing occupational dysfunction. Plans could then be enacted. The Lifestyle Redesign Program stressed the ways in which experience could create radiating change. For instance, venturing out to travel on a newly operating train system for the first time has many implications—that of being an urban traveler, learning transportation skills, developing a positive self-image of one who can meet challenges, and developing a sense of social connectedness.

Participants were encouraged to use small steps in overcoming risks. All of these can ultimately benefit well-being and health. Understanding the elements of occupations helped enable older individuals to have a tool kit to redesign their lives. Participants learned that flow (a positive psychological state that results when the person engaged in occupation is challenged carefully to match his or her ability level) can provide meaningful occupations. Finally, it is occupation that is an impetus that propels individuals forward. Through narrative (occupational storytelling and occupational storymaking) life events are made meaningful. Thus, the individual participant, through occupation, is enabled to move forward to greater levels of accomplishment and challenge.[3]

Lifestyle Redesign: Implementing the Well Elderly Program offers a pragmatic approach for interested practitioners to implement their own programs as well as promotes a theoretical basis for providing such a program. This excellent source book and manual lists at least 34 themes and presentations (e.g., stress management through an active body; mental challenges and games; deciphering food labels; adaptive equipment in the home; home safety-body mechanics; energy conservation, fall prevention, and joint protection; and community safety—guest lecturer from the police department).[3] Well written and precise with knowledgeable content modules and module handouts, this resource is an outstanding find for any therapist. It is a vital program in enabling elderly persons to remain independent in the community as long as possible.

In conclusion, the results of the USC Well Elderly Study demonstrated that occupational therapy intervention was highly successful. Subjects who received occupational therapy experienced more positive gains and fewer declines than did the subjects in the social activity and no program groups. In the area of limitation in work activities due to physical health problems, the occupational therapy group demonstrated an increase of 1% while the control groups declined by 13%. In the increase of vitality, the occupational therapy group demonstrated an increase of 6%; the control groups declined by 2%.[3]

First and foremost, the research of this study demonstrates that occupational therapy can help older adults remain independent and healthy for a longer period of time. Second, the study indicates that the morbidity and the effects of disability can be reduced and that health care costs can be driven down. The U.S. Government currently spends 60% of its Medicare budget on nursing home care. Third, the findings of this study suggest that "keeping busy" is not enough. Professional direction is needed in producing therapeutic effects that can result from engagement in activity and meaningful occupation. Finally, the positive results show that occupational therapy has a new frontier—that of prevention.[3] This excellent resource points to scientific research that is dedicated to helping the practitioner with the complex challenges of an ever-expanding aging population.

One of the biggest problems of the 21st century will be how to enable the older population to remain productive and independent in the community as long as possible. Occupational therapy can become an important solution to this challenge. Trumpeting the call to therapists and assistants is only part of the answer. The call must be heard in the boardrooms of insurance companies and in congressional committees concerned with helping seniors and bringing health care costs down as much as possible. Most importantly, older adults themselves should hear it so that they will be able to learn how and why preventive occupational therapy is important to them. Older persons are interested in health care and are, for the most part, one of the most active age groups that vote. Their interest in having occupational therapy help them remain independent and stay optimally healthy for as long as possible is a vital concern to us all.

ALTERNATIVE APPROACHES IN GERONTIC OCCUPATIONAL THERAPY

Besides the exciting research that is coming from USC, there are other approaches to wellness that therapists are currently using. Ann Burkardt reports that wellness has become an important priority of United States' governmental policy. The Public Health Service of the U.S. Department of Health and Human Services, Office of Disease Prevention and Health Promotion developed an initiative known as Healthy People 2000. In a recent meeting in New York City, representatives from national, state, and local governments, as well as health care professional associations and cultural and community organizations, met to discuss health care policy for the year 2000 and plan others to guide our society toward health care in 2010. The goals of Healthy People 2000 were to reduce health delivery disparities, to increase the life span, and to achieve access to prevention services for all Americans. Indeed, the arena of prevention lies before us.[42] Please see Appendix E for the newest information of Healthy People 2010.

Swarbrick and Hettinger (therapists working with smoking cessation activities to promote good health) outline the ABCs of wellness as affirming:[43]

1. An attitude that promotes satisfaction and quality of life and seeks wellness.

2. A balance of positive social support, emotional expression, environmental interactions and factors, and productive activity.

3. The controlling (taking charge) of one's health through education about behaviors that can lead to a state of wellness.

Mary Roth (occupational therapist and coordinator of the Senior Health Programs at Rush North Shore Medical Center) is a promoter of her organization's Good Health Program. The model used is one of collaboration of an interdepartmental team to influence wellness within their own community. The major focus is to enable individuals to change personal habits so their quality of life and personal habits can be enhanced. This program is also involved in an initiative to demonstrate how primary prevention can lessen illness, reduce health care costs, and reduce mortality.[42]

Burkardt informs us that at the Wellness Exchange in Chicago (American Occupational Therapy Association 1996 Annual Conference in Chicago) many therapists reported using complementary approaches in leisure time activities. Half of the occupational therapists who attended the Wellness Exchange stated that they used tai chi or chi gong within their practice. This approach can easily be incorporated into leisure and/or spiritual pursuits that can then become a part of one's activities of daily living routine.[42]

Some cultures (such as Chinese) harness their social beliefs to promote wellness throughout their life span. From my own personal experience, I can state that when touring China (at every city, town, and hamlet) I witnessed from 7:00 a.m. to 9:00 a.m. elderly Chinese people outside in public parks and streets performing tai chi or chi gong. Many had tape recorders of Chinese music playing as they participated. Some came in groups with fans or colorful swords to enhance the movements. As a part of Chinese culture, these activities are seen as ways of maintaining and promoting good health.

THE COMMUNITY-BASED OCCUPATIONAL THERAPIST AS A SERVICES COORDINATOR

Womack reports that she has used the concepts of the well elderly program to enhance a new job opportunity.[3,44] In May 1998, noting that there was a lack of traditional job situations, she responded to an advertisement for a resident services coordinator in housing for low-income residents. The Vanderbilt Apartments (of Asheville, NC) advertisement was searching for an individual who had a background in human services (preferably a public health nurse or social worker). Duties of the job were manifold. They consisted of the ability to assist in assessing and finding community resources, the possession of experience and knowledge with issues relating to older adults, the ability to address health and wellness needs, and the ability to facilitate the development of a sense of community within the apartment complex.[44]

The Vanderbilt Apartments house 158 older adults whose income falls below the federal poverty guidelines. The residents represented a wide variety of individuals who were retired professionals, homemakers, blue collar workers, military personnel, and those individuals who had difficulty working at all due to disorders such as substance abuse, mental illness, or physical disability. The Vanderbilt is funded by grants for the initial 3 years by a variety of services and sources, two national endowments, and three regional philanthropic organizations. The grant funds included $60,000 that may be used for special financial assistance to the Vanderbilt residents (e.g., purchasing medicine, supplying durable medical equipment, and assisting with transportation). This allows a great deal of accessibility to the residents as time is not spent dictated by third party payers.[44]

Initially, residents spent little time interacting with each other. They often sat in silence side-by-side in the lobby, checked their mail without looking at their neighbor, and rode elevators without speaking to each other. This represented an extremely impoverished social environment. The concept of building a sense of community became a major focus. Activity opportunities were structured to promote a greater sense of "coming together" among the residents and also to promote the role that each individual had within the community.[44]

The Vanderbilt program has a threefold focus (often these areas overlapped). First, there is the concept of intervening with the residents. This includes assistance with a variety of individual concerns (medications, household items, and durable medical equipment; accessing community agencies; obtaining transportation on an individual basis; budgeting on a fixed income; promoting and enhancing cooking skills for individuals who may be living alone for the first time in many years; dealing with the functional implications of living with low vision; and household safety) that were addressed as needed. Residential interventions in this setting assumed a humanistic approach. Womack states that she took a reflective stance toward the resident's viewpoint and approached each individual with care, respect, and empathy. The role of maintaining a formal professional distance was not utilized. Creating opportunities for occupation became Womack's skill. This required rapport and knowledge of the individual client and a desire to enable that person to bring forth his or her highest level of competence and creativity to meet challenges.[44]

The second approach is to develop and maintain the concept of community. Group opportunities for residents to engage in meaningful occupations, encouraging awareness of neighbors' needs and strengths, and caring for the physical environment are ways that community is promoted in the Vanderbilt Program. The Resident Services Program—decorating for the holidays, taking trips, and developing a weekly group modeled after the USC Well Elderly Study—promoted community.[3,44] After inception of these interventions residents had begun to interact, on their own, in the lobbies and in other communal areas. "Parallel lives" had developed into community responsiveness.[44]

The third area of concern of the Vanderbilt Resident Program was the development of a comprehensive focus. This involved collaborating with community agencies and partnering with the residents' friends and families to achieve positive outcomes. Other components included promoting goodwill among downtown businesses that serve the residents, identifying alternative funding sources for the program, and diversifying the coordinators' community involvement. Community networking was an essential part of this facet of the program.[44]

This exciting program should make us think about how rich and flexible our profession is. Womack sums this up best in her closing remarks: "The roots of occupational therapy grow deep, and, in my experience, will sustain us as we branch out into the community, where a multitude of needs, under the guise of many different names, await us all."[44]

THE OCCUPATIONAL THERAPIST AS ERGONOMIST AND ENVIRONMENTAL SPECIALIST

Donna Hoelscher and Sallie Taylor describe how they established an ergonomics consultation business entitled Safesite Ergonomic Consultive Services in St. James, MO. They sought to provide a service that examines the relationship between task demands and worker capabilities in the workplace.[45]

With the numbers of workers expecting to decline in the future, it is highly suspected that employers will try to lure well-trained and educated older workers back to the workplace—or to prolong retirement with incentive packages, flexible hours, and part-time opportunities. Certainly, for this group of workers, ergonomics will provide a special need to accommodate any accompanying disabilities and chronic diseases.

Service objectives of this consultation business included:[45]

✧ Improving and promoting health, safety, and comfort at work sites

✧ Preventing work-related musculoskeletal disorders

✧ Promoting early return to work after illness or injury

✧ Optimizing on-the-job work flow and productivity

✧ Facilitating employment and retaining employees with disabilities

✧ Identifying and then designing reasonable workplace accommodations

The major service focus required Safesite to establish a broad base of preventive services. First and foremost, evaluative services were offered: Occupational Safety and Health Administration (OSHA) 200 log analysis, job tasks analysis, functional job descriptions that met Americans with Disabilities Act standards, and worker symptom analysis and survey represented the basic evaluation criteria.[45]

Therapeutic interventions included work task modification as needed, equipment and tool design and modification as needed, the recommendation and implementation of administrative and engineering controls to minimize or eliminate risk factors associated with musculoskeletal disorders, and company-wide understanding and development of the ergonomics process. Training involved dividing supervisors, managers, workers, and company officials into ergonomics teams and educating them in the ergonomics process and principles.[45]

Marketing strategies included speaking to groups, referrals from satisfied clients, and marketing calls with follow-up appointments. In all of these approaches the goals during the initial contact were to help evaluate a company's level of risk and to determine if the company would benefit from Safesite services.[45]

The benefits of ergonomic consultive services can readily be addressed. Reducing the incidence and severity of illnesses and injuries results in fewer days lost and lower company medical costs. The employer, then, is able to minimize the cost of worker's compensation insurance premiums. Also, ergonomic improvements in the workplace can favorably affect worker morale, worker comfort in the workplace, job turnover rate, and productivity. All of these factors benefit the employer, the workers, and the workers' families.[45]

In the spring of 1999, Safesite developed a second component—that of establishing a network and support system to other occupational therapists interested in this area of practice. Safesite presently provides therapists with information tools and techniques in business systems (establishing effective and accurate accounting systems and understanding tax obligations). Another area of information is how to perform and develop a marketing survey in a local area to identify potential clients (customized mailers, brochures, proposal outlines, and letterheads are discussed). The third focus includes developing service delivery tools (checklists, forms, and reports that provide comprehensive ergonomics consultative services to industry and business) in an effective and efficient manner. Any questions regarding Safesite can be addressed by emailing SafeSite99@aol.com.[45]

This remarkable program demonstrates the flexibility to serve occupational therapy clients in new, entrepreneurial, and ever-expanding conduits of care and concern.

THE HOME ENVIRONMENT AS AN AREA OF CONCERN IN THE COMMUNITY

This is a splendid arena for occupational therapy primary prevention, as the elimination of architectural barriers, planning housing for older adults, and promoting safety and efficiency in the home can decrease factors that cause accidents, disabilities, stress, and illness.

Environmental modifications are helpful in enabling older adults to lead productive and meaningful lives in the community as long as possible. The husband and wife team of Shoshana Shamberg, occupational therapist, and Aaron Shamberg, landscape architect, suggests the following innovations for housing of the present and for the future. Open halls, wide doorways, and non-slip flooring are major elements of barrier-free designs. Slide-down cabinet interiors and adjustable-height countertops are helpful solutions in the kitchen. Persons with hand or visual problems can readily utilize large numbers, tactile indicators, and an enlarged thermostat. Suggestions for those with visual impairments include a variety of recommendations:[46]

 ⬥ Increase lighting—high-wattage or multiple bulbs may be used.
 ⬥ Non-glare lighting is essential (covers like shades and sconces are helpful).
 ⬥ For close-up work, halogen lighting is recommended.
 ⬥ Task lighting should be used in work areas where extra illumination may be required.
 ⬥ Switches that can provide adjustable intensity and light for difficult tasks are highly recommended.
 ⬥ Window treatments that permit light filtering and adjustment should be installed.
 ⬥ Awnings should be placed on outside windows where direct sunlight is most intense.
 ⬥ Contrasting color surfaces that define spaces and objects such as background and foreground are essential (e.g., wall and floor spaces, countertop sinks, step edges and step surfaces, light switch covers, and walls).
 ⬥ Voice output on controls, raised letters and signs, and tactile indicators are helpful sensory tools that can provide cues for dangerous situations and also provide direction.
 ⬥ The elimination of low-profile furniture (or at least moving it against walls out of the way of major access routes) affords a safe environment.
 ⬥ Grab bar systems in the bathroom that contrast in color from the wall should have a non-slip surface and at least be 1.5 inches in diameter to provide the greatest protection from accidents.

✧ Illuminated switches (for lights, appliances, and other electrical equipment) and large non-slip knobs and handles that have contrasting colors demonstrate good safety and efficiency.

For those with hearing impairment, the Shambergs suggest:[46]

✧ Writing implements and paper should be available for communication.

✧ A fax machine, a telephone relay system, and telecommunication devices for the deaf for telephone-enhanced communication.

✧ Visually alerting and vibrating signal devices are helpful when used on alarm clocks, smoke alarms, telephones, and doorbells.

✧ Furniture should be arranged so that individuals are facing each other when they are seated.

✧ Lighting should be adequate in social spaces so that the client can make use of visual cues when conversing.

There are numerous other recommendations that are helpful in the home. The use of ramps, stair glides, and outdoor chair lifts can help to create a "no-step" entrance. When doorways need to be widened, swing clear hinges can be applied, which can increase the door's clearance by 2 inches. Wall ovens can be installed at an appropriate height, which will aid in providing easy access. Bidet hygienic devices attach to standard toilet bowls and allow the user to be washed and dried. Anti-scald devices in the bathroom and kitchen guard against burning. Carpeting should consist of tight, short loops to prevent tripping. No-threshold shower stalls that use shower curtains instead of sliding glass or Plexiglas promote accessibility and safety.

In the kitchen, some items are useful in promoting a safe working environment. Pull-out shelves or cutting boards beneath a wall oven can provide a stable surface for transferring hot substances. All sinks and appliances should have counter space on both sides so that items (especially those that are heavy) can be slid from one place to another in order to avoid excess lifting.[46] These recommendations are useful in ensuring improved and safe activities of daily living performance in elderly persons.

THE OCCUPATIONAL THERAPIST AS HOME SAFETY CONSULTANT

Joan Sevigny, who has been a practicing home health occupational therapist for the past 10 years, came to realize that much of her work involved home safety. She is currently creating a new business into which she is integrating her occupational therapy skills with alternative interventions. Safety management is a prime factor—not only in the home but also in assisted living facilities, senior housing complexes, and retirement communities. Sevigny contends that as home safety therapists and managers, practitioners will be able to expand the scope of occupational therapy in the community wellness mode.[47]

In her article, "The Value of OT in Home Safety: More Than Just an Assessment," Sevigny divides her therapeutic approach into three areas. First, there are five key components of possible problem areas. These are environmental, cognition, sensory, physiological/neuromuscular, and psychological. Next she lists her concerns and then provides occupational therapy insight (interventions or strategies). The following serve as examples of her therapeutic approach.[47]

An *environmental* component might involve the problem or concern of accessibility to enter the home from the outside (or vice versa). The occupational therapy insight into this situation would be to ensure that the ramp is appropriately aligned. In the *cognitive* component area, the client might be confused. The occupational therapy insight would involve incorporating visual cues throughout the environment to deal with that concern. The *sensory* component might include loss of hearing that could cause frustration for the client. Occupational therapy insight in dealing with this concern could involve instructing the client and others who have contact with the client to establish eye contact before initiating a conversation. In the *physiological/neuromuscular* component the concern might involve problems with dynamic standing and sitting balance. Occupational therapy insight could include establishing a level of safe mobility while performing daily tasks. Then work could be done on exercises related to functional reaching to be able to retrieve items on a shelf in the kitchen. The last component includes *psychological* issues. A concern might include a client having difficulty coping with changes in the home (e.g., adaptations in the bathroom). A solution (occupational therapy insight) could involve providing adaptations slowly.[47]

Fall prevention and safety issues are prime concerns of practitioners and clients. Sevigny briefly describes a fall prevention situation. Occupational therapists understand the use of adaptive equipment such as the appropriate size of a bath bench for a specific client. In one instance a client had been ordered a bath bench (from an agency without an occupational therapist's evaluation as to the appropriateness of the equipment) where the client's feet were 6 inches off the floor when she was sitting on the edge of the bench. Clearly, this was unsafe. It wasn't until the occupational therapist had been called in on the case that safety measures were enacted. The occupational therapist contacted the durable medical equipment provider to replace the larger bench for a smaller version. Thus, a "safe" intervention was provided, and the client could begin instruction in safe transfer in and out of the tub.[47]

Sevigny instructs us that "we must look for situations in which safety is an issue. Many times we do not focus on what lies right before us. Safety is a concern in all environments."[47, p. 13] Safety is certainly an area ripe for occupational therapy intervention and consultancy practice.

OCCUPATIONAL THERAPISTS COLLABORATING WITH ARCHITECTS REGARDING HOUSING AND INSTITUTIONAL NEEDS

We have seen how occupational therapists have become advocates for improved design in the workplace and in the home setting. Occupational therapists are now becoming actively involved in co-designing a variety of living arrangements with architects.

The following quote from a publication entitled *Design for Aging: Strategies for Collaboration Between Architects and Occupational Therapists* very aptly describes occupational therapy's special attributes as applied to older adults and housing: "Occupational therapists are one of the professional groups to which architects can look for knowledge about aging as it applies to built environments."[18, p. 12]

This very interesting resource describes ways in which occupational therapists acted as design consultants for a variety of settings. Some examples included a design for an assisted living facility, and an interior design for the renovation of the psychiatric ward and bone marrow transplant unit of a tertiary care teaching hospital with a large percentage of elderly users.[18]

Specifically, occupational therapists have participated and collaborated in a variety of projects by providing:[18]

⬦ Planned adjacencies for ideal wheeling and walking distances
⬦ Determined room configurations based on objective pattern-of-use data
⬦ Appropriate adaptive devices (e.g., adjustable height kitchen surfaces based on how older adults manipulated and maneuvered objects whether they were progressively frail or well)
⬦ Designed ramp and stair surfaces and configurations for mobility needs
⬦ Clarified performance criteria for bathrooms and kitchens
⬦ Appropriate color schemes for signage and legibility
⬦ Optimized acoustics for noise abatement and lighting for glare reduction; optimal continuity regarding appropriate lighting

In the existing home setting or care facility requiring modification, an occupational therapist's consultation usually begins with the observation of a specific individual's daily activities and an assessment that identifies environmental problem areas. Some areas of observation (involving the answering of specific questions) are:[18]

⬦ The Three-Dimensional Environment
    ▲ Are stepping and balance use of entries and doorways appropriate?
    ▲ Are lifting arm, reaching, and finger dexterity adequate when using light switches?
    ▲ Are reaching and bending needs met when utilizing outlets?
    ▲ Are reaching needs for closets, cupboards, and grab bars appropriate?
    ▲ Do rails (that involve support, steps, and ramps) provide appropriate safety?
    ▲ Are grasping needs met for hardware?
⬦ The Lighting Environment
    ▲ Does the lighting level provide visual adequacy and is placement adequate regarding the lighting level?
    ▲ Do lighting features control glare?
⬦ The Home Furnishings
    ▲ Are furniture edges and features protecting the individual from bruising and bumping?
    ▲ Are placements of cords protecting the older person from tripping and providing adequate circulation?
    ▲ Are rugs and flooring safe from tripping or sliding?
    ▲ Are chairs adequate for older individuals when seated (regarding positioning and comfortable seating) and when rising?

Many solutions to these problems may be relatively inexpensive and small scale. Some intervention strategies could include grab bars, non-slip floor surfaces, placement of fixtures, and easily reachable storage arrangements.[18]

With new construction projects occupational therapists have the opportunity to expand their scope considerably. Consider that occupational therapists can affect decisions about site planning, room size and configuration, and the development of space requirements by dealing with circulation layouts (e.g., as needed by wheelchair use) and defining adjacencies.[18]

Occupational therapy's involvement with the community has a new and expanding focus dedicated to the needs of promoting wellness for as long as possible and providing late life adults with new methods, plans, and adaptations to improve productivity, meaning, and quality in their lives.

UNIT 1 REFERENCES

1. Neistadt, M.E., Crepeau, E.B. (1998). *Willard and Spackman's occupational therapy* (p. 5). Philadelphia: Lippincott.

2. The American Occupational Therapy Association. (1994). *Occupational performance areas as defined by the American Occupational Therapy Association's uniform terminology*: Bethesda, MD: The American Occupational Therapy Association, Inc.

3. Mandel, D.R., Jackson, J.M., Zemke, R., Nelson, L., & Clark, F.A. (1999). *Life style redesign: Implementing the well elderly program* (pp. 6-70). Bethesda, MD: The American Occupational Therapy Association, Inc.

4. Foti, D. (1996). Gerontic occupational therapy: specialized intervention for the older adult. In K.O. Larson, R. G. Stevens-Ratchford, L. Pedretti, & J. L. Crabtree JL (Eds.), *The role of occupational therapy with the elderly* (pp. 25-33). Bethesda, MD: The American Occupational Therapy Association, Inc.

5. Scwartz, K.B. (1998). The history of occupational therapy. In M. E. Neistadt, E. B. Crepeau (Eds.), *Willard and Spackman's occupational therapy* (p. 854). Philadelphia: Lippincott.

6. Barton, G.E. (1919). *Teaching the sick: A manual of occupational therapy as re-education* (p.10). Philadelphia: W.B. Saunders.

7. Hopkins, H.L. (1983). An historical perspective on occupational therapy. In H. L. Hopkins & H. D. Smith (Eds.), *Willard and Spackman's occupational therapy* (6th Ed.). Philadelphia: Lippincott.

8. Lewis, S. (1989). *Elder care in occupational therapy* (pp. 8-11, 56-74, 224-226, 231-237). Thorofare, NJ: SLACK Incorporated.

9. Dunton, W. R., Jr. (1919). *Credo. In Reconstruction Therapy.* Philadelphia: W.B. Saunders.

10. Hildenbrand, G. (1947). Geriatrics and occupational therapy. *Am J Occup Ther, 1,* 159-161.

11. Willard, H. S. & Spackman, C. S. (Eds.). (1963). *Occupational therapy* (3rd Ed.). Philadelphia: Lippincott.

12. Davis, L. J. & Kirkland, M. (Eds.). (1986). *The role of occupational therapy with the elderly (ROTE).* Bethesda, MD: American Occupational Therapy Association, Inc.

13. Larson, K. O. (1998). Section 2: Conceptual models of practice and frames of reference. In K. O. Larson, R. G. Stevens-Ratchford, L. Pedretti, & J. L. Crabtree (Eds.), *The role of occupational therapy with the elderly (ROTE)* (pp.109-116). Bethesda, MD: American Occupational Therapy Association, Inc.

14. Allen, C. K. (1985). *Occupational therapy for psychiatric diseases: Measurement and management of cognitive disabilities.* Boston: Little, Brown and Company.

15. Ludwig, F. M. (1988). Anne Cronin Mosey. *Six perspectives on theory for the practice of occupational therapy* (pp. 41-64). Rockville, MD: Aspen.

16. Van Deusen, J. (1988). Mary Reilly. *Six perspectives on theory for practice of occupational therapy* (pp. 143-163). Rockville, MD: Aspen.

17. Kielhofner, G. & Burke, J. (1980). A model of human occupation, part one: Conceptual framework and content. *Am J Occup Ther, 34,* 572-581.

18. Ware, C. (Ed.). (1993). *Design for aging: Strategies for collaboration between architects and occupational therapists* (pp. 4, 12-35). Washington, DC: Aging Design Research Program—The Administration on Aging.

19. Vitez, M. (1999, December 19). Longevity. *The Philadelphia Inquirer Magazine, 21-22.*

20. Sokolove, M. (1999, December 19). Demography. *The Philadelphia Inquirer Magazine, 21-22.*

21. David, D. (1966). Section 1: Gerontology: the study of aging and older adults. In K. O. Larson, R. G. Stevens-Ratchford, L. Pedretti, & J. L. Crabtree (Eds.), *The role of occupational therapy and the elderly* (pp. 15-19). Bethesda, MD: The American Occupational Therapy Association, Inc.

22. American Occupational Therapy Association. (1991). *1990 Member Data Survey.* Rockville, MD: The American Occupational Therapy Association,Inc.

23. Schuster, C. S. (1992). The holistic approach. In C. S. Schuster & S. S. Ashburn (Eds.), *The process of human development: A holistic life span* (pp. 24-29). Philadelphia: Lippincott.

24. Kohlberg, L. (1973). Stages and aging in moral development: Some speculations. *Gerontologist, 1*(3), 497-502.

25. Cipriani, J. (1996). Section 3: Maturation: Development of the older adult. In K. O. Larson, R. G. Stevens-Ratchford, L. Pedretti, & J. L. Crabtree (Eds.), *The role of occupational therapy with the elderly* (pp. 47-51). Bethesda, MD: The American Occupational Therapy Association, Inc.

26. Fidler, G. (1996). Life-style performance: From profile to conceptual model. *Am J Occup Ther, 50,* 139-147.

27. Schwartz, A.N. (1974). A transactional view of the aging process. In A. N. Schwartz & I. Mensh (Eds.), *Professional obligations and approaches to the aged* (pp. 25-29). Springfield, IL: Charles C. Thomas.

28. Davis, L. J. (1986). Gerontology in theory and practice. In L. J. Davis & M. Kirkland (Eds.), *The role of occupational therapy with the elderly* (p. 34). Rockville, MD: American Occupational Therapy Association, Inc.

29. Mish, F. C. (Ed.). (1983). *Webster's ninth collegiate dictionary* (p. 1358). Springfield, MA: Merriam-Webster.

30. Barron, M. L. (1961). *The aging American: An introduction to social gerontology and geriatrics.* New York: Thomas Y. Crowell.

31. Hey, R. P, & Barry, P. (1999, December 4). Animosity politics: 1999's missed opportunities. *AARP Bulletin, 40,* 4.

32. Macrae, N. (1991). The older worker. In K. Jacobs (Ed.), *Occupational Therapy: Work-Related programs and assessments* (2nd Ed., pp. 358-364). Boston: Little, Brown and Co.

33. Ludwig, F. M. & Kornblau, B. L. (1996). Evaluation and intervention for work and productive activities. In K. O. Larson, R. G. Stevens-Ratchford, L. Pedretti, & J. L. Crabtree (Eds.), *The role of occupational therapy with the elderly* (pp. 705-722). Bethesda, MD: The American Occupational Therapy Association, Inc.

34. Mish, F. C. (Ed.). (1983). *Webster's ninth collegiate dictionary* (p. 1007). Springfield, MA: Merriam Webster.

35. Kerr, T. (1998, July 27). Occupational performance in retirement. *Advance for Occupational Therapy Practitioners, 25-26.*

36. Glantz, C. H. & Richman, N. (1956). Evaluations and intervention for leisure activities. In K. O. Larson, R. G. Stevens-Ratchford, L. Pedretti, & J. L. Crabtree (Eds.), *The role of occupational therapy and the elderly* (p. 729). Bethesda, MD: The American Occupational Therapy Association, Inc.

37. Pedretti, L. W. (1996). *Occupational performance: A model for practice in physical dysfunction* (4th Ed., pp. 3-11). St. Louis: Mosby-Year Book.

38. House Select Committee on Aging, Subcommittee for Health and Long Term Care. (1985, May 10). Elder abuse: A national disgrace (executive summary). Washington, DC: United States House of Representatives.

39. Larson, K. O. (1996). Section 8: The social environment. In K. O. Larson, R. G. Stevens-Ratchford, L. Pedretti, & J. L. Crabtree (Eds.), *The role of occupational therapy and the elderly* (pp. 278-287). Bethesda, MD: The American Occupational Therapy Association, Inc.

40. Holland, L. R., Kasraian, K. R., & Leonardelli, C. A. (1987, Spring). Elder abuse: An analysis of the current problem and potential role of the rehabilitation professional. *Phys and Occup Ther in Ger, 3,* 41-49.

41. Aitken, M. J. & Lohman, H. (1996). Health care systems: Changing perspectives. In K. O. Larson, R. G. Stevens-Ratchford, L. Pedretti, & J. L. Crabtree (Eds.), *The role of occupational therapy with the elderly* (p. 58). Bethesda, MD: The American Occupational Therapy Association, Inc.

42. Burkhardt, A. (1997, June). Occupational therapy and wellness. *OT Practice, 6,* 28-35.

43. Hettinger, J. & Swarbrick, P. (1996, September 12). The wellness connection. *OT Week, 12,* 12-13.

44. Womack, J. & Farmer, P. (1999, November 22). Strong roots, flexible branches: Community-based occupational therapy at the Vanderbilt Apartments. *OT Practice, 4,* 17-21.

45. Hoelscher, D. & Taylor, S. (2000, January 3). Ergonomics consultation: An opportunity for occupational therapists. *OT Practice, 5,* 16-19.

46. Shamberg, S. & Shamberg, A. (1996, June). Blueprints for independence: Carefully planned environmental modifications can improve functional performance. *OT Practice, 1,* 22-29.

47. Sevigny, J. (2000, March 13). The value of OT in home safety: More than just an assessment. *OT Practice, 5,* 10-13.

CASE STUDIES

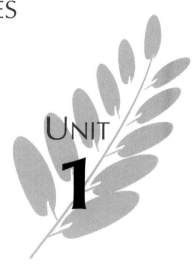

UNIT

1

CASE STUDY 1

Community-Based Occupational Therapy Focusing on Healthy Living/Wellness

Womack provides a well-thought-out and well-integrated community-based case study that appeared in the November 1999 issue of *OT Practice*. This case review summarizes her intervention approach.

Ms. P is a resident of the Vanderbilt Apartments where Jenny Womack, MS, OTR/L served as a resident services coordinator from July 1998 to September 1999. The Vanderbilt is a high-rise apartment building that houses 158 older adults whose income falls below federal poverty guidelines. In her article, "Strong Roots, Flexible Branches: Community-Based Occupational Therapy at the Vanderbilt Apartments," Womack describes, through Ms. P's own words, how this client was helped by occupational therapy intervention.

Ms. P was diagnosed initially with post-traumatic stress disorder (almost 10 years ago when she admitted herself into a psychiatric hospital). Ms. P was later diagnosed as bipolar. There had been a long period of depression, suicide attempts, a failed marriage, and washouts of confidence and self-esteem. It was during that hospitalization that Ms. P first became involved with occupational therapy. Although uninterested at first, she later learned that occupational therapy provided an outlet for her anger, and as such helped to channel destructive behavior into constructive activity. Occupational therapy also helped to awaken problem-solving skills and taught Ms. P strategy and planning techniques.

Womack's program at Vanderbilt provided numerous opportunities for occupation. Ms. P considered these opportunities (both those she created and those created within the program) as a way to balance her "fixed daily routine" (such as taking medications, keeping doctors' appointments, getting physical and mental exercise, and sticking to her diet) with that of "daily abandonment" (spontaneous, creative, and community activities—such as building things, painting, photography, and community events).

In her own words Ms. P told us, "Occupational therapists have helped with daily routines ranging from finding someone to assist with bathing and picking up medications, to getting to doctor's appointments. They strengthen us with exercise classes, lead walking groups... sponsor specialists in various areas of health care and care for safety."[1]

Ms. P further illustrates occupational therapy's roles at Vanderbilt when she relates that occupational therapists also made available opportunities through classes that encompass healthy living, community meals, communication skills, stimulating discussion on a variety of topics, as well as dramatic and musical entertainment. Occupational therapy is instrumental in "creating an environment that affords maximum potential for healthy living."[1]

CASE STUDY 2

Case Discussion Involving Safety Intervention in the Community

The reader is advised to review Chapter 4, under "The Occupational Therapist as Home Safety Consultant," where a case discussion is referenced regarding the use of appropriate bath equipment in order to prevent falls.

REFERENCE

1. Womack, J. & Farmer, P. (1999, November 22). Strong roots, flexible branches: Community-based occupational therapy at the Vanderbilt Apartments. *OT Practice, 10,* 17-21.

UNIT 2

LIFE SPAN CHANGES AND THE ELDERLY, DEATH, AND DYING

Biological, Psychosocial, and Cognitive Considerations in Aging

5

The life span changes that occur over one's lifetime are varied and individualistic. Human beings are influenced by their environment, intrinsic factors, and ethnic heritage. Aging involves three major components: the biological factor, the psychosocial aspect, and the cognitive element. These three major components are, in turn, affected by a variety of disease states that can be encountered during the aging process.

The Biological Factor

Physical maturity, in most individuals, is reached approximately between ages 18 and 22. At that time, many researchers believe, the biological changes that occur with aging become a continuation of a decline that will proceed throughout the life span of an individual. Other elements, such as those that are a result of environmental and physical conditions (e.g., obesity, nutrition, environmental toxins, economic advantage, physical activity, traumatic events, diet, hereditary factors, and lifestyle choice) can definitely affect the pace of aging. Biological aging can also be the result of an increased vulnerability to stress and disease.[1]

It should also be noted that within each person biological change can take place at different rates and times and in different cells, organs, and tissues. Besides the biological changes and declines in old age, 85% of adults over the age of 65 experience at least one or more chronic conditions. Despite these facts it is interesting to note that limitation in activities of daily living is only experienced by 23% of the population over 65 (14% of those between the ages of 65 and 74, 29% of those between 75 and 84, and 34% of those 85 years and older).[2] This speaks to the endowment of the human body to provide elaborate compensation systems and a vast amount of functional reserve when encountering the changes that aging brings.[1]

THE GENE REVOLUTION IN MEDICINE

Before discussing the biological changes and subsequent diseases associated with aging, it is paramount to briefly discuss the scientific revolution that is taking place in the area of genome research and its relevance to aging and disease. The genome is basically an instruction manual that contains the 100,000 or so genes that govern human development, maintenance, and operation. Deficits in various genes can contribute to or cause almost all human disease. Competition in gene research has become intense because the stakes are high. Companies that are the first to develop useful drugs from genomic information may have the opportunity to develop an eventual gold mine.[3]

On June 26, 2000, in front of television cameras (on all three major American networks), it was announced that the genetic code of human life had been broken. It was a great moment, and I felt fortunate to be able to witness this live television moment. Dr. Francis S. Collins, head of the Human Genome Project, and Mr. J. Craig Venter, head of Celera Genomics, announced that they had finished the first survey of the human genome. The human genome contains the genetic material that is encased in almost every cell of the human body. It is at least some 3 billion chemical letters long. Now that the human genome has been mapped and codified, the difficult task of putting it to work is at hand.

According to scientific reports, genes are believed to be responsible for gray hair, wrinkled skin, osteoporosis, and certain types of organ failure. Research in gene activity over a lifetime has become more advanced due to the recent advent of "gene chips" (DNA-coated microchips the size of postage stamps), which allow scientists the opportunity to trace the activity of tens of thousands of genes individually over time. Also, with the development of high-powered computers, patterns can be more readily detected.[4]

It has been reported that from infectious disease to oncology, science is transforming and revolutionizing medicine. For instance, a hereditary condition known as *hemochromatosis* (in which the body stores iron at dangerous levels) can now be identified through a DNA test that can spot it in a drop of blood. Clients can then be treated by a weekly regimen of blood lettings (which reduces the iron level). Formerly individuals with this condition died of organ failure in their mid 40s. Dr. Francis Collins of the National Human Genome Research Institute predicts that by the year 2010, DNA-based screening tests will enable the individual to gauge his or her unique health risks.[5]

Genetic discoveries will most likely trigger an avalanche of new pharmaceuticals that will be aimed at treating the disease rather than at disease symptoms. Depending on a client's genetic profile, physicians will be able to prescribe custom-made medications. Collins believes that by the year 2050 many potential diseases will be able to be cured at the molecular level before they have an opportunity to arise.[5]

Scientists are pursuing an array of varied gene-based interventions. Useful genes can be utilized to make medicinal proteins in a culture or introduced directly into the body. At the same time researchers are also learning to stifle or block the activity of harmful genes by interfering with a gene's production of proteins or by inhibiting the action of those proteins.[5]

In the future, genetic knowledge may be harnessed to slow aging as well as to cure diseases. The Genome Project was designed to unlock an organism's complete genetic code, which can determine whether a fertilized egg develops into a fly, a human, a mouse, or another living species. As an example of the sensitivity of this process, a simple misspelling in a gene can bring havoc, causing a normal cell to become cancerous. Genes also have an influence over our behavior and personalities.[6]

On May 4, 2000, *The Wall Street Journal* reported that gene therapy was beginning to show promise in some cancer trials. Though still in its nascent state, researchers and clinicians are testing gene intervention on several tumor types. For instance, Ms. Patricia Aneff had been treated as a test subject for a lung tumor. A test demonstrated that she had a defective gene, known as p53. The function of p53 is to break runaway cell growth. When physicians injected her tumor with sound copies of p53, it shrank into a small ball. This enabled surgeons to readily remove it. Previously, the tumor's tentacles had made surgery out of the question. She now appears to be free of cancer.[7]

The future lies before us with real hopes of slowing aging and battling disease with a new zeal that is girded by advanced genetic technology. However, Robert Sapolsky reminds us that despite the new gene age, genes and the environment interact. A particular gene can be affected differently depending on the environment. Although there is genetic vulnerability, it may not lead to inevitability. Genes may be turned on and off through environmental factors. For example, if a college student has a miserably stressful day of exams, his or her immune system may be suppressed with a resultant cold. Dr. Sapolsky believes that the more scientists learn about genes, the more they will learn about the importance of the environment.[8]

Now that some major aspects of the genetic revolution in medicine have been described, it is time to discuss an overview of age-related biological changes that have a particular relevance to practitioners working with older persons. This discussion will first describe progressive physiological changes in organ systems and review specific disease entities as related to those systems.

THE CARDIOVASCULAR SYSTEM

The cardiac cycle within the heart is responsible for coordinating the volume and direction of blood flow. It is through this process that the heart regulates body core temperature in order to maintain hemostasis, delivers oxygen to vital tissues and organs, and removes carbon dioxide and other byproducts.[9]

The heart is a four-chambered pump. The right side of the heart, containing the right atrium and right ventricle, collects blood and delivers it to the lungs. There, it can be reoxygenated. The left side of the heart (the left atrium and the left ventricle) collects blood from the lungs and delivers it for circulation throughout the body. There are four heart valves that assist in the direction and passage of blood flow within the heart. The opening and closing of these valves is dependent upon pressure and volume changes on the papillary muscles and within the heart.[9]

There is a specialized nervous conduction network within the heart. The coordinated sequence of depolarization and contraction is initiated by the pacemaker of the heart (known as the *sinoatrial* or *SA node*). From the SA node the impulse travels to the ventricles through the *atrioventricular* (AV) *node*, then through the bundle branches and the *Purkinje fibers*. Because depolarization is an electrical cellular process, it can be studied by *electrocardiogram* (EKG). Physicians, then, are able to study normal or abnormal conduction status through the use of this diagnostic tool.[9]

The cardiac cycle adjusts and maintains cardiac output. This cycle occurs in two phases (input and output). The *input phase (diastole)* occurs when the input valves (known as the *mitral* and *tricuspid*) are open, and the *output valves* (*aortic* and *pulmonary*) are closed. When the input valves are closed, the first heart sound is heard. When the pressure rises in the ventricles, the output valves will open. The numerical value assigned to the pressure that is required to open the output valves is the *diastolic pressure* (bottom number of a blood pressure reading).

The *output* (*systole*) occurs when the aortic and pulmonary valves are open. At that point the ventricles will continue to contract, and the pressure will continue to climb into the ventricles. The peak pressure generated when the ventricles eject blood is the *systolic blood pressure* (the top number of a blood pressure reading). When the ventricular pressure falls, the output valves will close, and a second heart sound is created. During one contraction the total amount of blood ejected is called a *stroke volume*. The amount of blood that is ejected per minute is known as *cardiac output*.[9]

The following discussion includes the structural and functional changes that occur in the heart during aging as well as disease entities within the heart and vascular system. There are a number of structural changes that occur as one ages without an identifiable pathology. These include:[1]

  ✧ The heart muscle becomes fattier (usually due to accumulating amyloid deposits). Both the heart volume and mass increase.
  ✧ There is hypertrophy of the left ventricle of the heart that may be attributed to an adaptive mechanism to maintain cardiac wall stress.
  ✧ The heart's muscle fibers become stiffer and less elastic due to an increase of collagen around the muscle fibers and the valves causing a decrease in the relative amount of heart muscle.
  ✧ The electrical conduction system becomes altered in that the pacemaker cells of the ventricles become infiltrated with fat and connective tissue. This produces *dysrhythmias* (SA and AV node dysfunction).

Pacemakers can be utilized to improve malfunctions in the impulse-conducting system.

These structural changes result in a number of functional changes. Because there is a decreased compliance of the blood vessels, blood pressure (both diastolic and systolic) may increase as we age. There is a decline in cardiac output and myocardial contractility. Stroke volume is diminished, and there is an overall decline in resting cardiac output. There is a decrease in the maximum heart rate (from 190 in an individual in his or her 20s to 130 in his or her 70s). There is a general reduction of oxygenated blood supply to various organs, tissues, and muscles often resulting in fatigue, decreased work capacity, limited endurance, and a gradual reduction in exercise tolerance.[1]

HEART DISEASE AND RELATED CONDITIONS

Although the number of Americans affected by heart disease has declined in recent years (from a high in 1963), it still remains the number-one killer in the United States.

Coronary Artery Disease

Coronary artery disease can most commonly be seen in *atherosclerosis* (a blocking of the coronary artery through the development of fibrofatty plaques within the vessel intima that causes the arterial lumen to narrow) and *arteriosclerosis* (a change in the extracellular material of the arterial walls that decreases the compliance of the vessels), causing the arterial walls to harden and thicken.[10]

Hypertension

Hypertension, commonly identified as high blood pressure, is a leading factor that can produce myocardial infarction, stroke, kidney failure, vascular dementia, peripheral vascular disease, congestive heart failure, and angina pectoris.[1,10] Physicians now believe that both the systolic and diastolic blood pressure should range no higher than 140 mmHg/90 mmHg. The wider the spread is between the numbers, the greater the risk is to the client.[11] Hypertension and heart disease, in general, call for utilization of drugs that control blood pressure (there are about 60 such drugs on the market at present); usage of cholesterol-reducing drugs (that keep cholesterol at 200 mg/dL or less and that maintain LDL [the bad cholesterol] as far below 130 as possible); utilization of drugs that prevent clotting (as needed); initiation of substances that reduce the homocysteine level (high intake of folic acid and B vitamins); utilization of a controlled diet that is low in cholesterol and saturated fats; participation in exercise at least 30 minutes three times a week; utilization strategies that combat stress; and the elimination of smoking.[12,13]

New Weapons Against Heart Disease

No discussion concerning heart disease would be complete without a review of the technology that is currently being employed to counter this condition. The ultrasound probe or the noninvasive *magnetic resonance imaging* (MRI) can be used to ferret out "vulnerable plaques" (killer plaques that are hidden and expand when the fibrous tissue holding them lets go). These are plaques that do not show up on a traditional angiogram. Statin drugs are helpful in shrinking these vulnerable plaques.[13]

There are a number of cutting-edge surgical interventions for heart disease that are allowing older individuals to live longer lives, and at the same time improve the quality of those lives. One such is an *off-pump coronary bypass* (OPCAB). In this procedure, surgeons open the chest (as in ordinary bypass surgery), but do not use a heart-lung machine. Instead, operations are carried out on a beating heart with the aid of instruments that hold portions of the heart steady. Sections of blood vessels are then taken from other parts of the body and are grafted to create detours around the blocked arteries. Another surgical alternative, *angioplasty*, in which a catheter is inserted through an artery in the groin and snaked into the coronary artery to the narrowed area, utilizes a tiny inflated balloon to squash fatty plaques against the artery wall. Often a mesh cylinder, known as a *stent*, is inserted to prop and keep the channel open. Another technique, known as *angiogenesis*, utilizes *capsules* (made from a basic fibroblast growth factor) that are implanted into the heart wall alongside the diseased artery to spur the growth of new arteries.

Other approaches include the punching of new channels into the heart wall. A method known as *percutaneous myocardial revascularization* (PMR), involves a laser-tipped catheter that is guided to a blood-starved part of the heart wall. Quick blasts from a laser drill of 20 or more tiny holes, most of the way through the wall, cause tissue damage that appears to stimulate new blood vessel growth. Yet another technique uses radiation to supplement angioplasty. With this intervention (known as Beta-Cath), tiny radioactive pellets are sent through a catheter to the blockage and held in place for several minutes and then removed. The radiation inhibits scar tissue that could result in new blockages. This technique is in the early stages, and studies are being conducted to review the long-term effects of this type of radiation therapy.[13]

A final surgical procedure, which may prove useful in the 21st century, is bypass surgery done by robots (termed *minimally invasive telerobotic surgery*). This procedure is really in a nascent stage at this writing, but it does bring another new and exciting method to the operating room table. With this experimental robot-assisted surgery, physicians are able to get deep inside the body by means of tiny incisions that are no larger than pencil holes. This allows for a shorter recovery period. At the end of the robot's fingers are tiny metal fingers with rotating wrists that hold a minuscule instrument, a light, and a camera. These arms and fingers are actually controlled by a surgeon sitting at a computer console in a corner of the operating room. The controls, designed to look and feel like traditional instruments, allow the surgeon to readily adapt to the system. Each movement is processed by the computer's system. Interpretive algorithms help to eliminate the natural tremor of the human hand.[14]

One more intervention aspect being studied by researchers is that heart disease may actually be caused by infection, specifically *Chlamydia pneumoniae*. This particular microbe is often found in the artery-clogging plaque that is associated with atherosclerosis. It is postulated that the infection could cause inflammation within the arteries, allowing them to be vulnerable and ripe for plaque formation. Three major clinical trials are now underway in the United States testing the effectiveness of antibiotics with heart patients.[13,15]

The following information deals with a discussion of disease states within the cardiac framework.

Ischemic Heart Disease

Ischemic heart disease (also known as *coronary artery disease*, or CAD) is a chronic condition that may produce symptom-free periods for prolonged periods. These can alternate with acute symptomatic episodes that may lead to *angina pectoris* or *acute myocardial infarction* (heart attack). An imbalance of oxygen supply and demand created by arteriosclerotic narrowing of the coronary arteries is responsible for this condition.[9]

Angina Pectoris

Angina pectoris is characterized by a feeling of pressure or severe midsternal chest pain that occurs upon exertion and is alleviated by nitroglycerin and rest.[9]

Myocardial Infarction

Myocardial infarction (MI) occurs when there is severe ischemia that lasts longer than 20 to 30 minutes. MIs are described by their size and their location. *Infarction* (tissue death) results from inadequate blood flow.[9]

The primary symptom of MI is pressure-like chest pain that is severe and unrelenting. The pain, usually located substernally, can radiate to the back, arms, or upper jaw. Secondary symptoms include *dyspnea* (shortness of breath), vomiting, feelings of anxiety, nausea, and confusion.[16]

Medications are used during the acute hospitalization phase to relieve anxiety and pain, prevent complications, and limit the extent of heart muscle necrosis (death). The most common groups of medications include nitrates, β-adrenergic blockers, calcium channel blockers, and inotropic agents.[16] Surgical interventions have been described in the preceding section entitled "New Weapons Against Heart Disease."

Congestive Heart Failure

Congestive heart failure (CHF) occurs when the heart muscle is unable to maintain adequate output. It can also be manifested by ischemia, which may be due to diseases of the heart vessels, the heart valves, and the heart muscle itself. If the left ventricle is unable to move blood out of the lungs, pulmonary venous congestion will occur and fluid will accumulate in the lungs. If the left heart failure should continue, the system will continue to back up further, and the right ventricle will fail, causing the legs to become edematous. When both sides of the heart fail, there may be *oliguria* (decreased urine output) during the day and *nocturia* (excessive urine output) at night, shortness of breath, edematous feet, weakness, and loss of energy. Digitalis is often used to improve heart efficiency and reduce excess fluid from body tissues. Other medications include diuretics and angiotension-converting enzyme (ACE inhibitors). Heart failure can increase one's vulnerability to pneumonia and influenza, phlebitis, and clots in the lower extremities.[10,16]

Aortic Stenosis

Aortic stenosis (calcification) affects cardiac output. When the left ventricle hypertrophies, the following symptoms can occur: arrhythmias, cerebral insufficiency resulting in confusion, *syncope* ("blacking out" when exerting effort), and dizziness due to a drop in blood pressure. These clients are at risk for sudden death and may require surgery.[9]

Cardiac Arrest

Cardiac arrest occurs when an arrhythmia is produced by prolonged myocardial ischemia that disrupts the pumping of the ventricles. Ventricular fibrillation produces an uncoordinated quivering of the ventricles and can cause sudden death.[1]

Peripheral Vascular Disease

This disorder occurs as a result of inadequate blood supply to the extremities. Pain in the calves of the legs and a feeling of coldness or numbness in the feet are often symptoms. Gangrene and tissue necrosis may result.[10]

Cerebrovascular Accident

Cerebrovascular accident (CVA) or *stroke* is the second most significant cardiovascular disease in older adults. This condition is the third most common form of death in the United States and most other industrialized countries. It is surpassed only by heart disease and cancer.[17]

Stroke can be defined as a rapid onset of neurological deficits that persist for at least 24 hours or more. It may be a result of:[18]

1. *Intracerebral hemorrhage* (leak of blood from the vascular system)
2. *Thrombosis* and/or *embolism* (obstruction of blood flow through the vascular system)
3. Vascular insufficiency

These conditions lead to the infarction of brain tissue.

A major stroke can be preceded by *transient ischemic attacks* (minor strokes). These attacks (known as TIAs) are clearly a warning sign that oxygen and blood supply are temporarily insufficient. The symptoms resemble that of a stroke but are less severe and last for a brief period. These include confusion, deafness or ringing in the ears, slurred words, temporary nausea, fleeting blindness in one eye, hemiparesis, sudden severe headache, sudden falls, unsteadiness, and aphasia.

Controlling the risk factors is highly important in prevention and intervention of TIAs and stroke. The most common risk factors are high blood pressure, high cholesterol level, sedentary lifestyle, high salt intake, high stress levels, cardiac disease, obesity, smoking, and diabetes. Intervention frequently used to combat this condition includes anticoagulant drugs, utilization of diuretics, removal of plaque from affected arteries, bypass surgery, changes in diet, weight control, and exercise, and a healthy lifestyle in general.[10] Many of the risk factors and the medical intervention for stroke are similar to that of heart disease.

The most common permanent impairments in stroke are *hemiparesis* (weakness on one side of the body), *hemiplegia* (paralysis on one side of the body), and *aphasia* (decreased language ability associated with left hemispheric lesion). The most common forms of aphasia include non-fluent and fluent. *Non-fluent* aphasia is often divided into global aphasia and Broca's aphasia. In *global aphasia* there are no consistent language skills in any modality. Non-purposeful parts of words such as "mammi" and "mommi" may be used. In *Broca's aphasia* clients exhibit slow, hesitant, labored speech with the frequent misarticulation of the first sounds of words.

Wernicke's aphasia is a prime example of *fluent aphasia*. In this condition speech is easily produced and fluent. However, the language is often circumlocutory and lacks content. There frequently are sound substitutions, inappropriate word substitutions, nonmeaningful jargon, and nonmeaningful combinations of real words. In *conduction aphasia* the verbal expression is similar to Wernicke's, but the client has good comprehension. In *anomic aphasia* the client demonstrates word retrieval problems (in the context of grammatically correct, usually fluent, and easily articulated output), and speech tends to be empty and circumlocutory.

Other language difficulties include *right hemispheric language dysfunction* (deficits in the efficient and effective use of language), *paraphasia* (inconsistent sound substitutions), and *dysarthria* (oral speech production impaired). Other impairments characterized by stroke include bilateral planning deficits, *apraxia* (inability to plan voluntary motor movements), *unilateral visual perceptual neglect* (the individual neglects visual stimuli on the impaired side of the body), *homonymous hemianopsia* (visual field neglect—most clients with this condition are generally able to compensate with little demonstration of visual neglect), and *dysphagia* (swallowing disorders).[1,10]

Vascular Dementia

Vascular dementias are the result of the additive effects of multiple small infarcts. Vascular dementia is most likely to occur when the back of the brain is damaged. Emboli from the heart or within other parts of the vascular system as well as hypertension are often the cause of this condition. Controlling blood pressure is an important form of intervention. Symptoms are demonstrated by a sudden and/or abrupt onset and a step-by-step deterioration that follows a fluctuating course. Emotional lability frequently accompanies this disorder.[10,19]

THE CENTRAL NERVOUS SYSTEM

There are a variety of physiological and anatomical changes that occur in the brain as one ages. There is a decrease in the number of nerve fibers and cells in various portions of the brain as well as a decrease of approximately 10% in weight. Studies have demonstrated a loss of neurons that vary from 20% to 50% in areas of the cerebellum, the cerebral cortex, and the hippocampus. The cerebral ventricles can enlarge three to four times from age 30 until age 90. From the 30s to the 70s, the blood flow to the brain decreases by 13% to 20% (as measured by electroencephalogram).

There is a slowing to the response of stimuli. At times neuronal functioning can be compromised by the obstruction of the cytoplasm and neurotransmitters from cell bodies and the axons and dendrites. This is thought to be due to deposits of *lipofuscin* (aging pigment) in nerve cells, deposits of *amyloid* (aging protein) in the blood vessels and cells, the appearance of senile plaques, and the development of neurofibrous tangles. As a result, the transmission of information from one neuron to another becomes slower as we age. Concentrations of neurotransmitters generally decline with aging.[1]

However, some of these changes can be mitigated. First, the human brain possesses many more nerve cells than are needed. Second, compensatory mechanisms can be developed if the brain becomes damaged. Finally, it is now believed that the brain possesses more plasticity at the nerve cell level than was formerly thought.[1]

Memory: A Function of the Brain

Before reviewing disease states involving the brain and the nervous system, it is important to consider memory as an entity in itself, as it represents the highest order of human functioning.

Memory is a basic cognitive function that incorporates attention and executive cognitive functions (i.e., reasoning, planning, problem solving, learning social awareness, abstraction, judgment, and basic activities of daily living).[20]

According to the *information-processing* memory model, memory involves the processing of information through the sensory-perceptual memory system. Next involved is the short-term memory system, then on to the long-term memory system. Thoroughly processed information becomes a part of the long-term memory system and can be reactivated at any time.[21,22]

The handling of information into each of these three stages of the memory system is processed much like a computer. First, there is *encoding information* (experiencing, gathering, and representing information into a form that can be stored in memory). Next, there is *storage* (maintaining or holding information that is to be later remembered for immediate or later use). Third, there is *retrieval* (accessing information when it is needed).[20,21]

It is important to note the difference between learning and memory. *Learning* involves the acquiring of new information, and *memory* involves the retention of that information.[20] Each stage will now be more fully explored.

SENSORY-PERCEPTUAL MEMORY

Sensory-perceptual memory involves memories that are stored according to the sensory modality that receives it. This type of memory has a large storage capacity and a registration period that lasts no longer than 5 seconds. Information can be retrieved by paying attention to it. It is then transferred into the next stage—the short-term memory store.[21,22]

SHORT-TERM MEMORY

Short-term memory (also known as *active memory*) represents conscious awareness. It is used to process information from either sensory memory or long-term memory (to help interpret and understand incoming information). It consists of two component memory systems—primary memory and working memory. *Primary memory* represents the storage component of short-term memory (reflects recently experienced information that can be consciously held in the mind and recalled immediately). *Working memory* involves holding information in the mind and also being able to process the information to discern its underlying meaning. Working memory is highly correlated with executive functions. Short-term memory encodes information by means of images, sounds, and semantic codes (more complex and based on meaning). However, most information in short-term memory is encoded as sounds. In contrast to sensory-perceptual memory, short-term memory has a small storage capacity.[22] Nevertheless, this short-term storage capacity is helpful for thought as it narrows down information to manageable limits during comprehension. *Chunking*, the ability to group individual bits of information into smaller chunks, is a way to increase the amount of information that can be stored within short-term memory.[20,22]

Retrieval for storage in short-term memory, like in sensory-perceptual memory, is very short. Information is lost if attention is lost. In short-term memory, there are two strategies that the brain uses to retain information for longer than 30 seconds. One is *maintained rehearsal* (repeating the information to oneself) and the other is *elaborate rehearsal* (actively organizing the information and then associating it with other relevant information that is stored in long-term memory).[20,22]

The hippocampus, currently viewed by scientists as a kind of automatic station for short-term working memory, is now believed to be the primary site of short-term working memory.[23]

LONG-TERM MEMORY

Long-term memory involves any information that is no longer in conscious awareness or short-term memory. It includes information that is of remote long-term memories as well as those memories that were recently transferred. Not only are human beings able to recall memories at will, but individuals are able, when learning a new skill or basic information, to transfer relevant associated knowledge from long-term memory to working memory to enhance and better use the new information.[20,24]

Information in long-term memory is encoded in the form of abstract concepts. These concepts are in verbal, motor, visual, or auditory codes that are organized for eventual retrieval either by meaningful relations (semantic memory) or by time and place (episodic memory).[24,25]

The storage system of long-term memory is divided into two systems:

⬧ *Declarative* (or *explicit*), which is comprised of episodic and semantic memory

⬧ *Nondeclarative* (or *implicit*), which is comprised of procedural memory

Episodic memory is involved in the memory of personally relevant events and facts (e.g., faces, names of past presidents, birthdays, weddings, where one puts his or her eyeglasses). Episodic events and facts are the least durable of all types of memory. Retrieval from episodic memory depends upon one's ability to reconstruct the context of the original experience (by using contextual cues such as place and time).[20,25]

Semantic memory builds on episodic memory. It is complex and tightly integrated and involves a synthesis of facts that provides judgment, insight, and knowledge. It is more durable than episodic memory and is retrieved by associated concepts and meanings. Semantic memory is primarily generated by language, but it also includes symbols and concepts not associated with words (for instance, understanding nonverbal communication).[20]

Procedural memory, the most durable and basic type of memory, is believed to reside in the basal ganglia. Procedural memory involves motor, cognitive, and perceptual skills that are associated with the acquisition of movement-based information. After procedural memories are acquired they become automatic and evolve into routines that do not require conscious effort (e.g., how to throw a ball or ride a bicycle, typing, tying shoes, and brushing one's teeth).[20,26] Levy notes that procedural memory bypasses the need to devote a great amount of attention to a task and can reduce the demand on the limited capacity of short-term (working) memory.[20] This skill can become helpful and serve as a pivotal source of cognitive ability that can be capitalized on in rehabilitation when working with elderly individuals with dementia.[20]

Long-term memory (episodic, semantic, and procedural) is stored in an organized manner as it involves the storage of millions of pieces of information. New information is associated with information that is already stored in long-term memory (as one constructs his or her own understanding of material from working memory).[20]

Elaboration, organization, and environmental context are important storage strategies used in long-term memory. *Elaboration* involves the addition of new meaning to information through its connection with knowledge that already exists. *Organization* is characterized by placing a concept into some organizing structure (e.g., a guide to direct one back to individual parts of information when it is needed). *Environmental context* is a strong determinant for episodic memory encoding and storage, as it involves the *contextual* (e.g., setting, time, day, and companions who were with the individual when the information was retrieved) element for a given memory.[20]

Spread of action is the term used to indicate the retrieving of long-term information and the transferring to short-term (working) memory.[27] There are two ways in which long-term memory is retrieved. First, there is *recall*. This involves retrieving a particular piece of information by means of a conscious and deliberate search of long-term memory storage. *Recognition*, on the other hand, utilizes the ability to match information that is presented to one with information from long-term memory storage. It is an association process that makes use of externally provided associated cues that are processed directly into the long-term storage. Therefore, recognition memory tasks significantly reduce the retrieval demands of memory tasks.[20] Levy informs us that during the rehabilitation process occupational therapy clinicians can capitalize on this type of retrieval capacity by providing the appropriate psychological, physical, and social environmental cues.[20]

Intellectual Functioning

Memory is an important aspect of intellectual functioning. However, it is also important to explore other facets of intellectual status. Two very different types of intellectual function are associated with intelligence and knowledge. *Crystallized intelligence* consists of abilities learned through experience and education. It is the intelligence of wisdom, culture, or judgment. This becomes optimized (at the very least stabilized) with experience and age. Contrarily, *fluid intelligence,* involving the mechanics of thinking (such as reaction time) declines with age. Specific examples of these two differences are noted in the fact that vocabulary and other verbal abilities change very little with age. On the other hand, the search time for a visual symbol increases as one ages. With aging it takes a longer time to perceive and interpret stimuli appropriately, and then act on them.

The Wechsler Adult Intelligence Scale (WAIS) has long been used to measure intelligence in the United States. It includes both a verbal and performance scale that is timed. The WAIS tests clients in four major areas:[10]

1. Abilities learned through experience and education

2. The ability to cope with novel tasks

3. The ability to shift from familiar to unfamiliar tasks that require visual-motor coordination

4. The ability to process visual materials

Since the WAIS measures aspects of areas where older adults demonstrated decline (e.g., visual-motor flexibility), this has been interpreted by some professionals to mean that as one ages, intellectual function declines. Conversely, we know that crystallized intelligence involving wisdom and judgment does not usually decline with age. In fact, judges (who must deal with issues such as justice and wisdom) are often older adults.

Dementia Associated With Organicity

Organic brain syndrome (OBS), commonly referred to as dementia, may be divided into two types—*acute* (reversible) and *chronic* (irreversible). Characteristics or symptoms of these conditions can include: impairment of intellectual functioning, impairment of memory, impairment of orientation, impairment of judgment, and shallow or labile affect (often including behavioral changes).[10]

Acute Dementia

Acute dementia episodes can be due to decreased oxygenation of the blood (e.g., pulmonary disease, anemia); increased cerebral oxygen requirements (i.e., those found in thyrotoxicosis and febrile states); insufficient supply of necessary substances (e.g., thiamine, appropriate vitamin, mineral, and nutrition intake); disruption of cerebral metabolic processes (e.g., manifested by head trauma, endocrine disorders, fluid and electrolyte imbalance); and impaired cerebral blood supply (e.g., as manifested by hypertensive encephalopathy, decreased blood volume, and cardiac disease).[10] Careful screening and evaluation are essential in determining the cause (infectious, degenerative, vascular, toxic, metabolic, trauma, alcoholism) of dementia so that appropriate intervention can be rendered.

Chronic Dementia

NORMAL PRESSURE HYDROCEPHALUS

With this disorder the client presents with gait disturbance, urinary incontinence, and a slow progressive dementia. In normal pressure hydrcephalus, the cerebral ventricles become enlarged, and the pressure of the cerebrospinal fluid is normal. Intervention usually consists of *shunting* (placement of an artificial device in the brain cavity that assists in the drainage of the cerebrospinal fluid).[10]

General Considerations

When considering dementia, it is imperative to distinguish between dementia, delirium, and depression. In *delirium,* the disturbance in consciousness is manifested by a decreased awareness of the environment. Symptoms can include loss of the ability to focus, shift, or sustain attention; disorientation; memory impairment; and perceptual disturbances involving poor sensory judgment and visual hallucinations. The onset of these symptoms may be due to renal disease, metabolic disorders, and systemic infections.[28]

Depression and pseudodementia can manifest as a dementia and will be discussed in the section concerning psychosocial disorders.

Alzheimer's Disease (Degenerative Causation)

When the German psychiatrist Alois Alzheimer first discovered this disease in 1906, it was rare. Life expectancy was much shorter (47 years at that time); it has now increased to 77 years in the United States. The incidence of Alzheimer's disease has risen accordingly. About 4 million Americans are now afflicted, and by mid-century it is estimated that 14 million persons will have developed Alzheimer's disease. At present, 19% of individuals between 75 and 84 have Alzheimer's; 50% of those who are 85 or older are affected by this disease.[29] This condition is the major cause of cognitive impairment in late life adults.[17]

In Alzheimer's disease the clients' brains are littered with sticky amyloid deposits known as *plaque,* and their neurons contain twisted protein filaments that are commonly called *tangles.* These tangles actually exterminate brain cells. Researchers now suspect that the process of tangle formation begins when amyloid plaques press up against a neuron's outer surface—thus, initiating a cascade of chemical changes within the neuron. Harvard researchers have demonstrated that tangles are produced by an enzyme called cdK5. Other factors that have led to the development of Alzheimer's involve the concept that clients with Alzheimer's have a genetic makeup that makes them more susceptible to environmental triggers. Persons with one affected parent are three times more likely to develop Alzheimer's than those with no familial history. People with head trauma and those individuals with a poorly nurtured brain (e.g., childhood deprivation—low educational stimulation; those with more than five siblings in a family) may be at risk for Alzheimer's.[29]

Birnesser describes a variety of areas of the brain that can be affected by Alzheimer's. *Granulovacuolar degeneration,* affecting the neurons in the hippocampus, attacks the cytoplasm of the cell.[28] Thick granular material fills the vacuoles that cause swelling of the cell's cytoplasm. The hippocampus portion of the brain may then become smaller. Brain cell degeneration is often the result.[28] Some researchers believe that deficiencies in the immune system, the development of a very slow infection virus (such as in Kuru or Creutzfeldt-Jacob disease), or possibly toxins may be the root of the problem.[28]

In general, Alzheimer's appears to be a disease that is the result of a *degenerative process* (characterized by cell loss from the cerebral cortex with concomitant enlargement of the ventricular system). During the course of this disease process, the cortex becomes atrophied and shrunken and loses approximately one-third of its volume.[1]

Determining if a person has Alzheimer's disease often involves a process of elimination. The Positron Emission Tomography (PET) scan can assess brain function by showing metabolic activity in different brain regions, and in clients with late Alzheimer's a dramatic loss of brain function can actually be demonstrated using PET technology.[29] An extensive history and physical examination are essential for appropriate diagnosis. Clinical psychiatric and neurological evaluations should include areas such as memory, praxis, visuospatial behavior, affective state, delusional beliefs, and anxiety level so that a comprehensive review of the client's status may be rendered.[10,28,29]

Recently, a double-blind clinical trial involving more than 200 clients has confirmed that AD7C (Nymox, Rockville, MD), a urine test for Alzheimer's disease, is highly accurate and has significant clinical usefulness in helping physicians determine if Alzheimer's is present.[29] This product is currently in the development stage, but its promise looks very helpful in establishing an accurate marker for Alzheimer's.[30]

Alzheimer's disease progresses through stages of mild memory loss, then to significant impairment, and lastly to exceedingly serious confusion that eventually leads to the loss of all verbal abilities and motor skills. At this point the client is no longer able to command the body (e.g., there is incontinence of urine and feces; the individual can neither feed him- or herself nor swallow).[1,10,20]

While there is no known cure at present, scientists are at work with new research outlooks. A major interest is how to combat key enzymes that contribute to the disease. Researchers are now developing techniques that use enzyme-blocking therapy. Another development is the use of human gene therapy to revitalize damaged brain cells. Yet another area of research includes the possibility of developing a vaccine.[31]

Parkinson's Disease (Degenerative Causation)

In 1817, Dr. Parkinson, an English physician, first characterized this disorder and termed it the "shaking palsy."[10] It is a progressive neurodegenerative disease and is the most common degenerative disorder of the central nervous system after Alzheimer's disease. Nearly 1 million Americans are affected (most are over the age of 60).[10,20,32,33]

The cardinal features are:

❖ *Tremors*. These occur in relaxed limbs. They are suppressed during activity and absence of sleep. Initially, it involves the flexion and extension of the thumb and index finger and results in what is commonly known as "pill rolling." The tremor can be more pronounced on one side.[10,32,33]

❖ *Bradykinesia*. This involves slow, incomplete movement. There is a great deal of difficulty initiating movement. In the early stages of the disease, the gait is slow and shuffling is noted. There is reciprocal loss of arm movements. In the more advanced stage, the steps become smaller. Eventually fine motor control becomes severely impaired.[32,33]

✧ *Rigidity*. Muscles and joints become stiff and sometimes lock, causing the client to become frozen and unable to move. Both flexor and extensor muscles are affected. The rigidity is comprised of two forms: *cogwheel* (movement is performed with a jerky, intermittent manner leading to an impairment of fine motor movements of the upper extremity; handwriting becomes small and cramped); and *leadpide* (there is an increased resistance throughout the entire range of motion when the lower and upper extremities are moved passively).[32,33]

✧ *Postural instability*. This involves loss of coordination and balance. The individual might lose his or her protective rigidity reactions and become unable to maintain a standing balance or be unable to right oneself when falling down.[32,33]

✧ *Cranial nerve dysfunction*. The ocular, facial, and oropharyngeal nerves cease to function appropriately. This can produce a mask-like face (decreased facial expression), difficulty swallowing or chewing, ocular fixation in one position for a prolonged time period, and speech dysfunction (lowered voice volume, monotonous tone, poor enunciation).[32,33]

Impotence, depression, and some cognitive impairment occur in a large percentage of older adults with Parkinson's. A full 30% of late life adults affected by this syndrome are also diagnosed with dementia.[1,32,34]

Parkinson's disease is believed to result from cell death. The exact reason for this remains unknown. Neurons, based in the substantia nigra, facilitate movement when dopamine is fired into the striatum. Parkinson's develops when approximately 80% of these neurons die. The nigral neurons produce dopamine, and the striated neurons receive dopamine. Normal movement requires the transfer of dopamine between the cells. This process becomes erratic or poorly developed in Parkinson's and is thought to be caused in part by abnormalities in the motor circuit from the basal ganglia to the thalamus.[32,35,36]

The symptoms of a newly diagnosed individual who is medically well-managed are most often not readily apparent. The client may be able to continue to fulfill family, social, work, and community roles. This period of disease control normally lasts from 4 to 8 years.[35,36]

Most Parkinson's clients are managed by drugs. Levodopa (L-dopa) can mask symptoms for approximately 5 years. L-dopa is clearly related to dopamine, but unlike dopamine it can freely pass from the bloodstream into the brain. Sinemet (DuPont Merck, Wilmington, DE), an oral medication that combines L-dopa with carbodopa (buffering agent), is commonly used today. However, after about 5 years usage of increasing amounts of L-dopa, side effects consisting of drug-related dystonia with sustained muscle contractures, repetitive or twisting movements, abnormal postures, and sudden nonpurposeful movements (dyskinesias) may develop.[35] Another medication group, dopamine agonists, mimics the effects of dopamine but does not boost the body's production of this substance. It is often used to postpone levodopa's side effects. monoamine oxidase (MAO) inhibitors are yet another group of drugs that are used with Parkinson's. First, they enhance the effect of dopamine by interfering with its breakdown within the brain, and, second, they may help to prevent further damage to the cells.[32]

There are three major types of surgical procedures that are normally used to lessen symptoms when drug intervention is no longer effective. *Ablative* surgery destroys a small mass of cells within one of three brain structures (the thalamus, the globus pallidus, and the subthalamic nucleus). *Deep brain stimulation* (DBS) involves placing a small electrode in the brain and wiring it to a battery-powered stimulator that is manipulated near the client's collarbone. Electrical current can silence errant cells (uses the same brain structures as ablative surgery). Some risks are involved as the electrode to the stimulator can cause infection, and changing the battery requires minor surgery. The third surgical procedure involves the implanting of fetal dopamine-producing cells into the striatum. If these cells become visible, they will survive to produce a continuous supply of dopamine and have the ability to alleviate symptoms.[32]

Researchers are working with transplanting fetal brain cells from pigs. Another group of scientists is focusing on cultivating huge populations of undifferentiated stem cells in laboratory dishes. They plan to use various signaling molecules to guide their development. The hope is that the stem cells will eventually develop into replicas of human nigral cells, thus replacing the dead nigral cells found in Parkinson's.[32]

The Hoehn and Yahr scale, frequently used by neurologists, describes five states of Parkinson's disease going from minimal impairment associated with unilateral involvement only to confinement in bed or in a wheelchair.[36]

Care partner instruction is essential. The basics involve enabling the client (and the household) to plan a routine that includes a balance of rest, exercise, adequate diet, and enables the client to experience emotional health.[35]

Networking and the use of support groups is an excellent way to combat isolation and inactivity and at the same time allow for regular problem discussion, brainstorming, and a forum for speakers.[35]

The American Parkinson Disease Association (116 John St., New York, NY 10038) offers many booklets on parkinsonian management and is a useful resource for the client and families.

THE SENSORY SYSTEM AND THE AGING PROCESS

The senses provide us with information about our environment; alteration to the sensory experience can produce restriction on the impact that is necessary to appropriately interpret, perceive, and respond to the world outside of the human organism.[10]

The Visual Sense

One in four adults over the age of 80 have a visual impairment that is so severe that they are not able to read standard print. Vision loss is the third largest disability among older adults after cardiac and arthritic problems.[37]

During the aging process most individuals experience a slow, steady loss of visual efficiency. This includes:[1,10]

✧ Diminished acuity (reduced ability to discriminate fine details).

✧ Accommodation becomes diminished (reduced ability to focus on an object at varying distances).

✧ Visual field narrows.

✧ Decreased light sensitivity (reduction in the ability to adapt to the dark, reduced ability to recover from glare, and an increase in lumination needs; most older people require increased illumination for close visual tasks). Some of these changes are due to the fact that the size of the pupil diminishes with age and this, then, restricts the amount of light that is able to reach the retina. Other physical changes, such as the thickening of the lens; an increase in light scatter (due to opacities and reduced lens transparency); and smoky and less translucent cornea are responsible for reduction in light sensitivity.

◆ A decrease in the ability to discriminate colors (especially violet, blue, and dark green) due to the thickening of the lens.

◆ Difficulty with the perception of ambiguous figures.

◆ An increase in the susceptivity to the perception of geometrical optical illusion.

◆ Increased difficulty perceiving figure-ground organization.

◆ Increased difficulty perceiving visual closure.

◆ A slower response to tasks that involve spatial ability.

◆ Decrease in low vision ability (difficulty perceiving frowns, smiles, gestures or even recognizing faces) can decrease an individual's ability to appropriately interact with others.

◆ Decreased depth perception.

Mary Warren, MS, OTR divides visual impairments into two categories—ocular impairment and visual processing impairment. *Ocular impairment* involves structures that are anterior to the retina and the retina itself. Symptoms of this dysfunction involve decreased acuity and contrast sensitivity function, poor ocular motor control, and possible visual field deficits. Persons with ocular impairment have difficulty with a low-contrast or high-visual-detail activity such as determining when water is boiling.[37] *Visual processing impairment* involves structures that are posterior to the chiasm of the optic nerve and the central nervous system. Clients with visual processing deficits exhibit difficulties using vision in an effective manner and experience problems in trying to adapt to their surroundings. Deficits can be observed in visual scanning, visual attention, visual memory, pattern recognition, and complex visual processing (spatial analysis and figure-ground perception). In general, persons with visual processing deficits exhibit a visual field deficit, which is the diminished ability to organize and effectively understand visual information.[37]

THE LENS

As an individual ages the following structural changes occur. At about the mid 40s the lens begins to lose its elasticity. The ability to focus, the speed of focusing, and near vision become compromised. Most older adults experience *presbyopia* (farsightedness) and require bifocals for close work (such as reading or sewing). The lens is also developing opacities due to the fact that the cells at the center of the lens atrophy and harden. This thickening of the lens, reduced transparency, and increased opacities result in the fact that many older adults are required to have increased illumination, glare, and brightness control. Therefore, a balance between appropriate lighting and glare control is recommended within the older person's home.[1,10]

CATARACTS

A *cataract*, which is a product of the clear lens opacifying, leaves the older person with hazy, distorted, dim, and/or blurred vision. This process begins at the lens' periphery and gradually spreads to the central portion. Intervention involves the surgical removal of the lens. This is known as an *intracapular lens removal* and requires an intraocular lens implantation.[1,10]

ARCUS SENILIS

The *arcus senilis* (the development of an opaque ring just inside the border between the cornea and the sclerotic coat) can cause reduction in peripheral vision.[10]

The cornea thickens and becomes less transparent. This produces poor light transmission, and light scattering becomes more pronounced. The cornea also flattens and results in an astigmatism that further distorts the perception of the relationship between objects and depth perception.[1,38]

GLAUCOMA

The *aqueous*, a fluid that is continually in flux, lies directly behind the cornea. It nourishes and cleanses the lens. In *glaucoma,* the drains for intraocular fluid are blocked. This results in increased intraocular pressure and results in reduced blood flow to the optic nerve and the retina. This leads to a loss of peripheral vision and the visual fields. Blindness can eventually be the result. Most often glaucoma begins in mid-life. Its progression can be slowed by medical intervention (usually eye drops) or laser glaucoma surgery.[1,10]

Another physical change of the eye that occurs with aging is the loss of water in the scleral tissue. Fatty deposits increase and cause a yellow coat and decreased opacity. When this occurs, images tend to wash out. Striking color contrasts help to promote adequate visual discrimination.[1,10]

VITREOUS HUMOR

The *vitreous humor* tends to shrink with age. This can cause traction on the retina. It also can become more liquid, and increased densities (termed *floaters*) may appear. These are distracting black spots or small lines within the field of vision.[1,10]

RETINA

The *retina* exhibits several physiological changes during aging. First, both venous and arterial occlusion can occur in retinal blood vessels. This vascular insufficiency can result in: spotty visual fields, portions of objects may become indistinct, a gradual decease in the size of the visual field may occur, the size of the macular blind spot (located in the center of the retina) may increase, and the retina also becomes less sensitive to low levels of illumination. Learning to scan the environment is helpful to attain peripheral vision. The use of magnification and the avoidance of glare or lighting extremes are helpful in combating some of these changes.[1,10]

AGE-RELATED MACULAR DEGENERATION

Age-related macular degeneration (ARMD), a disease affecting the retina, is the leading cause of vision loss in people over 60.[39] With this disease entity the center area of the retina (termed the *macula*) is affected. The center point of the macula is called the *fovea*, which allows for detailed vision (e.g., the most precise visual tasks such as writing, reading, setting an oven dial, and sewing). In ARMD the macula gradually deteriorates causing the central vision to be lost and leaving the peripheral vision intact.[40]

The exact cause of ARMD is not known. However, the following are thought to be contributing factors: exposure to ultraviolet light without protection, an inadequate intake of carotenoids (leafy green vegetables such as collard greens, mustard greens, turnip greens, and spinach), smoking, and uncontrolled blood pressure.

There are two types of ARMD—dry and wet. With *dry (*nonexudative*)* ARMD there is the presence of scar tissue or drusen deposits on the retina (in the pigment epithelium of the macula). With time the drusen deposits may enlarge, increase in number, and calcify. Vision can become distorted. There is no known intervention or cure at the present time.[40]

*Wet (*exudative*)* macular degeneration is the more common form of ARMD. It is characterized by the abnormal growth of blood vessels that are beneath the macula from the *choroid* (a thin layer of vascular tissue that provides the retina with nutrients). This network of new blood vessels is termed *neovascularization*. These newly developed fragile vessels may leak blood into the macular region. In many instances laser intervention can be performed to cauterize the neovascularization and retard its growth, but it cannot completely stop its progression.[40] Early detection and intervention is the key for slowing this disease process. There is a new option called *photodynamic therapy*. In this procedure a low-power laser is combined with an injectable drug that attacks the vessels when activated by the laser. Physicians are also testing surgical procedures that transplant fresh cells into the damaged retina or remove the faulty blood vessels.[39] The warning signs of ARMD include: skewed depth perception, blurred vision, glare sensitivity, and difficulty with color and light contrast.[39]

Some tools and resources that are helpful to these clients are:

✧ Telesensory Corp.
This company sells video magnifiers and equipment that scans print and reads it back.
1-800-804-8004

✧ American Foundation for the Blind
11 Penn Plaza, Suite 100
New York, NY 10010
212-502-7600

✧ Light House Low Vision Products
1-800-648-2266

✧ Independent Living Aids
1-800-537-2118

✧ *Reader's Digest* (Large Print)
1-800-877-5293

✧ *New York Times Weekly*
(Large Print)
203-438-7471

The three general variables that can most easily be utilized for the benefit of ARMD clients include the use of contrast, increased lighting, and increased magnification.[40]

DIABETIC RETINOPATHY

This condition occurs in elderly persons who exhibit long-term, poorly controlled diabetes. Blood vessels in the eye can rupture causing *scotoma* (blind spots) in the central visual fields. Repeated bleeding can cause blindness. *Retinal detachment* is another consequence of this condition (scar tissue forms near the retina and can detach it from the eye. Early diagnosis and laser therapy are important in preserving vision.[1,10]

THE PUPIL

During aging, the pupil's diameter and maximum pupillary opening decrease. This limits the amount of light reaching the retina and affects the slowing of the time for the eye to adapt to change in illumination.[1]

Amber-colored lenses have been helpful for cutting glare when driving at night.

Exotropia, a condition caused by muscle weakness, results in a decreased ability to rotate the eye upward. An outward deviation of the eyeball is the result.[1]

As one ages the eyelids tend to droop (*ptosis*). This further narrows the visual field. There may also be an overflow of tear formation (causing dryness and irritation).[1]

Audition (Hearing)

Thirty-three percent of all older adults are affected by hearing loss between the ages of 65 and 74. This rises to 75% in those individuals between the ages of 75 and 79.[2]

Hearing impairment in older adults is often so gradual that the older person might not be aware of the change. This decrease in hearing loss can affect the elderly individual in a number of ways. First, it can be dangerous and promote a loss of a sense of security (e.g., the individual may be unable to hear the whistling of a tea kettle, to detect the approach of a car, or to hear a fire alarm). Second, it can lead to social isolation (such as day-to-day conversations, and an inability to understand others). This in turn can lead to frustration, anger, misperceptions, disorganization, embarrassment, depression, fearfulness, feelings of rejection, suspiciousness, and even paranoia. Third, basic sounds that connect an individual to life's happenings (such as the patter of rain, the rustling of leaves, and the flowing of a brook) are lost.[1,10] Hearing loss is considered to be one of the most devastating of the sensory losses because it isolates older individuals from their environment.[1]

HEARING LOSS

Hearing loss can be divided into three categories: conductive, sensorineural, and mixed. In *conductive* hearing loss there is a lack of acoustical energy that can be caused by excessive wax plugging the outer canal, the calcification of the ossides or the dislocation of the bones, and/or fluid immobilizing the middle ear. Sound has difficulty reaching the cochlea, and there is a loss of perceived intensity. On the other hand, *sensorineural* hearing loss is due to damage within the inner ear (i.e., within the cochlea, any damage to the basilar membrane or damage along the auditory nerve). It is sensorineural hearing loss that is most characteristic of the type of degeneration that occurs during the aging process. *Mixed* hearing loss is a combination of sensorineural and conductive hearing loss.[10]

PRESBYCUSIS

Presbycusis is the most frequent cause of sensorineural hearing loss in elderly persons. Damage occurs within the cochlea. There are four major types of presbycusis. *Sensory presbycusis* first appears in middle age and results in the loss of high frequency hearing (a direct consequence of the degeneration of the basal end of the organ of corti).[1,38]

Neural presbycusis, associated with the progressive degeneration of the auditory neurons in the auditory pathways of the cochlea, is characterized by losses in speech discrimination but does not occur in pure tone thresholds. The onset of this condition occurs in late life.[1,38]

Mechanical presbycusis (also known as *cochlear conductive presbycusis*) results from the stiffening of the basilar membrane. This interferes with the vibratory mechanisms of the cochlear duct. This condition can lead to an increasing hearing loss from low to high frequencies which could readily affect the ability to understand speech.

High-frequency sounds (such as the consonants f, g, s, z, and t) become difficult to hear. The low-frequency sounds (most often vowels) are more readily heard. Lowering the voice and decreasing background noise can help the older individual's ability to hear more clearly.[1,38]

Metabolic presbycusis is the result of the atrophy of the blood vessels found in the cochlea's wall. It is believed to be caused by arteriosclerotic vascular changes. This leads to deficiencies in the biochemical and bioelectric properties of the lymph fluids that are responsible for supplying energy to the sensory organs. With the metabolic presbycusis there is a relatively uniform reduction in pure tone sensitivity for all of the frequencies that are accompanied by an abnormally rapid increase in loudness as the sound intensity increases (known as *recruitment*).[1,38]

TINNITUS

Tinnitus, a type of hearing disorder that involves ringing in the ears, is also found in late life adults. Devices such as tinnitus maskers can provide some relief.[10]

DEVICES AND STRATEGIES

There are a variety of interventions for the hearing impaired. The most common one is the hearing aid. This device amplifies existing sounds, but it does not correct speech discrimination problems and needs to be prescribed judiciously. Lip reading and sign language are other strategies. *Assistive listening devices and systems* (ALDS), in which a signal is picked up by a microphone and amplified through a loop, wire, IM signal, or infrared wave to the listener, have been successfully used in public theaters. *Integrative strategies* (modifications of the older adult's social and physical environment) can aid in helping the hearing impaired elder to improve communication with others (e.g., dampening ambient sounds by means of carpets and wall-to-ceiling coverings, the appropriate use of light and furniture so that the hearing impaired elder can observe facial and gestural cues).[41,42]

Gustation (Taste) and Olfaction (Smell)

GUSTATION

Taste receptors, located in the taste buds, are found on the sides, back, and tip of the tongue. Taste nerve fibers have been known to project to parts of the limbic system. As one ages, the tongue itself contains only about 50% of the taste receptors that were present when one was young. Many late life adults lose the ability to discriminate and perceive taste sensations.[10]

There is also a decrease in saliva flow associated with aging. This can aggravate an already dulled taste sense. The decline in the ability to taste sweet substances in older adults is pronounced. Therefore, many late life adults will try to compensate for this decline by increasing the amount of sugar in their food or beverage intake.[1,10] Likewise, older individuals experience an increased threshold for salt. Thus, more salt is perceived as being needed to satisfy this taste sensation.[1]

OLFACTION

It is estimated that two-thirds of taste sensations depend upon *olfaction*. The receptor sites of smell are located in each side of the olfactory cleft on a piece of tissue called the olfactory epithelium. The olfactory process is initiated when gaseous airborne particles reach the olfactory epithelium by means of eddy currents.[10] There is an age-related decline in the ability to smell. This change may be due to a decline in the olfactory tracts and bulb, nerve damage, parietal lobe cellular degeneration, and a variety of obstructions of the nasal passage such as nasal polyps, swelling of the mucus lining of the olfactory epithelium, and acute sinusitis.[1,10]

It should be noted that many late life adults experience difficulty enjoying food the way they once did. This in part is due to a decline in the taste and smell receptors. Older adults should be encouraged to use spices to enliven food and provide thoughtful food presentation and production (food color combinations in a prudent and/or artful manner, setting the table in a neat and attractive manner, use of flowers on the table as appropriate, the use of food textures to enhance the sensation of food) to make food more interesting and enticing.[1,10]

The Vestibular System

The *vestibular system*, which is associated with balance, exhibits a decline with aging. There is a loss of sensory receptor organs and their supporting organs. For instance, studies have indicated that there is a 40% decline of hair cells in the semicircular canals and a 20% reduction of hair cells in the saccule and utricle.[1,43]

Presbyastasis, an age-related disequilibrium when there is no known pathology, is believed by some researchers to be associated with the degeneration of the mechanoreceptors of the spinal apophyseal joints (secondary to spondylosis).[1]

Kinesthesia, the ability to perceive changes in position and space and body orientation, declines with aging. This sense is closely related to balance and the vestibular system. These kinesthetic changes often occur in the lower extremities, and many researchers believe they are the result of neuromuscular and neurological strength and tone dysfunction as well as disturbances of the vestibular system.[10]

The consequences of disequilibrium are even more compromised by the reduction in vision, declines in the sense of position, reductions in muscle strength, and changes in blood pressure and central nervous system processing. All these factors, coupled together, can result in an increased risk for falls in elderly individuals.[1] It should be noted that falls cause 12% of all deaths for persons 65 years of age or older. This makes falls the sixth leading cause of death among older adults.[44] Modification of living areas (i.e., secure all rugs, provide non-skid floor waxes) and the promotion of appropriate exercise and good nutrition are strategies that can be used to help offset this situation.

Skin, Hair, Nails, and Subcutaneous Tissue

As aging occurs the sweat glands, sebaceous glands, and hair follicles decrease. This often leads to the reduced ability in older persons to perspire. The skin's epidermis thins, and the dermis becomes less elastic (causing wrinkles), dehydrated, and weaker. A variety of hyperplastic and neoplastic occurrences take place (such as senile keratoses or benign waxy lesions). The skin frequently darkens in splotches or spots. This is believed to be due to the melanocytes' loss of ability to distribute pigment evenly.[10]

The skin disorder most frequently found in older persons is *basal cell carcinoma*. In this type of cancer, the basal cells become uncontrolled, and there is excessive growth and reproduction of these cells. The cause of basal cell cancer is the sun's cumulative ultraviolet (UV) rays. Prevention calls for a sun protection factor of at least 15, avoiding exposure between 10:00 a.m. and 3:00 p.m., wearing sunglasses that absorb UV rays, and wearing a protective hat and clothing whenever possible.[10,45]

Characteristics of basal cell carcinoma include open, oozing sores, crusts, or bleeds that last more than 3 weeks; a reddish patch that lasts 3 weeks or more; or a smooth shiny growth with a border that is rolled and elevated (with enlargement it can develop tiny blood vessels on three borders and produce ulceration). A scar-like area can develop that becomes white, yellow, or waxy.[10,45] Medical management calls for a variety of techniques to destroy the tumor: excisional surgery, *electrosurgery* (curettage and electrodesiccation), *cyrosurgery* (freezing with liquid nitrogen), *radiation therapy* (x-ray beams), laser surgery, and *Mohs' surgery* (tumor removed in layers microscopically so that it is certain that malignancy does not exist).[10,45]

The hair may recede and thin, causing balding in males. *Graying* (the loss of hair pigmentation) occurs in both sexes. At about 40, stiff hairs in the nose, ears, and eyelashes begin to appear in men. At the same time, women experience stiff hair growth on the upper lip and chin.[10]

Fingernail and toenail growth becomes more slowed with aging. They can appear dull, opaque, yellowish/greenish, or gray. The nail often becomes brittle and tough. Longitudinal ridges also develop.[10]

The subcutaneous tissues atrophy and cause a loss of insulator functions, which result in the loss in many older adults of being able to adapt to cold, cool, heat, and warmth changes and to regulate body temperature.[10]

Hypothermia and Hyperthermia

Two conditions, accidental *hypothermia* and *hyperthermia* (heat stroke) can be the consequences of poorly functioning subcutaneous tissues. In accidental hypothermia the following characteristics apply: the temperature drops below normal body temperature; there is an unusual change in behavior or appearance during cold weather; the heartbeat can become irregular or slow; the face may be bloated; the skin color can be strangely pink, pale, or waxy; there may be trembling on one side of the body or one arm/leg but no shivering; slurred speech may occur as well as very shallow breathing; and the individual may also exhibit sluggishness, drowsiness, confusion, and low blood pressure.[10] Intervention consists of warming the person under specially controlled conditions (no more than 1 degree per hour with the blood pressure held steady).

Besides those older adults whose body heat regulating systems are malfunctioning, there may be other people susceptible to hypothermia, such as those who are too poor to afford appropriate heating, those who take drugs whose side effects hamper the body to regulate temperature, those who live in substandard housing where the furnace does not work adequately, and those who do not or will not take the appropriate steps to keep warm. Preventive measures involve: keeping room heat at about 70°F, layering warm clothing, providing at least several blankets for the bed, ensuring appropriate nutritional intake, and not leaving susceptible individuals alone for long periods of time.[10]

Hyperthermia (heat stroke) is a condition where the body's temperature rises above 104°F (40°C). This is a medical emergency that requires immediate attention. The onset is sudden, and the individual may collapse in just hours. The mouth often becomes dry. Intervention calls for the following procedure to be administered by qualified personnel. Keeping the person as cool as possible on the way to the hospital is imperative. This involves removing the older adult's clothing, applying cool water to the face and body, and reducing vasoconstriction by massaging the limbs. Precautions to avoid hyperthermia include drinking plenty of fluids, avoiding alcoholic beverages, staying out of sunlight, avoiding strenuous activity, and wearing comfortable loose-fitting clothing.[10]

THE GENITOURINARY AND REPRODUCTIVE SYSTEMS

Within the urinary system there is a gradual glomerular filtration rate decline and a decrease of renal mass and loss of nephrons. The concentrating ability of the kidneys also declines. The residual urine volume increases due to a decline in the muscle tone of the bladder, ureters, and urethra. Bladder capacity declines by 50% or more. There is a deterioration of stretch receptors. A decline is noted of the normal cerebral inhibition of bladder contractions and emptying. At the same time, there is an increase in uninhibited reflex contraction. These changes result in increased night frequency.[10]

Urinary Incontinence

Urinary incontinence (UI), the involuntary loss of urine, affects 13 million people in the United States. This includes more than half of elderly persons in long-term care institutions and 30% of older adult Americans living at home. This condition negatively affects the psychological, physical, economic, and social well-being of elderly persons. There are many predisposing factors, causes, and variations associated with UI. Some risk factors include: urinary tract infection, menopause, genitourinary surgery, chronic illness, lack of postpartum exercise, and a number of pharmaceutical agents.[46]

✦ *Urge UI* is associated with a strong and abrupt desire to void. Often detrusor muscle over activity or involuntary bladder contractions prevent the individual from holding back the urine long enough to reach the toilet.

✦ *Stress UI* develops when the urethra cannot close enough to hold back urine when abdominal pressure is increased on the bladder (i.e., lifting, sneezing, coughing).

✦ *Mixed UI* is associated with the combination of urge and stress UI.

✦ *Overflow UI* develops when the bladder becomes over-distended and cannot empty properly (due to underactive contractions or obstruction).

✦ *Functional UI* most often occurs in frail elderly persons and is caused by factors outside the lower urinary tract. This condition may be due to chronic physical impairments or poor cognitive functioning.

✦ *Acute UI* is a transient state with a variety of factors, such as delirium or confused state; urinary tract infections; atrophic vaginitis or urethritis; diabetes; stool impaction; restricted mobility; pharmaceutical agents (such as sedative hypnotics, diuretics, anticholinergic effects from antihistamines, antidepressants, antipsychotics, opiates, antispasmodics, anti-parkinsonian agents, and calcium channel blockers); and stimulants such as those containing caffeine.[46]

Behavioral therapy has been helpful with UI. *Bladder training* (delay voiding; provide progressively large voiding volume; and longer intervals between voids) and *habit training* (timed voiding or toileting scheduled on a planned basis) are useful with urge and stress incontinence. Prompted voiding can be used with clients who experience cognitive impairments. Exercise that utilizes the strengthening of pelvic muscles are known as *Kegel exercises*. These are helpful in reducing stress and urge incontinence.

Vaginal cones (varying weights) may serve as an adjunct to pelvic muscle exercises. Biofeedback and proprioceptive neuromuscular facilitation (in the form of extension patterns—or stimulating the muscles of the perineal region during the performance of bilaterally symmetrical extension, external rotation, and adduction) are helpful in reducing both urge and stress incontinence.[46] Reichenbach believes that extension patterns can be successfully incorporated into many activities of daily living by occupational therapy clinicians (in the home setting, in long-term care institutions, and with many persons living in the community who are at risk).[46]

Kidney

The specific discussion of kidney changes in the elderly has previously been described. However, kidney cancer represents another area that has an impact on older persons.

Kidney cancer has recently been treated with a new technique involving an individual's personal vaccine in which the vaccine to treat the disease (by recruiting the immune system's material defenses to fight off unwanted invaders) has been helpful in shrinking and illuminating tumors in some clients. With this method cancer cells are extracted from a client's kidney tumor. Then the immune cells are extracted from a donor's blood. An electric current then fuses these two cells together. These "fusion cells" are then able to recruit the immune system's T-cells. Next, the cells are injected into the client. These cells have the capacity to instruct the T-cells to recognize the cancer as an invader that is foreign. At this point, when the T-cells encounter a tumor, they are able to detect the cancer and destroy the tumor. For many years researchers have been working on this type of approach to develop cancer vaccines. However, only recently have clinical trials begun to test their reliability with human subjects. This technique is still in a nascent stage—but its future looks promising.[47]

Prostate

The *prostate* is an apricot-sized gland involved in semen production. *Benign prostatic hypertrophy* is the result of the enlargement of the prostate (especially of the segment that contains the urethra). This condition, common in elderly males, can lead to the gradual obliteration of urine outflow. If this condition is not surgically corrected, it can lead to kidney and bladder infections and damage.[10]

Prostate cancer is the second most common type of cancer for males in America (just behind skin cancer). In 1999, approximately 37,000 men died of prostate cancer at an average age of 77. There is a 1-in-6 risk involved for males contracting this disease. Prostate cancer deaths rise sharply after the age of 65. Because impotence and incontinence can sometimes be the result, this is a disease that aims at the heart of human sexuality.[48-50] About three-quarters of men with prostate cancer have elevated levels of the protein prostate-specific antigen (PSA). Testing blood for PSA has become a standard screening for men (normal is below 4, and high is above 10). A digital rectal exam is also helpful in detecting prostate cancer. This condition can be detected, treated, and cured before it has begun to spread. Once it has spread beyond the prostate gland, it becomes incurable.

A diet low in fat and high in vegetables and fruit is highly recommended (especially tomatoes and soy products) as a preventative measure. Some studies have found that intake of vitamin E and finasteride (a dihydrotestosterone blocker) may be important factors in preventing prostate cancer.[51]

Intervention currently includes precisely targeted high-dose radiation. A new form known as *three-dimensional conformal radiation therapy* delivers very high doses while keeping other tissue damage to a minimum by aiming the radiation from many angles. Prostate surgery and radioactive seeds implanted directly into the diseased prostate are other options for combating prostate cancer.[48]

Drug therapy, at present, is in the experimental phase. Hormonal therapy (drugs that block testosterone) and exigulind (a drug that appears to block an enzyme that is unique to prostate cancer cells) are currently being tried for effectiveness in treating prostate cancer.[49,50]

Sexuality

In general, sexual capacity can continue for a lifetime even though older adults often experience a process of gradual slowing when it comes to sexual activity. As a consequence, there may be more time needed to become sexually aroused and achieve orgasm. However, this does not mean there is a loss of interest in sex, as many older partners are able to experience high satisfaction levels in sexual expression.[1]

With aging, the following physical changes occur in males. There is a decrease of seminal fluid production, ejaculatory force becomes diminished, the volume of ejaculate declines, while the refractory period after ejaculation increases. It is interesting to note that while sperm production decreases with age, males remain fertile until the end of life. Older men are often concerned about their ability to maintain sexual potency. For those who experience impotency, factors such as stress, tension, fatigue, depression, and illness may come into play. While impotence can occur from time to time, it is usually remediable.[1,10]

Menopause

In women, the major physiological change that occurs with aging is *menopause*. At that time estrogen production begins to cease. The discontinuance of menstruation is associated with the fact that females can no longer bear children. Menopause usually occurs at approximately 45 to 50 years of age. Some women experience "hot flashes" and "night sweats" during the beginning stages of menopause. The female ovaries shrink in size from that of a walnut to that of an almond. Post-menopausal women most often will experience a loss of lubrication and a thinning of their vaginal tissue. This, then, can lead to irritation or pain (especially during intercourse), a change in vaginal shape, and less acidic vaginal secretions that can result in a greater possibility of vaginal infections. The thinning of the vaginal walls can also lead to conditions such as cystitis. There is a reduction in clitoral size. There most often is a general diminution of muscle tone in breast and vaginal tissue. Estrogen replacement therapy can be helpful.[1,10] Because estrogen therapy alone increases the risk of endometrial cancer, women with an intact uterus are advised to pair progestin with estrogen to block the threat (known as *hormone replacement therapy,* or HRT). HRT is also helpful in reducing the risk of osteoporosis. However, recent studies raise the question that those women who use HRT develop a high risk for breast cancer the longer it is used.[52] As this book goes to press, *The New York Times* (Kolata, G., & Peterson, M. [2002, July 10]. Hormone replacement study: A shock to the medical system. *The New York Times,* A1, A16.) reported that findings in a recent study revealed that besides an increase in breast cancer, other risks (such as increases in heart attacks, strokes, and blood clots) outweighed the benefit of HRT.

Breast Cancer

In 1999, 43,300 women in the United States died of breast cancer, at an average age of 66. The lifetime risk of developing breast cancer is 1 in 8.[52] In general, cancer is a *malignant neoplasm* (proliferations of abnormal cells in the body). In breast cancer these cells usually form a solid mass known as a *tumor*. Malignant neoplasms invade surrounding cells and disrupt the function of those cells. There is life-threatening danger when malignant tumors metastasize (abnormal cells are sent to other body parts via the lymph or blood systems). These tumors, in turn, have a higher metabolic rate than normal tissue, which allows them to grow and replace themselves in a more rapid manner than normal tissue.[53]

Women are advised to perform a breast self-examination at home as often as possible (checking for lumps, swelling, changes in breast texture, tender areas, signs of irritation, puckering of the skin, unusual asymmetry, and supple secretions). Periodic physical examinations by qualified health professionals and mammography are also recommended for early detection. Medical intervention usually consists of surgical removal of the cancerous breast tissue, radiation therapy, and chemotherapy.[10] As a result of intervention, clients may experience limitation in mobility, lymphedema, scar management, alterations of body image, depression, adjustment disorder, and fabrication of cosmetic devices (when sort tissue is compromised).[53] Occupational therapy can be helpful in providing intervention in these areas (for instance, therapeutic exercise to promote greater mobility of the affected upper extremity or fabrication of adaptive equipment).

Prevention (wellness) strategies can be helpful in reducing the risk of breast cancer. It is advised that individuals cease smoking, develop stress reduction strategies, utilize nutritional diets, and eliminate drug and alcohol tendencies (if they exist). Occupational therapy clinicians can provide adaptive strategies in this area.[53]

Cervical Cancer

Because cervical cancer rarely has symptoms in its early stages, it is essential that healthy women of all ages have regular pelvic examinations and a PAP test at least yearly. Risk factors include having multiple partners, having been infected with human papillomaviruses, having had vaginal sexual intercourse (especially if initiated at an early age), and smoking cigarettes. Medical management usually involves surgery, radiation therapy, and chemotherapy.[10]

Cystocele, Rectocele, and Prolapsed Uterus

With *cystocele* there is a herniation into the anterior vaginal wall. *Rectocele* involves a herniation into the posterior vaginal wall. A *prolapsed uterus* is due to downward displacement of the uterus. Symptoms of these conditions includes a feeling of "heaviness" in the pelvic area and experiencing difficulty defecating and urinating. All three conditions are treated by surgical intervention.[10]

THE PULMONARY/RESPIRATORY SYSTEM

There is a significant overall decline in pulmonary respiratory functions with aging. Because of this decline, older adults are more vulnerable to respiratory illnesses than younger persons. At approximately age 55 respiratory muscle mass begins to decrease as well as strength. The chest wall stiffens and there is a decrease in the elastic recoil of the lungs. This is thought to be due to damage of the elastic fibers. This in turn increases resistance to airflow, reduces airway diameter, and reduces the alveolar surface area. In the alveoli, air can be trapped which can eventually lead to their collapse. The result of this is that there are fewer effective sacs, and the amount of oxygen getting into the blood becomes reduced. Breathing becomes less efficient (due to the outward pull of the stiffer chest wall and the reduced ability of the lung to pull inward as well as a reduced metabolic rate).[10,54] Particularly significant declines are noted in: (1) *vital capacity* (the air volume that the lung is able to hold after normal inspiration), (2) the *airflow rate* (forced expiratory volume in 1 second), and (3) gas exchange efficiency.[54] This results in a reduced capacity to consume oxygen. For instance, the vital capacity of a 65-year-old is about 77% of a person who is 25.[54] This general decline of the pulmonary system results in distressed breathing (especially upon exercise), a reduced ability to breathe deeply, a decreased capacity to cough, and increasing susceptibility to respiration complications involving pneumonia and surgery.[54] Instruction in appropriate exercise (especially including appropriate breathing techniques) is helpful.[1,10]

Lung Cancer

Lung cancer is the United States' leading cause of cancer deaths. Approximately 157,000 Americans die of this disease per year. The 5-year survival rate is just 14%.[55] In this disease state, malignant tumors invade healthy lung tissue, eventually metastasizing to other parts of the body. If detected early, the diseased area can be removed. However, many clients are not aware of any symptoms in the early stages. It is usually a persistent cough that drives the individual to find an answer to the problem. Most often, by that time, the tumor may have become too invasive to treat.

Smoking and environmental pollutants (including secondary smoke as well as airborne carcinogens) are the most common causes of this type of cancer. For those individuals who are or were former smokers, routine chest x-rays are recommended. However, with the advent of the *spiral CT* (computerized tomography), physicians are now able to scan nodules as small as the diameter of a soda straw (compared with the quarter-sized tumors seen with conventional chest x-rays). Former smokers are now clamoring for this new test. Whether such early detection makes a difference has not yet been established.[55] Usually, as in most cancers, early detection can lead to early intervention and possible cure. Time will tell if this powerful new tool will be helpful.

Intervention usually includes chemotherapy, radiation, and surgery. *Gene therapy* (utilizing sound copies of p53) has been recently introduced by researchers as an experimental factor in reducing "runaway" cancerous cell growth with some lung tumors.[7] Instruction in energy conservation, work simplification, and situational coping are some ways in which occupational therapy can serve these clients where fatigue is often a major symptom.

Chronic Obstructive Pulmonary Disease

Chronic obstructive pulmonary disease (COPD) is a general term embracing a spectrum of clinical syndromes (chronic bronchitis, emphysema, bronchiectasis, and asthma) that are involved in chronic airway obstruction (limited airflow in and out of the lungs). These disease states (usually interacting with each other) result in airway collapse (inflammation), airway *bronchospasm* (swelling), and excess mucus. COPD often advances insidiously. When significant symptoms do appear, lung function has usually become compromised and results in irreversible airway damage.[1,10,56]

This condition affects 16 million Americans of all ages and is the fifth leading cause of death in the United States. It is 1.8 times more prevalent in males than females and affects approximately 10% of the elderly American population.[1,56,57]

The primary cause for COPD is smoking. It usually presents with *dyspnea* (difficulty breathing, expiratory wheeze, and morning cough). In the later stages of the disease, breathlessness prevents those with advanced COPD to even lie down.[56] As the disease progresses, the right side of the heart is required to produce high pressure to force blood through the narrow blood vessels of the lungs. Eventually this causes the right chambers of the heart to thicken and enlarge. The right ventricle of the heart hypertrophies and results in right heart failure (*cor pulmonale*). Pulmonary insufficiency and respiratory failure accompany this condition.[1,56]

Modalities useful in treating this disease include:[10,56]

1. The cessation of smoking
2. Instruction in general health education (such as avoiding exposure to dust and fumes and avoiding extremes in temperature and humidity)
3. The use of pharmacological therapy (bronchodilators to open air passages, corticosteroids to reduce inflammation, antibiotics to treat infection)
4. Utilization of supplemental oxygen
5. The use of nutritional therapy
6. Participation in prescribed exercise programs
7. Participation in intermittent positive pressure breathing
8. The use of postural drainage
9. Participating in pulmonary rehabilitation (of which occupational therapy is an important team member)

THE GASTROINTESTINAL SYSTEM

In general the most significant age-related change in the gastrointestinal system is a decrease in motility.

Within the oral cavity a number of changes can be observed. Deterioration of dental pulp is noted as well as an increase in fibrous tissue deposition. There is more dentine displacement, cracking, and deposition. Many older adults experience resorption of gum and root tissue. As one ages there is an increase in periodontal disease, and teeth frequently become more worn.[10] It is very important that older adults seek dental help to remediate these conditions. Poor gum and tooth care can directly affect food intake as well as increase vulnerability for bacterial-caused infections that can become systemic.

In the esophagus there is reduced motility (known as *peristalsis*), and the peptic and mucous glands of the stomach experience an increase in atrophy that is responsible for a decrease in motility. Transit time through the colon is increased while at the same time peristalsis of the colon is usually decreased. Due to smooth muscle and gastrointestinal changes, many older adults experience increased heartburn, *flatus* (gas), and constipation.[10]

A number of pathological changes occur within the gastrointestinal tract. Most hemorrhoids involve enlarged veins in and around the rectum and anus that can become inflamed. Blood clots and bleeding may occur. Pharmacological therapy and surgery are common interventions for this condition.[10]

Diverticulosis and Diverticulitis

Diverticulosis occurs when small sacs form on the wall of the large intestine. Some pain is often experienced in the lower left side of the abdomen. When these sacs become infected, a condition known as *diverticulitis* occurs. Symptoms include inflammation, the individual may become feverish, and pain is experienced in the lower left side of the abdomen. Intervention for diverticulosis calls for a high fiber diet and generous amounts of liquid. Intervention for diverticulitis usually involves antibiotics and bedrest.[10]

Colon Cancer

Colon cancer is probably the most grave of the disease entities within the gastrointestinal system. The United States is considered to be a high-risk country for colon cancer. Many scientists believe that diet can be a contributing factor (intake of high-fat foods; not enough intake of high-fiber foods; exposure to carcinogenic matter as found in charcoal-broiled food and highly processed foods; deficiencies in vitamins A, C, E; and deficiencies in selenium and calcium). Other risks factors include colonic polyps, a family history of colon cancer, and a personal history of longstanding ulcerative colitis. Both males and females are equally at risk for acquiring this disease. Early detection of polyps in the colon and their subsequent removal can prevent this disease from occurring. Once someone has acquired colon cancer, surgery, radiation, and chemotherapy are the most common intervention choices.[10]

The Pancreas and Diabetes

The pancreas, a fist-sized gland lying behind the stomach, secretes digestive enzymes and the hormone insulin. In normal individuals the pancreas secretes insulin as a response to a rise in blood sugar (often after a meal). The insulin molecules, in turn, bind to receptors on muscle cells. This prepares them to absorb glucose from the blood. The muscle cells, activated by insulin, create portals that glucose molecules can enter. The glucose is then converted into energy. As the glucose is burned and absorbed by the muscle cells, the glucose level in the bloodstream is able to quickly return to normal.[58]

Diabetes mellitus type 2 is usually a late adult onset condition, although a growing number of Americans are acquiring this disease at earlier ages. It is estimated that 15 to 16 million Americans are afflicted by diabetes mellitus type 2. In the United States, there are 195,000 diabetic type 2 related deaths annually.[58,59] Type 1 diabetes, considered to be an autoimmune disease, is marked by a shortage of insulin. It is relatively uncommon.

Type 2 diabetes is a complicated disease affecting the pancreas, the liver (which stores and releases glucose), muscles, fat cells, nerves, arteries, kidney function, vision, and the brain. In type 2, overworked muscle cell receptors become less responsive to insulin. These resistant cells are not able to create the portals needed to absorb glucose from the blood. Consequently, glucose builds up in the bloodstream. Vital processes are thwarted, and aging vessel walls are damaged.[58] Uncontrolled type 2 diabetes can have devastating results. Diabetes is the leading cause of new cases of blindness (often termed diabetic retinopathy) in persons whose ages range from 24 to 74. Nearly one-half of all new cases of end-stage kidney disease stems from type 2 diabetes. Eight percent of type 2 diabetic males experience impotence. Diabetic type 2 individuals suffer from two (males) to four times (females) more of the usual rate for cardiovascular disease. Many type 2 diabetics are afflicted with nerve damage (termed diabetic peripheral neuropathy). As a result these clients often require leg amputation (most commonly due to gangrene and severe foot ulcers). Uncontrolled diabetes can lead to diabetic coma (*diabetic ketoacidosis*) or death.[10,58]

Several factors play a role in acquiring this condition. Genetics is one of those factors. A team at the Whitehead Center for Genome Research identified a variant form of the gene on the human chromosome 1. This appears to increase the risk of type 2 diabetes by about 25%. Lack of exercise and poor nutritional intake (diets high in fat, calories, and carbohydrates) are considered to be prime causes of this type of diabetes.[58]

Symptoms of this disease include fatigue, nocturia, unusual thirst, sudden weight loss, urinary tract and gum infections, slow-healing infections or sores of the skin, and blurred vision. Diagnosis is usually confirmed by urine and blood tests.[10]

Intervention involves the following recommendations: appropriate exercise; appropriate diet (low fat, low calories, low carbohydrates); meals that are spaced throughout the day; limited alcohol intake; appropriate skin care; proper foot and dental care (diabetics do not heal easily); the monitoring of sugar levels in the blood and urine through home tests and by physician monitoring; stress control strategies; and intake of medicines designed to improve the metabolization of carbohydrates within the body (such as oral medications and insulin intake, including insulin pumps).[10,58] Stimulators (such as Glucotral that prompt pancreatic cells to make increased amounts of insulin); sensitizers (such as Glucophage [Bristol-Meyers Squibb, Princeton, NJ] and related interventions that enable cells to be more responsive to whatever amounts of insulin present in the body); and carbohydrate blockers (such as Precose and Glyset [Bayer Corporation, West Haven, CT] that help regulate blood sugar levels by slowing the breakdown of carbohydrates that are in the digestive tract) represent a new arsenal of pharmaceuticals that are available to fight this disease.[58]

Researchers have recently developed even more startling methods of treating type 2 diabetes. At the University of California at San Diego scientists reported that they have developed in the laboratory a line of human cells that can make insulin. These cells, transplanted into rodents, were able to function like normal insulin-producing cells (termed *beta cells*). The impact of this is enormous, as hopefully in the future clients will be able to make their own healthy, insulin-producing cells without waiting for organ donations.[59] At the same time, researchers at the University of Alberta (in Edmonton, Canada) were able to successfully transplant insulin-regulating islet cells (which contain beta cells) that were harvested from donated organs in seven clients.[59] While the large-scale production of genetically engineered islet cells is in the nascent stage, the future looks hopeful in enabling type 2 diabetics to find a new source of help in battling this disease.

THE SOMATOSENSORY SYSTEM (TOUCH AND PAIN)

Age-related changes in the somatosensory system include declines in sensitivity to pinprick sensation, light touch, position sense, vibratory sensation (especially in the lower extremities), and deep pain. With aging there is a loss, microscopically, of the integrity and number of peripheral receptors and nerve fibers. These are thought to raise sensitivity thresholds for temperature, perceived movement, and pain. These changes, then, are also instrumental in increasing the risk of mechanical and thermal injury.[1,60]

Some of the direct consequences of these somatosensory changes are manifested by older adults experiencing difficulty maintaining constant body temperature and intolerance for extreme temperatures (as evidenced by many elderly being vulnerable to such conditions as hypothermia and hyperthermia). Older individuals also experience change in skin elasticity as more pressure is needed to mechanically deform tissue and stimulate the sense receptors that lie beneath the skin. The loss is particularly pronounced in the skin of the sole of the foot and the palm of the hand.[10]

THE MUSCULAR SYSTEM

With age there is a decline in strength and the presence of a slow, progressive muscle wasting (*sarcopenia*). Evans notes that in healthy young adults 30% of the body weight is muscle; 20% is *adipose* (fat) tissue, and 10% is bone. When one reaches 75 about 15% of the body weight is muscle (muscle mass has decreased by half), 40% is adipose tissue (twice as much fat tissue is produced in late life), and 8% is bone (a loss of 2%). This decrease in muscle mass is a direct result of: (1) a reduction in the number and diameter of *type 1* (slow twitch) muscle fibers (responsible for endurance) and *type 2* (fast twitch) muscle fibers (associated with speed and power); and (2) a reduction in the size of each alpha-motor neuron. There is an additional increase in fat content between muscle fibers and *connective tissue* (fibrin) deposits. A direct relationship exists, in old age, of muscle mass reductions as related to reductions in muscle strength.[61]

It should be noted that in aging not all muscles decline at the same rate. Decline first appears in the lower extremity flexor muscles, and the decline is more pronounced than in upper extremity muscle groups.[61,62] In general, the effects of deconditioning (as associated with restricted mobility or bedrest) become accentuated in late life adults.[1]

There is evidence that physical exercise has a direct positive effect in maintaining physical function and strength of older adults in their 80s and 90s.[62] Studies with frail elderly nursing home residents have manifested that when high-intensity weight training is involved, the result is a significant improvement in muscle size and strength as well as improvement in balance, bone density, mood, and functional mobility (including those up to the age of 96).[62] A 10-week strengthening program involving frail elders resulted in a 100% increase in muscle strength.[62,63]

Polymyalgia Rheumatica and Polymyositis

Two muscle disease states that are often associated with elderly persons are polymyalgia rheumatica and polymyositis. In *polymyalgia rheumatica,* pain, weakness, and stiffness occur in the proximal muscles of the upper extremities. The average duration of the disease is approximately 1 year. The pathology is unclear. In the majority of clients, intervention includes steroids.[1]

Polymyositis is considered to be an autoimmune disorder due to its association with systemic lupus erythematosus. It is manifested by an inflammation of the muscles. Characteristics include hip girdle and shoulder weakness, joint or muscle pain, and a skin rash. Steroids are the drugs of choice.[1]

THE SKELETAL SYSTEM

Loss of skeletal mass is a common characteristic and consequence of changes that are associated with aging. In old age women lose approximately 35% of their *cortical bone* (outer shell of the bone) mass and 50% of their *trabecular bone* (responsible for forming the internal latticework) mass. Men, on the other hand, lose about 20% of their cortical bone mass and 35% of their trabecular bone mass.[64] The strength of the skeleton to withstand trauma without fracture directly depends upon the percentage of bone mass within the skeleton.[10]

With aging the vertebral discs atrophy and the vertebral column becomes shorter, compressed, and less flexible. Changes occur within the temporal mandibular joints, and there is often a loss of teeth which can cause difficulty with eating and speech.[10] Tooth implants may help to remedy this situation.

Aging also manifests cartilage tissues (those that line the joints) that lose collagen due to enzymatic degradation. Degeneration takes place, and the ability to protect the ends of the bones from repetitive stress is compromised. At times the cartilage can split, and the bone underneath thickens and produces extra calcium. The joint becomes enlarged, and there is a proliferation of *osteophytes* (bony outgrowths) in that specific area. It is this cartilage deterioration that helps to contribute to what is commonly known as shrinking as well as the thinning and deterioration of the vertebral discs.[1,10]

Osteoporosis and Osteoarthritis

The two most common diseases associated with aging and the skeletal system are osteoporosis and osteoarthritis.

Osteoporosis is characterized as a disease in which bone mass decreases. When this occurs there is an increased bone porosity, a decreased mineral content, and a decreased resistance to fracture.[10] In fact the *fracture threshold* (a point at which bone can break when exposed to mild stress) occurs in approximately 50% of all women at age 65. On the other hand, 2% of men reach this threshold by age 70.[1,65] This means that by age 65 at least one-half of all women have developed some form of osteoporosis.[1] Fracture risk is directly related to the degree or amount of osteoporosis that exists within the individual. Clients who are most liable to fracture are those with the most severe loss of bone.[10] The most common fracture sites that are associated with osteoporosis are the neck of the femur; the *distal forearm* (known as a Colles' fracture), the vertebrae, and the pelvis. Fractures of the femur are the most serious, as death can occur from shock, hemorrhage, and other complications.[10] Falls cause about 12% of all deaths for individuals over the age of 65, and this makes falls the sixth leading cause of death among older adults.[66]

Bone density can be measured by a highly technical machine, the photon-bone densitometer, and specialized CAT scans. Not only can these technologies determine if a person has osteoporosis, but they can predict, at current rate of bone loss, when an individual will reach a fracture threshold.[10]

Other characteristics of osteoporosis are back pain, loss in height, multiple vertebral crush fractures, and *dorsal kyphoscoliosis* (also known as dowager's hump). As the disease progresses, seemingly benign activities such as picking up a bag of groceries, coughing, or picking up a fallen item can produce fractures.[10]

Although no specific cause of osteoporosis is known there are a large number of risk factors. These include being post-menopausal; being female; being Caucasian; insufficient amount of weight-bearing exercise; inappropriate nutrition (e.g., limited vitamin D, avoiding food with high amounts of calcium such as cheese, milk, tofu, yogurt); inappropriate magnesium intake; excessive protein intake; a family history of osteoporosis; excessive consumption of alcohol and caffeine; cigarette smoking; prolonged immobility; and long-term use of corticosteroids.[1,10]

The use of HRT, commonly known as a standard dose of Premarin (Wyeth Pharmaceuticals, Richmond, VA), which includes estrogen and progestin, was highly recommended by many physicians for post-menopausal women. However, extreme caution is now given, as there is a risk of developing breast cancer with this pharmaceutical.[52] In fact, *The New York Times* (Kolata, G., & Petersen, M. [2002, July 10]. Hormone Replacement Study: A Shock to the Medical System. *The New York Times,* A1, A16.) recently reported that there were also increases in heart attacks, strokes, and blood clots. Fosamax (Merck, Whitehouse Station, NJ) and Calcimar (Rhone-Poulenc Rorer, Bridgewater, NJ) are other drugs that are helpful in increasing modest amounts of bone density.[1] Evista (Eli Lilly, Indianapolis, IN), a new medication, has been recently approved to treat and prevent osteoporosis.

Other intervention strategies involve adequate calcium intake; appropriate magnesium intake; weight-bearing exercise (such as walking) at least 20 minutes three times weekly; adequate vitamin D, C, and K intake; and lifestyle changes that include eliminating alcohol and caffeine intake and cessation of smoking.[10]

Osteoarthritis, a degenerative joint disease, is manifested by cartilage deterioration.[1,10] There is loss of density in the cartilage. Increased erosion can cause the body to produce extra calcium known as *osteophytes* (bony spurs).[10] Joints can ultimately become damaged to the extent that fusion or subluxation can occur.[1] The most affected areas are the weight-bearing joints such as the knees, hips, and lumbrosacral spine. Other joints involved include the distal metacarpals of the thumb and fingers (known as Herbeden's nodes), joints around the base of the thumb, the lower cervical spine, and the base of the big toe.

In *cervical spondylosis* osteophytes can compress the peripheral nerves and the spinal cord causing additional neurological dysfunction. There may be a tingling of the fingers and difficulty performing fine motor tasks. In later stages of this condition the client may experience decreased sensation in the feet and weakness in the legs.[1]

Spinal spondylosis (usually occurring in the lumbar spine) is characterized by pain, weakness, and numbness in the thighs, buttocks, or legs upon walking or standing. This can often be alleviated by sitting. Both spinal spondylosis and cervical spondylosis are treated by surgically decompressing the spinal cord.[1] Arthritis, when it extends to the weight-bearing joints (the knees specifically), is the leading cause of physical disability in late life adults.[2]

Although the exact cause of osteoarthritis is not known, obesity and misuse of joints (such as performing repetitive motions for prolonged time periods) are considered predisposing factors. Common complaints include joint pain (especially upon rising), limited range of motion in the affected joints, stiffness after immobility, and reduced mobility.[1,10]

Medical management includes chemotherapy (anti-inflammation medications, analgesics); modalities such as paraffin, heat, and interferential electrical stimulation; specific exercises to correct muscle atrophy and provide muscle strengthening; and correcting anatomical changes by means of surgical intervention. The surgical procedures most often used are debridement; *arthrodesis* (joint fusion); *arthroplasty* (new prosthetic articulating surface); *osteotomy* (a new section of bone is used to alter the weight-bearing surface); and total joint replacement. Crutches, canes, walkers, and local support (as used in splints) can also be helpful in alleviating some of the symptoms of osteoarthritis.[1,10]

MENTAL HEALTH CONCERNS

6

MENTAL HEALTH AND PSYCHOSOCIAL DISORDERS IN OLDER ADULTS

Only the mental health disorders that most affect older adults will be discussed in this chapter.

LATE LIFE DEPRESSION

Depression is the most frequently occurring mental illness in older adults. Late life depression may be due to a number of changes such as: the loss of a spouse, the loss of peers, social isolation, stress of concurrent illnesses, retirement, the loss of one's home, and drug interactions. With normal aging there is a decline of neurotransmitters such as serotonin and dopamine. This decline may serve as a vulnerability factor for biological depression.[67]

Suicide rates rise in late life adults. Clinical depression is a co-factor in at least 70% of these cases. Each year approximately 6,000 elderly individuals take their lives (approximately 17 per day). White males age 80 and over have the highest suicide rate.[67] Risk factors for suicide include: being male, being widowed or divorced, increasing in age, being socially isolated, abusing alcohol or drugs, impulsive character trait, chronic disease, and the perception of hopelessness (i.e., the individual believes that he or she will never get well).[67]

The essential characteristic of a major depressive episode is a period of at least 2 weeks duration in which there is a loss of interest or pleasure in almost all activities and/or a depressed mood.[68] The client must also experience at least four additional changes in the following areas:[68,69]

⬧ Changes in weight or appetite
⬧ Changes in sleep (insomnia or hypersomnia)
⬧ Changes in psychomotor activity
⬧ Feelings of guilt or worthlessness
⬧ Decreased energy (fatigue)
⬧ Difficulty concentrating or thinking
⬧ Difficulty in making decisions
⬧ Recurrent thoughts of suicide ideation or death
⬧ Suicide attempts

In the elderly, depressive syndrome often presents in a variety of ways such as non-specific somatic complaints (e.g., pain, constipation, ill-defined dyspnea, apathy, memory or concentration problems) rather than with a depressed mood.[69]

Depression is a treatable disorder that is often under-treated and under-recognized in older adults.[70] Intervention usually consists of serotonin uptake drugs such as Prozac (GlaxoSmith Kline, Research Triangle Park, NC) and Paxil (Eli Lilly, Indianapolis, IN), electroconvulsive therapy for intervention resistant depression; identifying coping strategies in therapy sessions; and the provision or identification of a social support network.[67]

Dementia Syndrome of Depression (Pseudodementia)

Dementia syndrome of depression (also known as pseudodementia or depressive pseudodementia) is a treatable disorder that is often confused with true dementia.[71] It is a cognitive impairment that appears in depressed adults.

In dementia syndrome of depression the onset is subacute, and there is a relatively rapid progression. It is a treatable disorder that can often be confused with true organic dementia. In dementia syndrome of depression there is often a history of loss or some stressful life event that can be elicited. The client emphasizes his or her failures and tends to be anhedonic. Remote and recent memory are severely impaired on an equal basis. Daily mental status examinations tend to fluctuate. The client can often become very difficult to handle (angry or irritable). Mental status examinations are internally inconsistent. This condition is most effectively alleviated with intervention that is appropriate for depression.[10,71,72]

Somatization (Formerly Known as Hypochondriacal Neurosis)

With this disorder the client is over-concerned with his or her own well-being. The individual will often complain of a variety of bodily ailments for which no actual physiological basis exists. These ailments might serve the individual's psychological needs (for instance, as a way by which the individual can identify with a deceased loved one who might have experienced similar symptoms or as a displacement for anxiety). Common clinical presentation can include ulcers, hyperventilation, urinary, and colon (often constipation) disturbances, sleep problems, or diminished energy levels. With these individuals it is helpful to improve their environmental support and physical health as much as possible.[10]

ALCOHOL ABUSE

It is estimated that approximately 10% of older adults suffer from alcohol dependence.[73] Many older adults are retired and may live alone. Consequently, they usually drink in the privacy of their home and are less likely to be disruptive or noticed in public.

Characteristics of older adults suffering from alcohol abuse:

- ✧ Divorced persons, men who never married, or widowers
- ✧ Frequent falls
- ✧ Confusion
- ✧ Malnutrition
- ✧ Suffering from the effects of exposure
- ✧ Depression
- ✧ Poor personal hygiene

Alcohol abuse often presents with liver disease; cancer (especially the larynx, esophagus, and mouth); and cardiovascular disorders such as stroke, hypertension, and cardiomyopathy.[71]

Another concern relating to this condition is that alcohol intake can cause serious problems as alcohol interacts adversely with many of the drugs and over-the-counter medications that older adults consume. Also, late life adults respond more quickly (quicker intoxication levels) to alcohol due to the number of age-related changes that they experience (e.g., decreased kidney and liver function, decreased lean body mass, and lower body water content) than do younger persons.[71]

SCHIZOPHRENIA

Primarily, *schizophrenia* is a chronic disease begun in the prime of life in which thought content is disturbed. These individuals misunderstand the meaning of real stimuli (e.g., a client may become convinced that a television announcer is mocking him or her). Many of these clients manifest a disturbance in perception such as hallucinations—affect is frequently blunted, flat, or inappropriate. Role functioning becomes impaired.[10]

The advent of neuroleptic drugs helped to propel the deinstitutionalization of former clients in state hospitals into the "community." Some of these elderly, former clients, can be seen on the streets (commonly known as "bag" men and "bag" ladies) of large urban settings. Many late life adults from state hospitals have been placed in boarding and nursing homes. While drugs help to manage some of the symptoms, there is at present no known cure for schizophrenia. It is a lifelong condition.

ANXIETY

Anxiety disorders in late life adults can often be misdiagnosed or overlooked. Older adults are very vulnerable to developing chronic anxiety due to the fact that they often face constant and changing stressors (such as decline of physical health, retirement, loss of resources for emotional and physical support, loss of a spouse or friends, relocation, and social isolation).[10]

Characteristics can include apprehension, a troubled state of mind, uncertainty, tearfulness, insomnia, helplessness, panic, and agitation.[10] Psychiatric care (medication, allowing for ventilation of fears and feelings and examining them), relaxation training, and environmental stability are some of the methods that can be used to combat this disorder.

SUMMARY

Occupational therapy, with its holistic approach to intervention, is a valuable resource in alleviating pathological symptoms. Grounded in the belief that a person's performance can be enhanced through individually planned adaptive techniques (for mental health disorders or physical disability), occupational therapy can provide innovative and meaningful intervention to elders in the 21st century.

DRUGS AND THE ELDERLY

DRUGS, SAFE DRUG MANAGEMENT, AND THE ELDERLY

Drug Management

The vast majority of older adults are consumers of medications (prescribed and over-the-counter). In most instances late life adults take two or three or more different types of medications.[10]

With age there is a decline of drug metabolism. There are also alterations in drug distribution in elderly clients. This overall effect results in an extension of pharmacological half-life and duration of action. Drug excretion or clearance also declines with age. Therefore, drug accumulation and toxicity is more pronounced in older clients than in younger (excluding infants and small children) clients.[10]

Drugs can also affect nutrition and cause nutritional deficiencies. Particular attention needs to be paid to combinations of drugs and food. Polypharmacy and the prescribing of drugs need to be appropriately and carefully monitored.[10]

Foti points out that some deficits such as poor vision, hand weakness, hearing loss, incoordination, sensory impairment, and perceptual deficits may adversely affect adequate medication management.[74]

Therapists and assistants are particularly trained to be aware of these problems and should seek to provide remediation methods for their clients.

If an individual has difficulty swallowing medications, they may need to be crushed and placed in pudding or applesauce.[74]

Instructions to clients should be simple and clear, and the drug's purpose should be well indicated. Adhering to written schedules of the times of day and when the drugs are to be taken (e.g., with meals/without meals) is essential. Side effects (and educat-

ing the older adult regarding the side effects of each drug) should be noted and immediately reported to the physician. Large print medication labels, color-coded containers, pill containers that organize weekly and daily doses, and pill splitters are important devices that can help late life adults manage their medications safely and appropriately.[10,74]

REVOLUTION IN THE DRUG INDUSTRY

The drug industry is presently undergoing a technical and scientific revolution in the
way that drugs are being manufactured. *Nanoresearch* (nanometers are 10,000 times
smaller than the diameter of a single hair from a human), scientists believe, offers better drug delivery and better diagnostic tools. The concept behind this is that new drugs
and devices can be made more targeted and effective by building them molecule by
molecule (much in the manner that organs and tissues develop in human beings).[75]

In using this technology, cancer cells could be destroyed early, before they become
life-threatening tumors. Dr. James R. Baker, Jr., at the University of Michigan, is presently designing a type of "smart bomb" that could read the chemical symptoms of cancer
cells and at the same time be small enough to penetrate an individual cell.[75]

In Charlton, MA, researchers are injecting goat embryos with strips of synthetic
human DNA. The results reveal that goats have the capacity to churn out 12 potential
drugs in their milk. These animals, then, are able to produce pharmaceuticals in their
milk. A new chapter in commercially producing drugs in transgenic animals is being
developed. There are also transgenic cows in Wisconsin and Virginia, sheep in New
Zealand, and rabbits in Europe.[76]

A further example involving gene research is the work being done at La Jolla, CA
(Johnson and Johnson Pharmaceutical). Scientists there have isolated H-3, a gene considered to be elusive, that helps to regulate the body's supply of histamine. This gene
carries the chemical blueprint for a protein that is commonly found in the brain. It is
there that histamine plays a critical role in functions such as attention, memory, and
wakefulness. Other pharmaceutical houses (e.g., Pfizer, Bristol Meyers Squibb, and
Glaxo Wellcome/SmithKline Beecham) are also in the process of developing block-
buster drugs.[77]

The magic of human technology, with its full use of computers and gene research,
lies before us. It will undoubtedly change our lives—especially our longevity.

DEATH, DYING, AND INTERVENTIONAL STRATEGIES WITH THE ELDERLY

8

DEATH, DYING, THE HOSPICE MOVEMENT, AND CARING FOR THE TERMINALLY ILL OLDER ADULT

Death

Death, the end of life, is part of the life cycle. Like birth, death is common to all creatures. Every human that is alive will experience death, and many may witness it. Writings from long ago remind us of our fragile nature set in the calendar of time.

- ✧ "What man shall live and not see death" (Psalm 89:48)

- ✧ "A season is set for everything, a time for every experience under heaven: A time for being born and a time for dying" (Ecclesiastes 3:1-2)

As technology has extended the human life span, the definition of *brain death* (cessation of brain functioning) has become a commonly used medical term. Prior to this the cessation of respiration and the heartbeat had been commonly used. But with new methodology in which the heartbeat and breathing can be artificially restarted and maintained, this older classification has become outdated.[10,78]

Dr. Kubler-Ross, a pioneer social scientist in the area of death and dying, postulated that there are six stages involved in the dying process. First, there is denial in which the individual, filled with disbelief and shock, denies impending death. The second stage involves anger in which the dying person expresses resentment toward others and external events. Third, there is bargaining in which the individual "asks" for extension in time. The fourth stage is concerned with organizing and completing unfinished business (e.g., making a will, giving away keepsakes to those who will cherish them). Stage five is enveloped by depression. At this time the dying person experiences an increasing number of losses of functioning and somatic symptoms. Depression occurs and is usually accompanied by a reduction of interests. Stage six, the final stage, deals with acceptance. At this point the individual has been allowed to grieve and has come to "terms" with the inevitable outcome. It usually can be a period of quiet expectation.[10,79] It should be recognized that not all individuals move through these stages in a linear fashion, and some persons may not even reach the acceptance stage.

Weisman affirms that death from terminal old age involves another set of characteristics. First, there is a repudiation of getting older and then the denial of the extensions of aging. There is often a denial of irreversible decline that is followed by impaired autonomy. This leads to a yielding of control and counter control. Last, there is the cessation of life.[10,80]

Trump points out that there are other excellent resources available which are helpful in assisting clinicians to understand the meaning of death.[81] One of these is *Tuesdays With Morrie* (a book by Mitch Albom that was recently made into a movie for television). The book and movie describe the last stages of life of an older man who is dying from amyotrophic lateral sclerosis.[82] Insight into the meaning of life and occupations is offered.[81]

Another resource, *Ethnic Variations in Dying, Death, and Grief,* involves religious and cultural issues and describes the meaning of death in both universal and diverse terms. How one expresses and deals with emotions involving death is culturally determined.[83] Therefore, it is important for practitioners to first understand their own religion and culture so that they can better understand the contexts in which their clients function.[81]

Trump beckons us to understand what death may mean to an individual client, as the terminal condition of the client will affect his or her sense of self. Trump aptly states, "Everyone has a desire to be a productive member of society, and at the end of our lives, we want to know that we made a difference. Clients need to know that their lives made a difference and that their death matters to someone."[81, p.2]

PHILOSOPHICAL CONSIDERATIONS INVOLVING DEATH

There is a growing number of individuals who advocate having some control over whether their lives should be burdened with the painful indignity that is often associated with artificially prolonging life. A host of documents such as "do not resuscitate" (DNR), health care proxies, and living wills have sprung up to answer these needs. It is important to note that legal documentations (also who should hold the documents and appropriate authorization) vary from state to state and from country to country.[78]

In Missoula, MT, Dr. Ira Byock has spearheaded the development of a community program concerning people's attitudes on dying—framed by the question, "How can we integrate dying into the ongoing life of our community?" The response for this dialogue with the community was overwhelming. At the initial meeting the conference room was packed, forcing many out into the hallway. A community survey designed to assess knowledge, attitudes, and experiences relative to death was distributed to a random sample of 999 county residents. The preliminary results of that survey revealed that the desires expressed by the majority of respondents were to have things settled with their families during the dying process and to be able to die in comfort, without pain.[84]

Also important were the responses of several task forces that had been initiated as part of this project. These included supporting and encouraging people to write their own life histories (or relate them orally); providing advanced care planning that included preparing living wills and paperwork for durable power of attorney for health care; and providing for an opportunity to enhance the sacred at the end of life via the faith community's task force (made up of 15 faith groups). Other aspects included involving the community schools. For instance, one high school teacher is including thanatology as part of a social studies/psychology course.[84]

There is another approach, the projected "care circles." These circles are centered around a caregiver and a recipient. In this project a team captain will know about a client's trajectory. He or she will know who is part of the caregiving circle and will be ready to deliver assistance and help as needed.[84] These projects and philosophy are promising in providing excellence in the care for those who are at the end of life.

In September 2000, PBS aired "On Our Own Terms: Moyers on Dying," a four-part series (by Bill Moyers and his wife, Judith) that focused upon the critical issues in providing care for those at the end of life in today's society. Provocative and meaningful, this series presented many avenues of thought and concern for the care of the dying individual.

EUTHANASIA

Euthanasia is the act of death that is carried out painlessly to end the suffering of another individual.[10] This is very controversial and has spurred many heated debates. While advance directives allow for terminating life-sustaining intervention, assisted suicide involves supplying the client with a prescription for life-ending medication. In physician-assisted suicide, the physician writes the prescription, and the client takes the lethal dose him- or herself. A few countries, such as Holland, and in America the state of Oregon have already established guidelines in which physician-assisted suicide can be carried out. Surrogates may request an end of life-supporting equipment, but to assist in a suicide can put one at risk for charges of homicide.[85]

Despite these legal difficulties, there are two English-speaking organizations (Exit in England and the Hemlock Society in America) that advocate euthanasia. These groups affirm that the quality of life is personal and can only be judged by the individual who is suffering.[78]

HOSPICE—THE EARLY YEARS AND PRESENT HISTORY

Originally hospice was a medieval term that meant a place where shelter, food, and care were offered to religious pilgrims and travelers who were on a long journey. In those days the crusaders used hospices on their way to the Holy Land. In 1846 in Dublin and later in 1905 in London, the Irish Sisters of Charity opened hospices that included many long-stay clients. Their special focus became working with the dying, and it was under their guidance that the term hospice became equated with this type of work.[78]

In 1969, Dame Cicely Saunders, MD, established the first modern hospice, St. Christopher's, in a suburb of London. It offered inpatient intervention for the terminally ill. Saunders advocated a model of palliative care.[78] *Palliative care* is intervention that alleviates or controls symptoms but does not cure the underlying disease.[79] Under Saunders' philosophy, care would be provided that would control and/or alleviate symptoms and pain, provide diagnostic honesty, provide caregiver support, tend to the client's quality of life, and provide bereavement services to the survivors. This model promotes the belief that death is a part of the life cycle. As such it need not be feared, frightening, or violent.[78,79]

In 1971, St. Luke's Hospice opened in Sheffield, England, under the direction of Eric Wilkes, MD. St. Luke's added home and day services to hospice care. Canada opened its first hospice in 1973 at the Royal Victoria Hospital in Montreal. This hospital is associated with a large research and training hospital.[78] The Connecticut Hospice of New Haven, CT established the first U.S. program in 1971.[78] Inpatient services were inaugurated at Bradford, CT in July of 1980. It was established as a free-standing unit offering inpatient and home care services. Through its institute the hospice offers courses for research, training, and education.[86] Hospice programs now exist in every state of the United States.[78]

Hospice care may be rendered in a freestanding structure; a program that exists within an institution; and in either a home-based agency or part of a consortium (this involves a central hospice organization that offers intake, assessment, and some direct care. Often the central organization may contract with home health agencies and inpatient units to provide needed hospice care).[10] In the United States, most hospice intervention takes place in the client's home. This can be a single home, an apartment, an assisted living facility, or a skilled nursing facility.[81]

In the last few days of life several symptoms or characteristics are noted. The client may become unwilling or unable to eat. This can actually have a protective effect as endorphins are released in the system, and they can contribute to a greater feeling of well-being for the client. A dying individual who is force-fed could become uncomfortable, and choking could result. Also, most dying persons do not want to drink in their last days. Again, this is a protective mechanism, allowing the release of helpful endorphins.

The client usually will fall into a drowsiness and unarousable-like sleep. However, during this time one should presume that the client is able to hear and understand everything that is being said at bedside or in the room. Symptoms of "terminal delirium" (agitation, restlessness, moaning, and groaning) appear when the client's consciousness level is markedly decreased and as the client is on the verge of death.[85]

In relation to aspects of communicating with the dying person, the following suggestions are offered so that therapists and assistants can share them with family and friends of the dying person.

♦ Sit close to and at eye level with the dying person. Do not be afraid to touch. Let the dying individual set the pace for conversation and allow for silence. Just the fact that the family member or concerned friend is present to be with the dying individual is valuable.

♦ Do not contradict a client who states that he or she is going to die. Acceptance is all right. Permit the dying person to express feelings of anger, guilt, and fear to surface without trying to ameliorate them. Empathy and active listening are important.

♦ Enable the client to enjoy as much decision-making power as is possible, for as long as possible. Allow the dying individual to talk about unfinished business.

✧ Encourage happy reminiscences whenever appropriate and possible.

✧ Never pass up the opportunity to express love or say goodbye. If there is no opportunity, remember not everything can always be worked through. Do the best that is possible.[85]

In the United States (under the Medicare hospice benefit) there are three major hospice criteria. First, the individual must have a medical prognosis of 6 months or less to live. Second, the person may no longer undergo any curative intervention. Intervention, then, must be palliative in nature. Third, and finally, both the client and family must be made aware of the diagnosis and must be enabled to understand the differences between palliative and curative care.[81]

Hospice policy recognizes that individuals who initially choose palliative care rather than curative (or vice versa) may change their minds without jeopardy. Therefore, they can be admitted and discharged upon their own request.[78]

Tigges and Marcil affirm that there are five basic tenets of hospice care: symptom and pain control, diagnostic honesty (answering the client's and family's questions honestly and openly), 24-hour care as appropriate, quality of life care so that life can be led as fully and comfortably as possible, and bereavement services (most hospices provide such services for up to 1 year as needed).[78]

A full service hospice in the United States is expected to offer an interdisciplinary team that is headed by a physician. This team includes specialists in nursing, occupational therapy, speech therapy, physical therapy, and social work; home care aides for personal care and homemakers for light housekeeping; counselors; pastoral support personnel; and psychologists.[10,85] Community volunteers who have been carefully selected, trained, and well-supervised can be utilized as well as primary caregivers who can be neighbors, family members, significant others, and friends.[10] Other services include drugs for pain relief and symptom control, medical supplies and equipment (there is a cap, temporary hospitalization during a crisis, respite care (brief noncrisis hospitalization to provide family caregiver relief for up to 5 days), and bereavement support for the family (includes counseling, referral to support groups, and period check-in visits during the first year after the death of a loved one).[85]

In terms of pain and symptom control, Tigges and Marcil describe four types of pain that many hospice clients experience. First, there is the pain of the disease itself, which can be accompanied by the second type of pain, that of the side effects of chemotherapy, medication, and radiotherapy. As a result of the hospice movement, pharmacological research has established protocols to successfully manage these problems.[78]

Next, there is the pain that is associated with the effects of bedrest or long-term inactivity. In this specific area occupational therapy can be very helpful. Frequently, poor positioning in a bed or wheelchair can be a result of long-term inactivity. This, in turn, can lead to neck, back, shoulder, hip, or knee pain. Contractures can develop in these areas if not attended to by a therapist. The clinician can provide intervention that may reduce the contractures, offer recommendations, and provide teaching to the team and family members in proper transfer and positioning techniques.[78]

The fourth type of pain, that of loss of role, is another area in which occupational therapy intervention can be utilized. It is during this time that the dying individual may be helped to realize his or her potential through examination and by providing supportive strategies for achieving activity that is meaningful to the client. In this way the quality of the life of the dying individual can be enhanced by means of providing opportunities to the dying person, so that he or she can make a contribution to him- or herself and others (be it in the realm of achieving a form of self-care, projects involving loved ones, or work and leisure pursuits).[78] "Quality of life rests with internalized feelings of positive self-esteem."[78, p.748]

THE ROLE OF OCCUPATIONAL THERAPY IN HOSPICE

Trump asserts that the primary goal of occupational therapy in the hospice setting is to assist the client to maintain independence for as long as possible and then to be able to help move the dying individual (with grace and without trauma) to interdependence, and finally to dependence as functional status declines. Occupational therapy is extremely useful in preventing premature dependence and providing assistance to care givers.[81]

Tigges and Marcil provide a number of questions both for the physician to ask the client and family members to consider. These questions can then serve as a screening to see if a client would need occupational therapy. Caregivers are asked questions that deal with their greatest concern (excluding symptoms and pain control) about the client and what activities they are allowing the client to do for him- or herself or if they are doing everything for the client. The client is asked questions that deal with: the most important thing that his or her illness has prevented him or her from doing, what presently gives the client the most pleasure, and what he or she would like to do tomorrow if he or she could.[78, p.753]

If the physician determines that an occupational therapy evaluation is appropriate, then a full review of the client's needs and goals should be undertaken.

Tigges and Marcil recommend a full occupational history that includes past occupational roles so as to determine what was significant and meaningful in the patient's life and what provided a sense of accomplishment and independence. Then an assessment of temporal adaptation that seeks to compare past and present routines of daily living activities should be initiated. Finally, a performance assessment can be utilized to determine the client's functional ability to perform what he or she would like to achieve before death. The choice of the type of functional assessment to use is determined by the client's wishes and goals, and these goals must be honed in reality (including the client's physical abilities and projected course of illness). Tigges provides an assessment, entitled "Occupational History—Occupational Inquiries" in which employment history; homemaking history; family history; leisure, sport, and recreation interests; temporal adaptation; and functional evaluation are included.[78, pp. 761-762] This is an exceedingly useful tool in the hospice setting.

Trump's recommendations for an occupational therapy evaluation focuses upon similar considerations as Tigges' but she intertwines other types of information as well. First and foremost, she posits that the most important thing to evaluate is the client's concept of what death means to him or her at the present time. It is of the utmost importance that the therapist and assistant understand how the terminal prognosis is affecting the individual's self-concept. A major way to determine this is to understand what roles the client values and how he or she defines his or her life.

Evaluating the individual's self-esteem (which is related to thoughts involving helplessness, hopelessness, and uselessness) is an important issue. Everyone has a need to feel and be productive. Self-esteem is indeed decreased when one can no longer be productive.[81] Assisting the client in redefining his or her role and life in a meaningful manner is a sensitive task.

Evaluating the needs of caregivers is also of paramount importance. Hospice care delivery focuses upon friends and family members that surround the client as well as the dying individual.[81]

In general, information regarding occupational history, the environment, social history, desired goals, observations of significant others and the client's involvement in occupations, and interaction are important aspects of any hospice occupational therapy evaluation. Goals should be set collaboratively with the client, significant others, and the interdisciplinary team.[81]

Trump affirms that when providing direct care (after an occupational therapy evaluation has been administered) occupational therapists need to "devise a treatment plan, and provide intervention as efficiently as possible to be cost-effective."[81, p. 2] This may include forming a team with occupational therapy assistants, training volunteers, instructing home health aides and family members to carry out unskilled interventions as well as providing techniques and ideas to the interdisciplinary team to augment their skills.[81]

Some of the basic concepts involving intervention and social interactions of the terminally ill client include the clinician as "active listener" and "advocate." The therapist must be able to attend to what the client and family or significant others are saying and conveying (through nonverbal communication as well). This means making certain that the client's and the significant others' wishes are listened to and enacted upon.[10]

In working with the terminally ill client, therapeutic intervention does not commence at 8:30 a.m. and cease at 4:30 p.m. The practitioner can be called in at any time there is an occupational therapy need to assist the family, the client, and significant others.[10]

Trump suggests that Reilly's occupational behavior frame of reference (with its emphasis upon developing competence to meet the needs and demands of occupations in which the client chooses to participate in) and the Model of Human Occupation, as developed by Kielhofner and Burke (with its emphasis upon the valued goals and roles of the client) are useful in treating the dying individual.[81,87,88] She also affirms that the cognitive disability frame of reference (as discussed by Allen, Earhart, and Blue) can be readily employed as many clients' cognitive levels decrease when approaching impending death. This model emphasizes altering the environment for maximal functioning.[81,89] Trump believes that occupational science with its focus upon daily occupations and its inclusion of cultural meaning can be utilized to understand how to adapt and select activities that can at best enhance the client's quality of life.[81,90] Thus, we have seen how several occupational therapy frames of reference and occupational science can be used to enable the dying person to achieve his or her own personally determined goals and fulfill his or her maximum functioning potential.

Physical adaptation is also useful to both the client and caregivers. The following suggestions offer examples of utilizing this modality. In reducing painful bilateral edema of the upper extremities, a family member can be provided with instructions in application and removal of bimanual pressure gloves (with physician's orders) when the client presents with edematous hands. The client and family can be educated in appropriate positioning of hands and arms to decrease edema. Retrograde massage can be taught to significant others, family members, or hospice volunteers to reduce edema. To encourage and assist a client who is not able to hold or manipulate a cup or drink water whenever he or she wishes, intervention could be used to adapt and stabilize a large insulated cup (filled with ice water) to the client's chair. A long drinking straw could be secured to the cup. This would permit the client to independently sip water whenever he or she desires.[78]

Other techniques and modalities in hospice intervention include *activities of daily living* (ADL) such as self-care and leisure activities. Educating the client in energy conservation, relaxation, work simplification, breathing techniques, coping, and time management are helpful both to the client and family (or significant others).[81]

The clinician must also address psychological issues. A number of meaningful activities useful in increasing self-esteem can include: making remembrances, writing letters to loved ones to be received after the client has died, and completing a life review.[81]

Since most hospice care in the United States is predominantly carried out in the home setting, practitioners have the opportunity to initiate a home safety evaluation. This is particularly useful for a client who lives alone or for one who has just left familiar surroundings to live with a loved one. Trump reminds us that a home that was safe for two young adults may need to be reconfigured when a late life adult with a walker or a wheelchair moves into their home.[81]

We have explored the history, both past and present, of the hospice movement as well as occupational therapy's significant role with the hospice team and the many interventions that can be provided by practitioners. Because our profession has always considered the variety of facets that contribute to an individual, we are well-endowed to offer integrated, valuable, and meaningful service to dying elders.

UNIT 2 REFERENCES

1. Levy, L. L. (1996). Health and impairment: The performance context. In K. O. Larson, R. G. Stevens-Ratchford, L. Pedretti , & J. L. Crabtree (Eds.), *The role of occupational therapy with the elderly* (2nd Ed., pp. 169-198). Bethesda, MD: The American Occupational Therapy Association, Inc.

2. National Center for Health Statistics. (1994). *Trends in the health of older Americans.* (DHHS Pub. No. [PHS95]-1424). Washington, DC: U.S. Government Printing Office.

3. Wade, N. (2000, May 7). Rivals on offensive as they near wire in genome race. *The New York Times*, 26.

4. Weiss, R. (2000, March 31). Are the effects of aging tied to a few dozen genes? The *Philadelphia Inquirer*, A1.

5. Cowley, G. & Underwood, A. (2000, April 10). A revolution in medicine. *Newsweek*, 58-61.

6. Roberts, L. (2000, January 10). The gene hunters: Unlocking the secrets of DNA to cure disease, slow aging. *US News and World Report*, 34-38.

7. Johannes, L. (2000, May 4). Second chance: Gene therapy, much maligned, is promising in some cancer trials. *The Wall Street Journal*, 1, A6.

8. Sapolsky, R. (2000, April 10). It's not "all in the genes." *Newsweek*, 68.

9. Matthews, M. M., Foderaro, D., & O'Leary, S. (1996). Cardiac dysfunction. In L. W. Pedretti (Ed.), *Occupational therapy: practice skills for physical dysfunction* (pp. 693-712). St. Louis, MI: Mosby-Year Book.

10. Lewis, S. (1989). *Elder care in occupational therapy* (pp. 73-117, 119-197, 199-218). Thorofare, NJ. SLACK Incorporated.

11. Marcus, M. (2000, May 15). The pressure is now on the top. *U.S. News and World Report*, 63.

12. Brink, S. (1998, September 7). Unlocking the heart's secrets. *U.S. News and World Report*, 58-66.

13. Comarow, A. (2000, March 13). Healing the heart. *U.S. News and World Report*, 54-62.

14. Kolata, G. (2000, April 4). Next up: surgery by remote control. *The Science Times of New York Times*, F1, F6.

15. Brink, S. (2000, March 13). The role of infection: Fight germs, fight heart disease? *U.S. News and World Report*, 62.

16. Ferraro, R. (1998). Cardiopulmonary dysfunction in adults. In M. E. Neistadt & E. B. Crepeau (Eds.), *Willard and Spackman's occupational therapy* (9th Ed., pp. 693-715). New York: Lippincott-Raven.

17. National Center for Health Statistics. (1994). *Trends in the health of older Americans*. (DHHS Pub. No [PHS95]-1414). Washington, DC: U.S. Government Printing Office.

18. Acquaviva, J. (1996). *Occupational therapy practice guidelines for adults with stroke*. Bethesda, MD: The American Occupational Therapy Association, Inc..

19. American Psychiatric Association. (1994). *Diagnostic and statistical manual of mental disorders* (4th Ed.). Washington, D.C.: American Psychiatric Association.

20. Levy, L. (1999, November). Memory: An overview for cognitive rehabilitation intervention. *OT Practice, 4*(9), CE1-CE7.

21. Martindale, C. (1991). *Cognitive psychology: A neural-network approach*. Pacific Grove, CA: Brooks/Cole.

22. Baddeley, A. (1992). Working memory: The interface between memory and cognition. *Journal of Cognitive Neuroscience, 4*, 281-288.

23. Parken, A. J. (1997). Human memory: Novelty, association, and the brain. *Current Biology, 7*(12), R768-R769.

24. Clark, J. & Paivio, A. (1991). Dual coding and education. *Educational Psychology Review, 3*, 147-210.

25. Schacter, D. & Tulving, E. (1994). What are the memory systems of 1994? In D. Schacter & E. Tulving (Eds.), *Memory systems*. Cambridge, MA: MIT Press.

26. Squire, L. (1987). *Memory and brain*. New York: Oxford University Press.

27. Anderson, J. (1993). Problem solving and learning. *American Psychologist, 48*, 35-44.

28. Birnesser, L. R. (1997, June). Treating dementia: Practical strategies for long-term care residents. *OT Practice, 2*(6),16-21.

29. Cowley, G. & Underwood, A. (2000, January 31). Alzheimer's: Unlocking the mystery. *Newsweek*, 46-51.

30. Anonymous. (1999, December 13). Advances in Alzheimer's: Reports on risk assessment, urine test for identifying disease. *Advance for Occupational Therapy Practitioners, 27*.

31. Eastman, P. (2000, January). Scientists piecing Alzheimer's puzzle: Scientists close in on Alzheimer's disease. *AARP Bulletin, 41*(1),18-19.

32. Cowley, G. (2000, May 22). The new war on Parkinson's. *Newsweek*, 52-58.

33. Davis, J. C. (1977). Team management of Parkinson's disease. *J Am Occup Ther, 31*(5), 300-303.

34. Friedman, J. (1995). Neurological diseases in the elderly. In W. Reichel (Ed.), *Care of the Elderly: Clinical aspects of aging*. Baltimore, MD: Williams and Wilkins.

35. Hooks, M. L. (1996). Parkinson's disease. In L. W. Pedretti (Ed.), *Occupational therapy practice skills for physical dysfunction* (pp. 845-851). St. Louis, MI: Mosby-Year Book: 845-851.

36. Hoehn, M. M. & Yahr, M. D. (1967). Parkinsonism: Onset, progression and mortality. *Neurology, 17*, 427-442.

37. Collins, L. F. (1996, January). Understanding visual impairments, *OT Practice, 1*(1), 27-29

38. Abrams, W. B., Beers, M., Berkon, R., & Fletcher, A. (1995). *The Merck manual of geriatrics*. Whitehouse Station, NJ: Merck.

39. Marcus, M. B. (2000, March 6). Vision loss in seniors: The future looks brighter. *U.S. News and World Report*, 55.

40. Toth-Riddering, A. (1998, January). Living with age-related macular degeneration. *OT Practice, 3*(1), 18-23.

41. Washburn, A. O. (1986, July). Hearing disorders and the aged. *Top in Ger Rehab, 1*(4), 61-70.

42. Falconer, J. (1986, Winter). Aging and Learning. *Phys and Occ Ther in Ger, 4*(2), 3-19.

43. Paparella, M. M. & Shumrich, D. A. (Eds.). (1991). *Otolaryngology* (3rd Ed.). Philadelphia: Saunders.

44. Walls, B. S. (1999, December 6). A dangerous secret: "I had a fall." *OT Practice, 4*(11), 13.

45. Ramsay, D. L. (1988, May 30). Summer skin alert: Basal cell skin cancer, health and fitness. *Newsweek,* 5-26.

46. Reichenbach, V. (1998, March). Incontinence. *Gerontology Special Interest Section Quarterly, 21*(3), 1-3.

47. Sobel, R. (2000, March 13). A tailor-made vaccine: Scientists try a new strategy to combat cancer. *U.S. News and World Report,* 53.

48. Duke, L. (2000, April 28). Giuliani has a very, very early stage of prostate cancer. *Philadelphia Inquirer,* A2.

49. Brink, S. (2000, April 3). Prostate cancer: Kinder cuts mean sharper dilemmas. *U.S. News and World Report,* 58-60.

50. Brink, S. & Fishman, J. (2000, May 22). Prostate dilemmas: Early detection is forcing more men to weight the difficult treatment options. *U.S. News and World Report,* 66-80.

51. Sobel, R. K. (2000, May 22). Greens (and reds) may cut risk. *U.S. News and World Report,* 79.

52. Begley, S. (2000, May 29). The risks of estrogen. *Newsweek,* 51.

53. Pizzi, M. & Brukhardt, A. (1998). Occupational therapy for adults with immunological diseases. In M. E. Neistadt, E. B. Crepeau (Eds.), *Willard and Spackman's occupational therapy,* (9th Ed., pp, 705-715). New York: Lippincott-Raven.

54. Sherman, C. & Shovrinski, T. (1995). Pulmonary problems in the elderly. In W. Reichel (Ed.), *Care of the elderly: Clinical Aspects of Aging.* Baltimore: Williams and Wilkins.

55. Kolata, G. (2000, June 21). Lung cancer test is much in demand, but benefit is murky. *The New York Times,* 1A, A16.

56. Johannsen, J. M. (1994). Chronic obstructive pulmonary disease: Current comprehensive care for emphysema and bronchitis. *Nurse Practitioner, 19,* 59-67.

57. Stump, J. B. (1999, July/August). Treating chronic pulmonary disease. *OT Practice, 4*(1), 28.

58. Adler, J. & Kalb, C. (2000, September 4). An American epidemic: Diabetes. *Newsweek,* 40-47.

59. Winslow, R. (2000, June 12). Scientists report diabetes-research advances. *The Wall Street Journal,* B2.

60. Kenney, R. A. (1989). *Physiology of aging—A synopsis.* (2nd Ed.). Chicago: Year Book Medical.

61. Evans, W. J. (1995). Effects of exercise on body composition and functional capacity of the elderly. *J Gerontol, 50*(A), 147-150.

62. Fiatrone, M. A., Marks E. C., Ryan, N. D., Meredith, C. N., Lipsitz, L. A., & Evans, W. M. (1990). High intensity strength training in nonagenarians: Effects on skeletal muscle. *JAMA, 263,* 3029-3032.

63. Fiatrone, M. A., O'Neill, E. F., Ryan, N. D., Clements, K. M., Solaris, G. R., Nelson, M. E., et al. (1994). Exercise training and nutritional supplementation for physical frailty in very elderly people. *N Engl J Med,* 330: 1769-1775.

64. Riggs, B. L. (1991). Overview of osteoporosis. *West J Med, 154,* 63-77.

65. Riggs, B. L. & Melton, L. J. (1992). The prevention and treatment of osteoporosis. *N Engl J Med, 327,* 620-627.

66. Walls, B. S. (1999, December 6). A dangerous secret: I had a fall. OT Practice *4*(11), 12-16.

67. Quinn, B. (1998, April). The aging of the brain; The aging of the mind (lecture). Chicago: Northwestern University School of Medicine.

68. American Psychiatric Association. (1994). *Diagnostic and statistical manual of mental disorders* (4th Ed., p. 134). Washington, D.C.: American Psychiatric Association.

69. Benedict, K. B. & Nacaste, D. B. (1990). Dementia and depression: A Framework for addressing difficulties in differential diagnosis. *Clinical Psychology Review, 10*, 513-537.

70. Callahan, C. M. & Wolinsky, F. D. (1995). Hospitalization for major depression among older Americans. *J Gerontol, 50*(A), M196-M203.

71. Levy, L. (1996). Mental disorders in aging adults. In K. O. Larson, R. G. Stevens-Ratchford, L. Pedretti, & J. L. Crabtree (Eds.), *The role of occupational therapy with the elderly.* (2nd Ed., pp. 221-229). Bethesda, MD: The American Occupational Therapy Association, Inc.

72. Ravetz, R. S. (1981, September). Depression and pseudodementia. *Geriatric psychiatry lecture series*. Norristown State Hospital.

73. Jink, M. & Raschko, R. (1990). A profile of alcohol and prescription drug abuse in a high risk community elderly population. *Ann Pharmacother, 24*, 971-975.

74. Foti, D. (1996). Evaluation and interventions for the performance areas—Section 1 Evaluation and interventions for the performance area of self-maintenance. In K. O. Larson, R. G. Stevens-Ratchford, L. Pedretti, & J. L. Crabtree (Eds.), *The role of occupational therapy with the elderly* (2nd Ed., pp. 648-649). Bethesda, MD: The American Occupational Therapy Association, Inc.

75. Kalb, C. (2000, January 1). The war on disease goes miniature. *Newsweek,* 89.

76. Knox, A. (2000, June 4). Cure of the future are growing on pharms today. *Philadelphia Inquirer,* 1A, 16A.

77. Winslow, R. (2000, May 26). Head Start: Johnson and Johnson finds an elusive gene and races to exploit it. *The Wall Street Journal,* A1, A8.

78. Tigges, K. N. & Marcil, W. M. (1996). Palliative medicine and rehabilitation: Assessment and treatment in hospice care. In K. O. Larson, R. G. Stevens-Ratchford, L. Pedretti, & J. L. Crabtree (Eds.), *The role of occupational therapy with the elderly* (2nd Ed., pp. 744-763). Bethesda, MD: The American Occupational Therapy Association, Inc.

79. Kubler-Ross, E. (1969). *On death and dying.* New York: Macmillan.

80. Weisman, A. D. (1972). *On dying and denying: A psychiatric study of terminality.* New York: Behavioral Pub. Inc.

81. Trump, S. M. (2000, June). The role of occupational therapy in hospice. *Home and Community Health-Special Interest Section Quarterly, 7*(2),104.

82. Albom, M. (1997). *Tuesdays With Morrie.* New York: Doubleday.

83. Irish, D., Lunquist, K., & Nelson, V. J. (1993). *Variations in dying, death and grief: Diversity in universality.* Philadelphia: Taylor and Francis.

84. Atcheson, R. (2000, September-October). The Missoula experiment: How a small town learned to make dying a part of life. *Modern Maturity, 43R*(5), 60-64.

85. Matousek, M. (2000, September-October). Start the conversation: The modern maturity guide to end of life care. *Modern Maturity, 43R*(5), 51-59.

86. (1980). *The Connecticut hospice: In serving Connecticut and the nation.* New Haven, CT: Sprint.

87. Reilly, M. (1969). The education process. *Am J Occup Ther, 23*, 294-307.

88. Kielhofner, G. & Burke, J. P. (1980). A model of human occupation: Part 1: Conceptual framework and content. *Am J Occup Ther, 34*, 572-581.

89. Allen, C. K., Earhart, C. A., & Blue, T. (1992). *Occupational therapy treatment goals for the physically and cognitively disabled.* Bethesda, MD. American Occupational Therapy Association, Inc.

90. Zemke, R. & Clark, F. (1996). *Occupational science: The evolving discipline.* Philadelphia: F.A. Davis.

CASE STUDIES

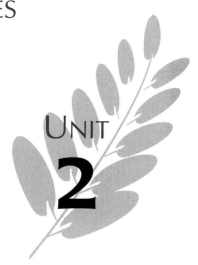

UNIT

2

CASE STUDY 3

Occupational Therapy Hospice Intervention Within a Hospice Setting

Tigges and Marcil provide an interesting and well-managed account of occupational therapy intervention in the hospice setting. This discussion summarizes their case review that appeared in the second edition of *The Role of Occupational Therapy With the Elderly*.[1]

Mr. J is a 65-year-old married man with a diagnosis of amyotrophic lateral sclerosis (ALS) who has recently begun hospice service. He lives with his wife, who is a nurse and is currently working due to financial difficulties incurred with Mr. J's present illness. They have four adult children who live nearby and visit often. Their home is a ranch house that has a ramp entrance in the rear. Mr. J's wife is his primary caretaker, and she would like to be able to shower him in the tub. Mr. J's wife had recently purchased a bathtub transfer bench for the purpose of being able to obtain her above-mentioned goal. However, at present, she is not able to transfer him. His wife also expressed an interest in having some personal time on weekends so that she can get her hair "done" and do some shopping.

Mr. J had worked for 25 years as a certified public accountant until 3 months ago. He is aware that he will not be able to return to work but would like to help his family and friends by preparing their tax returns. He is cognitively alert and mentally capable of performing this task.

Mr. J is dependent for all activities of daily living. Due to dysphagia, he is not able to eat solid food and is fed by means of a gastric tube. He is able to drink fluids but cannot hold or manipulate a cup. He is unable to perform a stand-pivot transfer and, instead, a hydraulic lift is utilized. Mr. J possesses enough finger movement to use the television remote control (although he does this with extreme difficulty). Most of his day is spent in a recliner.

Mr. J is nonambulatory, and he can only bear partial weight on his legs. He has no grip strength and poor-plus strength in both arms. On both hands he exhibits marked atrophy of the first dorsal interossei. Both hands are very painful to movement and touch and exhibit moderate edema. He has good head, neck, and trunk control. There are no visual-perceptual impairments, and all sensation is intact.

Mr. J is experiencing feelings of helplessness, hopelessness, and loss of control of his environment with minimal self-direction. He is depressed and at times emotionally labile.

A primary goal that Mr. J would like to achieve is first and foremost to be able to operate a computer. He would also like to independently be able to drink ice water when he wants and change the television station with more ease as his likes dictate.

After an initial evaluation with the occupational therapist, the findings were discussed with Mr. J and his wife. An intervention plan was developed cooperatively. This information and occupational therapy recommendations were relayed to the physician in charge and the team so they would be apprised of the findings and proposed program. Mr. J's occupational therapy intervention program focused on helping him be able to operate his computer independently. Mr. J would need assistive devices and environmental adaptations to facilitate and foster greater independence. Mr. J was provided with bilateral mobile arm supports to permit him to use minimal active movements of his arms. The client's computer table was raised 4 inches to permit complete wheelchair access. The work area was ergonomically arranged to allow for ease of access for all equipment. Next Mr. J was presented with and trained in the use of the mouth stick. This permitted him to operate the computer by depressing the keys.

The computer mouse was replaced with a track ball. This permitted him to move the cursor with less movements of his hands and arms.

Another goal, that of pivot transfer for bathtub use, was addressed. Both of the client's sons were instructed in stand-pivot transfer techniques by the occupational therapist. This was supervised by the occupational therapist until it could be performed safely.

A third goal dealt with minimalizing bimanual pain and edema. With physician's orders, bimanual pressure gloves were provided. The client's wife was instructed, by the occupational therapist, in application and removal of the gloves. Retrograde massage was provided to both hands. The client, his family, and a hospice volunteer were instructed by the occupational therapist in proper positioning of the arms and hands to decrease edema. They were also taught methods of passive bilateral upper extremity range of motion exercise designed to decrease joint pain on movement and maintain joint mobility.

A fourth area of concern for the client and his family was that he be able to drink water as he desired. In order to achieve this goal, the client's recliner chair was adapted and stabilized so that a large insulated cup (filled with ice water by caregivers throughout the day as needed) was made available. A long drinking straw was secured to the cup, allowing Mr. J to sip water as his desires dictated. The client had also expressed concern to be able to independently operate the television remote control with greater ease. This was achieved by the adaptation of the recliner with a bean bag tray and Velcro placed on the television remote and tray (so the remote would be secured).

Mr. J's wife's concern for more personal time was also addressed. The occupational therapist met with the hospice volunteer coordinator. This resulted in Mr. J having a volunteer for several hours on Saturday and Sunday (allowing Mrs. J to experience some personal time).

The case management of Mr. J's program involved the initial evaluation being conducted by a registered occupational therapist with a certified occupational therapy assistant present. The occupational therapy evaluation used in this case is the occupational history developed by Tigges and is based on the occupational behavioral model.[1,2] After the completion of the occupational history and discussion with Mr. J and his wife regarding the findings (with information and recommendations relayed to the physician to appraise), it was collaboratively decided that the occupational therapy program management would be as follows. For the initial 2 weeks, visits would take place five times weekly. Thereafter, visits would be scheduled three times weekly (for a period of 4 weeks). For the first week the OTR and the COTA would work together. Then the COTA would be responsible for executing the OT plan. Supervisory visits by the OTR were planned for every five visits.

In this case study we have seen how occupational therapy played a major role in enabling the client and his family to achieve goals that were valuable and meaningful to them.

CASE STUDY 4

Occupational Therapy Hospice Intervention Within a Home-Based Agency Setting

Trump aptly describes occupational therapy intervention within the home hospice-based setting. This review summarizes her case history analysis as it appeared in the June 2000 issue of *Home and Community Health Interest Section Quarterly*.

Mr. E was a 62-year-old male with a supportive wife. However, Mr. E's wife reported problems associated with stress that were related to caring for her husband. Mr. and Mrs. E lived in a ranch-style house with a ramp. Mr. E was very involved with his church.

Mr. E's past medical history included a right CVA that affected his left lower and upper extremities. Specifically, his left upper extremity gross motor coordination was intact, but he presented limited left upper extremity fine motor skills. Although he spent most of his time in a wheelchair, he was able to ambulate with occasional minimal assistance using a narrow-base quad cane. Mr. E's hospice diagnosis was end stage heart disease.

Mr. E's previous occupational pursuit was that of being a high school math teacher (recently retired). His primary leisure interest was woodworking.

At the initial occupational therapy evaluation, Mr. E presented with severely decreased overall endurance. He was not able to participate in any leisure activities, and he appeared to have a decreased awareness for safety.

Mr. E articulated one major goal—that of being able to ambulate down one flight of steps to his basement so that he could continue with his woodworking activities.

In order to enable Mr. E to meet his goal, the therapist first needed to increase his level of functional mobility and endurance. After Mr. E had developed an appropriate endurance level, the therapist and the client were able to navigate the stairs to the basement. Once in the basement, the sorting through of woodworking projects that Mr. E had started became a major focus. As the client began to participate in general woodworking activities, with hands-on supervision from the therapist, he gained strength and increased his safety awareness. Mr. E was then able to progress to working on his unfinished projects. The therapist introduced Mr. E and his wife to a volunteer who was an active member of the hospice team (and who also enjoyed woodworking). The therapist instructed the volunteer about Mr. E's precautions and abilities. After this initial meeting, Mr. E and the volunteer met weekly and worked together for many months. Utilizing the services of a volunteer was a cost-effective use of resources. At the same time it provided Mr. E with an opportunity to socialize and begin a new friendship as well as participate in a valued leisure occupation.

Mr. E became medically stabilized, and nursing staff visited him every couple of weeks to evaluate his status. Mr. E was extremely satisfied to once again be involved in his favorite leisure pursuit. He was able to decrease many of his medications, while at the same time, he became more independent for self-care. Due to this, his wife was able to resume her part-time job at a local church. After Mr. E's wife resumed her job, her initial complaints concerning stress in caring for her husband disappeared. Both husband and wife reported that they enjoyed quality time together.

This case study illustrates how occupational therapy intervention can enable a client to improve his physical well-being (including endurance and safety) as well as increase feelings of self-esteem.[3]

REFERENCES

1. Tigges, K. N. & Marcil, W. M. (1996). Palliative medicine in rehabilitation: Assessment and treatment in hospice care. In K. O. Larson, R. G. Stevens-Ratchford, L. Pedretti, & J. L. Crabtree (Eds.), *The role of occupational therapy with the elderly* (2nd Ed., pp. 758-762). Rockville, MD: American Occupational Therapy Association, Inc.

2. Tigges, K. N. (1993). Occupation therapy. In D. Doyle, G. Hanks, & N. MacDonald (Eds.), *Occupational textbook of palliative medicine* (pp. 535-543). Oxford, England: Oxford University Press.

3. Trump, S. (2000, June). The role of occupational therapy in hospice. *Home and Community Health Special Interest Section Quarterly, 7,* 1-4.

Unit 3

Occupational Therapy Work Settings, Documentation, and Intervention Approaches

WORK SETTINGS

9

Occupational therapists and certified occupational therapy assistants specializing in the care of older adults have many opportunities to work in a variety of settings. These settings may include (but are not limited to) the following services and programs:

✧ Community services (such as found in wellness programs, adult day care services, home health agencies, senior centers, and continuing care retirement communities)

✧ Acute care services (both physical and mental) such as those found in hospitals

✧ Rehabilitation centers

✧ Respite care services

✧ Subacute care

✧ Long-term care

✧ Hospice care

Clinicians may work as employees, consultants, private practitioners, private contractors, and be responsible for themselves (always), for their business, or for others as managers within an institution, company, or agency.

Information as to billing, Medicare requirements, and other pertinent information relating to reimbursement will be specifically discussed in a specialized appendix section entitled "Reimbursement Issues (Including PPS) in the United States."

The number of occupational therapists working with the elderly in the community has been increasing dramatically. Wellness, the concept of providing programs (such as smoking cessation, the use of joint protection and energy conservation, appropriate weight control, correct body positioning when performing functional tasks, ergonomically appropriate furniture and furniture placement, architectural adaptation in the home setting and work setting, and safety management in the home) that deal with the adoption of an appropriate lifestyle management, is rapidly becoming a major focus of occupational therapy expertise. Wellness and occupational therapy programs involving wellness concepts were discussed in Unit 1.

HOSPICE

Hospice, an area of practice that provides services to the terminally ill, is another setting in which clinicians can promote meaningful, appropriate, and thoughtful palliative intervention to the dying individual. Hospice's major mission is to provide quality of life care to the terminally ill person. Pain and symptom control play a major role as well as diagnostic honesty, caregiver support, and bereavement services. It is an around-the-clock service, as those working in hospice can be called at any time to provide care to the terminally ill person.[1] In the United States, individuals are usually admitted to hospice care if they have a prognosis of 6 months or less to live. Hospice, the hospice movement, and occupational therapy's role within the hospice setting have been specifically identified and described in Unit 2.

ACUTE CARE SERVICES

Acute care occupational therapy services (in the physical medicine setting) provide inpatient hospitalization. The older adult will usually have experienced an acute condition that may be due to an illness or an accident. These situations require the highly skilled care of a variety of professionals, x-ray, laboratory, and a host of other diagnostic and intervention services. Because the length of stay is often short, occupational therapists have learned to streamline the evaluation process, prioritize intervention, and articulate discharge-planning goals in an effective and succinct manner. In the United States, hospitals use 471 diagnostic-related groups (DRGs). Billing fees are prospectively based on pre-established rates that involve the type and amount of intervention needed for each diagnosis.[2]

REHABILITATION SETTINGS

Physical dysfunction rehabilitation occurs in rehabilitation units within community, teaching, or free-standing rehabilitation hospitals. Clients in this type of setting must be medically stable and able to tolerate 3 hours of intervention a day. Goals need to be measurable, and the client must be making progress for the duration of his or her stay. Many rehabilitation facilities make use of an integrated evaluation that is short, concise, objective, and clearly states the goals expected to be attained during intervention. Progress notes are usually written on a weekly basis with a daily log documenting daily attendance, interventions, and the response of the client. Outpatient rehabilitation may vary from daily to weekly notes. Like inpatient therapy, goals must be measurable, and the client must show progress while in the program.[2]

Common diagnoses for the older adult in the rehabilitation setting include (but are not limited to) orthopedic problems (most often hip fractures), cardiac conditions, respiratory conditions, cardiovascular accidents, arthritis, and cancer.[3]

In the outpatient rehabilitation setting, clients are expected to attend three times weekly. Home programs involving the client and the caregiver are exceedingly important in improving the status of the outpatient client.[4]

SUBACUTE SETTING

The subacute medical setting can be situated in nursing homes, acute care hospitals, and rehabilitation hospitals. This type of care fills the intervention gap between acute and long-term care. Subacute care is less costly than rehabilitation hospitals and rehabilitation units. Occupational therapy documentation includes evaluations with clearly stated, measurable goals. The client must be making measurable progress in order to remain in the program. Progress notes are usually written on a weekly basis, and a daily log is kept of specific intervention modalities and attendance.[2,4] In the United States, the prospective payment system has recently been initiated. For specific information about reimbursement and billing please refer to Appendix A, entitled "Reimbursement Issues (Including PPS) in the United States."

The most frequent diagnoses of clients in this setting is varied and most often include cardiac care, orthopedic care, neurological care, wound management, and ventilator care.[5]

LONG-TERM CARE

Nursing homes offer long-term care for frail elderly persons. Within the nursing home setting a variety of intervention and program options are offered. Some of these have already been described. These services may include any one or all of the therapies, respite care, a subacute unit, and hospice beds. Therapists and assistants working in long-term care may be hired directly by the nursing home, by agencies, and as private contractors or consultants. Clients can be admitted to nursing home facilities for rehabilitation, medical intervention, or custodial care.

RESPITE CARE

Respite care is planned, intermittent short-term care designed to provide periodic relief to the caregiver/family from the 24-hour continuous care of a frail older adult.[6]

Respite care services can be found in hospital units, through religious affiliated service and nonaffiliated service programs, through volunteer services which may be referred by some area offices on aging, in the elder's home, in special units or beds in nursing homes, in day care programs, and in assisted living facilities.

Respite care offers a health care option to frail elderly adults that can make it possible for them to continue to live in a familiar community setting. Some examples of occupational therapy involvement include providing interaction with stimulating activities such as reminiscing and promoting carry-over of self-care skills.[6]

ACUTE PSYCHIATRIC CARE

Practitioners also serve older adults in acute psychiatric facilities (mental health settings). Crisis stabilization is the most frequent goal for inpatients. Both group and individual intervention serves to help clients develop strategies that may be later used to prevent future crisis fomenting episodes. Stress management, anger management, task oriented groups, and self-esteem groups are some examples of intervention modalities that can be used in this type of mental health setting. Stays are short (anywhere from 7 to 15 days). Evaluations, intervention plans with measurable goals, notes to denote progress, and discharge planning are all part of the documentation process.[2]

LONG-TERM PSYCHIATRIC FACILITIES

Long-term psychiatric care is another area of employment for clinicians. A number of mentally ill frail older adults, who are unable to live in supported-living arrangements, are cared for in state hospitals. Many of these facilities have developed nursing home units to better care for these frail older individuals with chronic mental illness (who also have numerous medical conditions). At times, therapists may act as case managers within the team.[2]

Evaluations, intervention plans, daily attendance logs, and weekly progress notes (which clearly document the necessity for continuing intervention) based upon measurable goals are part of record requirements in this setting. Occupational therapy is frequently delivered via group programs.[2]

ADULT DAY CARE

Adult day care services offer community-oriented employment opportunities to practitioners. There are approximately 3,000 adult day care programs within the United States. Older adults in this setting may exhibit physical, mental, or cognitive limitations. These clients demonstrate a range of diagnoses such as cerebrovascular accident, Parkinson's disease, multiple sclerosis, Alzheimer's disease, and rheumatoid and osteoarthritis. Attendance by clients is on a planned basis during specific hours.[2] There are a number of objectives that adult care addresses:
- ⬦ The presence of peer social interaction in a safe and protected environment
- ⬦ The provision of respite care for caregivers
- ⬦ The provision of a variety of services involving care management such as health assessment, therapeutic diets, nutritional education, and access to community support services (e.g., lifeline, meals-on-wheels, and transportation)
- ⬦ The provision of health promotion, disease prevention, emotional and sensory stimulation, and socialization by means of structured groups (e.g., reminiscence groups, leisure activities, activities of daily living groups, exercise and health education groups, and community education groups)[4]
- ⬦ The improvement and maintenance or enhancement of functional abilities and the prevention of additional losses[2]

In adult day care, occupational therapy modalities involve enhancing perceptual, motor, psychological, and cognitive skills.[2]

HOME HEALTH CARE

Home health care is concerned with providing remediation, intervention, and health care services in the individual's place of residence. Care is provided by the intervention team, guided by the physician (who co-signs each intervention plan). Any number of professionals (social workers, registered nurses, occupational therapists, physical therapists, or speech therapists) may provide needed intervention. Home health aides are also part of the team, and occupational therapists, at appropriate times, may be involved in the supervision of these aides. In the United States, the individual must be homebound in order to receive payment (under Medicare and HMO sponsored Medicare programs).[4]

There are a variety of home health agencies. Some are part of the services of a hospital system. Others might be associated with a medical supply or pharmaceutical company. Still others may be free-standing or provide services to specific diagnoses.[4]

Occupational therapy services address those individuals who need assistance and instruction in performing self-care, home management, and leisure tasks as independently as possible and in a safe manner. Intervention frequently involves home modifications such as the installation of grab bars in the bathroom, the installation of appropriate lighting throughout the residence, the use of double-sided rug tape to hold a throw rug in place or elimination of the rug altogether, and the placement of non-skid surfaces in the tub. Instruction and procurement of the use of adaptive devices and equipment (e.g., sock donners, long-handled dressing sticks, long-handled shoe horns, long-handled sponges, button hole devices, use of the three-in-one commode, and safe transfer onto a raised toilet seat) is often practiced. Instruction in activities of daily living (e.g., dressing, bathing, cooking, laundry management) and home management (e.g., cleaning, shopping, money management) are sometimes taught.

Intervention may involve energy conservation and work simplification techniques associated with activities of daily living (e.g., rearranging of the most frequently used shelves in the kitchen or bedroom for easy access). Splint provision and modification for upper extremities, instruction in splint care, and instruction in upper body exercise improve upper extremity mobility, which in turn improves activities of daily living performance. Perhaps one of the most significant aspects of home health is the interaction, not only with the client, but also with the caregiver. The therapist frequently instructs the caregiver (and other family members or significant others) in home safety management, transfers in the bathroom area, use of adaptive equipment, care of the splint, or any other area of intervention associated with the client that is significant to the client's well-being and recovery.

The most frequent diagnoses in this health care setting include: hip fracture, shoulder dislocation and/or fracture of the humerus, wrist fracture, knee replacement due to arthritis, diabetes, cardiac impairment, change in mental status, cancer, cardiovascular accident, osteoarthritis in the upper extremities, Parkinson's disease, and chronic obstructive pulmonary disease.

Documentation requirements include:

1. An evaluation.

2. A intervention plan recommendation to the physician in charge of the case. This plan should include specific modalities; measurable long-term and short-term goals; time, frequency, and duration of the planned intervention; and the rehabilitation potential of the client.

3. Progress notes of each visit (indicating progress achieved and new short-term goals needed to achieve the major long-term goals).

4. A discharge note (usually involving a specific discharge form as well as a separate discharge note). The completion of intervention or discharge form needs to address the outcome (client's status at time of discharge, realization of goals); the modalities used, the number of interventions, and any recommendations issued

to the client and significant others caring for the client at time of discharge. The note or form also needs to indicate that the physician has agreed to the discharge (including time and date).

Therapists who work in this setting need to be flexible, possess excellent teaching skills, be well-organized and resourceful, be able to communicate effectively with the client and the team, and be tolerant, sensitive, and respectful to the cultural environment of the client.[4] Perhaps one of the most important aspects of home health occupational therapy is that of being able to problem solve at a moment's notice.

SENIOR CENTER PROGRAMS

Many multipurpose senior centers offer leisure, recreational, and educational programs that involve a variety of mentally stimulating activities. Health referral services, counseling, and wellness programs (many of which include nutritional education and a variety of physical fitness activities) are also available to participating older adults.[4] Clinicians have opportunities to serve as consultants on an as-needed basis in these facilities.

CONTINUING CARE RETIREMENT COMMUNITIES

These communities encompass a variety of living options. First, there is independent living in an apartment. Many of these facilities provide a congregant dinner hour. Breakfast and lunch services are usually optional, as residents have their own kitchens to prepare these meals. Social activities, interest groups, entertainment, and a variety of wellness programs are often offered. There is usually some form of health monitoring service by a nurse (either employed by the community or through a specialized visiting nurse program).

If a resident can no longer care for him- or herself independently, he or she may be transferred to an assisted living section. Assisted living involves providing care for; dressing and/or bathing as needed; daily monitoring of medication; provision of three nutritious meals daily; towel, linen, cleaning, bedmaking and laundry services; and the provision of socially, physically, and mentally stimulating activities. A nurse is usually on duty 24 hours a day, and physicians are available as needed. Besides assisted living programs in continuing care retirement communities, these services can also be found in independent free-standing facilities. Job opportunities for clinicians are available as consultants or through a visiting nurse agency (on a contractual basis) to assist elderly residents who are in need of remediation and who would benefit from professional instruction to improve their physical or mental status.

Finally, most continuing care retirement centers offer a medical center (acts as a nursing home) for residents who become physically frail or who are recovering from an illness or an accident. If a partner or a friend becomes incapacitated, the other partner or friend can readily visit on a daily basis due to the proximity of facilities and care levels.

Summary

The major gerontic occupational therapy work settings have been discussed. However, we live in an ever-changing world with ever-changing needs. Developing new ways of delivering services is a paramount issue in the 21st century. An entrepreneurial approach in which insightful professional programming and sound business management grow hand-in-hand is the "shaper" of tomorrow. Today's job is not forever. It will change, and we clinicians must be "ever-ready" to discern this change and seize the opportunity to serve.

WORK POSITIONS

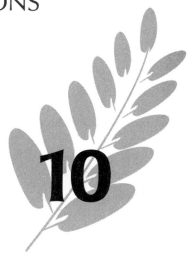

Occupational therapists and certified occupational therapy assistants seek employment in a variety of work positions.

THE EMPLOYEE

Clinicians working as employees have an assigned salary and assigned pay periods (usually every 2 weeks), assigned work day hours, an assigned lunch period, a job description, assigned holidays, and an assigned number of sick leave days and vacation days. Preparation and payment of all taxes (social security, state, and local) are performed by the employer. The employer may issue a written contract that also can include specific rules and regulations, health and medication benefits, credentialing qualifications, confidentiality requirements, the mission of the institution or agency, or any other segment of the job that the employer deems important.

THE CONSULTANT

As a consultant, the clinician is involved in raising concerns, identifying problems, giving opinions or advice, counseling, weighing alternatives, providing recommendations and suggestions, and sharing expert knowledge in a variety of areas to help the client (which could be an individual's intervention, a social support system, family members, or a residential support system) resolve problems in an efficient and effective manner. *Consultation* is the sharing of information and guidance that promotes the resolution of problems that relate to activities of daily living tasks, affect well-being, self-efficacy, life roles, life autonomy, and productive living.[7] The majority of consultants provide indirect services to clients, agencies, or groups.[8]

Consultancy can involve any number of resolutions involving environmental design, lifestyle design, specific intervention techniques, splint design and modification, use of adaptive equipment or adaptive techniques, providing appropriate positioning techniques, and instructing in energy conservation and work simplification as associated with activities of daily living. Actually, the list can be as long as is needed to resolve the problem.

In the nursing home setting, occupational therapy consultants work with the nursing home activity coordinator to help plan effective programs that meet the needs and interests of the residents of the nursing home. To accomplish this the consultant needs to possess:[8]

 ◇ Knowledge about the state and federal regulations and rules regarding activity programs in nursing home.
 ◇ An understanding of the particular nursing home environment.
 ◇ An awareness of the skills and knowledge of the activity coordinator.
 ◇ Knowledge of the needs and interests of the residents of that particular nursing home.
 ◇ Knowledge of various approaches to planning and implementing activities programming in the nursing home (e.g., use of community, social, and recreational opportunities; attendance of religious services for those who wish to attend).

Consultants may utilize a retainer fee, be paid a specific amount for a specific period of time (then be available for problem solving when needed), or receive a specific fee per incident of consultant usage. A contract that is agreeable to the specifications of the consultant and the person/facility/agency to be served is drawn up before initiation of services. The consultant is responsible for paying all of his or her taxes (federal, state, local), malpractice insurance, office expenses, recordkeeping, medical benefits, and any other business expense associated with the cost of running the consultancy programs. Fees are usually paid upon completion of the work assignment. The occupational therapy consultant can also work in the rehabilitation department of the nursing home (where his or her area of expertise will focus on physical rehabilitation).

THE PRIVATE CONTRACTOR

Private contractors specializing in the geriatric population often provide direct services in physical rehabilitation units (skilled care) that are found in nursing homes. They may serve on an individual basis with the nursing home or provide services through a rehabilitation agency. Private contractors are also involved in home health care and with the hospice setting.

In nursing homes and home health agencies, private contractors are involved in physical rehabilitation and skilled occupational therapy services to their respective clients. Hospice occupational therapy services are palliative. Specific functions of skilled occupational therapy services in the nursing home, home health, and hospice setting have been previously described.

The private contractor needs to draw up a contract that discusses and details a number of issues:[8,9]

1. The length of the contract (with terms of renewal that should include effective work dates and provisions for renegotiation and review)

2. Fee for service
3. Timely payment for services
4. Credentialing
5. Responsibilities of the agency/institution/facility
6. A statement of confidentiality of the client's records
7. A statement concerning assignability (subcontracting)
8. A statement concerning termination of services (usually 30 days written notice)

Other items that are a concern and agreeable to both parties may also be added.

Like the consultant, the private contractor is responsible for a variety of expenses such as self-payment for all taxes, recordkeeping, paying for malpractice insurance, and being responsible for all office and business expenses. As with consultancy, the responsibility for vacation time, sick leave, disability insurance, and medical benefits rests solely on the shoulders of the practice contractor.

THE PRIVATE PRACTITIONER

In the United States, the private practitioner wishing to serve adults 65 years or older must apply to the state Medicare certifying agency for participation in the Medicare program (known as the Provider Enrollment Office). In private practice, those working under Medicare guidelines are given a provider number. In general, occupational therapists in independent practice can also be reimbursed by other third party payers or by an individual.

Effective January 1, 1999, an occupational therapist in private practice (OTPP) bears the following description. An OTPP is an individual who meets all local and state licensing laws as an unincorporated partnership or unincorporated sole practice.[9] The OTPP may also be an individual who is "practicing therapy as an employee of an unincorporated practice, a professional corporation, or other incorporated therapy practice."[9]

Therapy services must be provided in the therapist's office or the client's home. An office is officially described as "the location(s) where the practice is operated in the state(s) where the therapist (and practice, if applicable) is legally authorized to furnish services during the hours that the therapist engages in the practice at that location."[9] The occupational therapist in private practice must meet all state regulatory and licensing requirements. Each therapist in a group must enroll "as an individual" with the appropriate carrier.[9] Aides and assistants must be personally supervised by the therapist and employed by either the practice to which the therapist belongs or employed by the therapist directly. Personal supervision, currently, requires that the therapist be in the same room during the time the service performance is rendered.[9]

Specific information regarding Health Care Financing Administration (HCFA), which is now titled the Centers for Medicare and Medical Services (CMS), forms and the application process in the United States can be found in Appendix A, "Reimbursement Issues (Including PPS) in the United States."

To be reimbursable, occupational therapy services must be provided to an older adult who is under a physician's care. The clinical record must show evidence of this care at least every 30 days. The intervention plan needs to include: the signature of the ordering physician and therapist; the amount, type, duration, and frequency of occupational therapy services that are expected to be rendered; anticipated goals; and statements about the client's diagnosis and prognosis.

Independent practitioners are responsible for providing payment of their own taxes, recordkeeping, paying malpractice insurance, all office and business expenses, their own sick leave, health benefits, vacation leave, disability insurance, and holiday leave. This has been true with all those who are self-employed.

THE PROS AND CONS OF SELF-EMPLOYMENT

Self-employment means being in business for oneself. It can take the form of consultancy, private practice, private contracting, or establishing a company. Clinicians engaged in self-employment need to be able to present their assets to prospective consumers in a positive and, at times, assertive manner.

⟡ *Pros*: Autonomy, flexibility, and "tax write-offs" are available in this type of setting. Income can be lucrative if the demand for services remains high, and the receivers of the services pay their bills.

⟡ *Cons*: Job security is risky, and cash flow might be irregular or erratic. The clinician who is in business for him- or herself must supply his or her own fringe benefits (e.g., health insurance, vacation time, holiday time, conference time, and reimbursement). Initial capital investment is usually needed (e.g., telephone, fax and copy machine, computer). No one is around to "fill in" unless prior arrangements have been made to cover illnesses or absences for other reasons. Like all businesses, unforeseen events or consequences can cause the therapist's practice to collapse unexpectedly.[10]

MARKETING OCCUPATIONAL THERAPY SERVICES

In initiating a business, there are a number of concerns. Knowing one's competition is essential in order to promote what is different about "your" business. Increasing one's visibility is a major goal. Hanna Gruen, OTR/L and president of Associated Occupational Therapists, Inc. (AOT) states, "I'm learning that you have to be visible, vocal, prepared to very succinctly tell people what you do, and you have to be prepared to talk about the importance and value of your field within the current system."[11] Visibility became such a major factor that of the three partners of the company, two are devoted to visibility. This meant knocking on doors, maintaining current contracts, and trying to establish new ones. Lists of frequently visited clients and colleagues are carefully kept (quarterly and semi-annually). Phone calls are made on a regular basis. Any problems are directly discussed with colleagues/clients (either through an arranged lunch or over coffee). The marketplace requires constant visibility.[11]

What is needed are marketing strategies. Gruen suggests the following key points:[11, p. 34]

1. Create an awareness of occupational therapy services (e.g., participate on committees and offer to speak).

2. Build a positive image of both the provider and the service.

3. Create consumer desire or need for services by public relations via the media and community visibility (e.g., billboards at malls, mailers, press releases, and newsletters).

4. Know the competition.
5. Train staff to be ambassadors. "A marketing plan should be a part of every growth-oriented business... It should be based on the strategic plan of the practice. It is a long-term, ongoing commitment and should include a business development or sales component."

Gruen reminds us, "We need to see those things that are distinctly OT. This total integration of mind and body that together allow us to perform our daily activities at our maximum—that's where we're so talented, and that's our uniqueness."[11, p. 34] When one thinks of the fact that people are now remaining at home longer and that they are working longer, there is a need for creating more community outpatient care. Third party payers are looking for good functional outcome that is achieved through an efficient and effective manner. Occupational therapy, with its emphasis upon the whole person, can offer a sound functional outcome achieved in a quick and cost-effective manner. Our product is highly marketable. The major question is how to best design this product and market it.[11]

A professional accounting firm, a marketer, and a public relations person all helped in the marketing process and in making AOT a successful company (growth from three partners to 80 employees in 17 years). One should never be afraid to seek professional help (who understand the marketing process). Flexibility and the willingness to understand and act on new and current needs was also essential to success. It took 13 months of hard work for the company to become a Blue Cross provider. Some managed care organization administrators told Gruen that they would prefer to refer a client to a physical therapy office that subcontracted with an occupational therapy group or an individual therapist. The company then collaborated with a number of physical therapy groups as subcontractors in order to deal with that specific reality.[11]

Marketing requires one to be assertive. It is definitely not for the overly sensitive, easily offended, or for those who are afraid of failure.[11]

THE CLINICIAN AS MANAGER

When a clinician assumes the responsibility of initiating and managing his or her own business (be it private practice, a business concern such as a company, or as a consultant or private contractor), he or she automatically becomes a self-manager (or a manager of others if the company or business has employees).

In the start-up phase it is necessary to determine the need for the services offered. Even when the business becomes ongoing, the wise manager is constantly reviewing current needs and discerning if past needs for the services should be adjusted, altered, or discarded in favor of new programs or services.

As a professional self-manager the clinician/entrepreneur is responsible for canvassing, advertising (e.g., brochures, business cards, video programs), and promoting the service or business. Networking with others can be helpful. Developing contracts and providing oneself with appropriate liability insurance is a major necessity. All licensing, safety, and health standards and requirements must be met (in the client's home or in one's own place of business).

Budget control and sound financial management (such as appropriate procurement of supplies and equipment and appropriate fee setting for services) are essential if one is to receive reimbursement for work that has been performed. Effective and efficient recordkeeping (such as copies of clients' records and reports that detail programs or services rendered) that is well-organized and readily available is necessary in maintaining good productivity.

Follow-up after the conclusion of a project or at termination of clinical services is helpful both from a public relations standpoint and in determining the effectiveness of the service or project over time.

The Clinician as Manager Within an Organization

When a clinician assumes a management position in an institution, agency, or company setting, his or her first responsibility is to fulfill the mission of the work setting. Many companies, institutions, and agencies expect the manager to know exactly what the mission is and to be able to translate this to supervisees. Productivity, efficiency, professionalism, and ethical behavior are requirements for maintaining an effective staff and providing good service delivery.

The manager is held responsible for seeing that supervisees under his or her management know their job responsibilities and are able to perform them in a satisfactory manner that meets all required standards. Some examples include: proficiency in performing modalities and interventions, ability to carry out all documentation as required by the organization, effectiveness in staff interfacing within the system, and the ability to practically apply the latest professional advances in intervention. Meaningful job descriptions that are well-organized and clearly stated can be helpful to new employees.

Most managers are required to assess, at least annually, a supervisee's progress. Management in this type of setting is the art and science of blending increased productivity through the involvement of supervisees with strategies that will enhance their performance.

A number of aspects of organizational management is described below. The manager's responsibilities can include:

◇ Respecting the organizational structure of the system (the chain of command)
◇ Respecting the worth and value of each supervisee
◇ Hiring new employees and when necessary terminating employees
◇ Providing troubled supervisees (e.g., alcohol abuse, drug abuse, and mental illness) with information as to where to seek help
◇ Dealing with union concerns (if the system is involved with a union)
◇ Ensuring that a safe, efficient, clean, and ergonomically sound environment is available for supervisees to work in (including such items as equipment and supplies, appropriate lighting, a non-faulty ventilation system, and clinic furniture that is ergonomically sound)
◇ Adhering to and "following up" on all licensure and credentialing requirements of supervisees and being involved in all accreditation processes
◇ Following established guidelines and regulations for any physically and mentally challenged supervisee
◇ Establishing a quality assurance program as required by the system to ensure good service delivery; this includes developing a program evaluation system
◇ Ensuring educational advancement opportunities (may be in the form of study groups, inservices on professional topics, courses, conferences, and workshops)

✧ Providing established inservices in fire and safety hazard procedures (e.g., bomb threats, hygiene, the use of gloves, fire safety routes)

✧ Controlling budgetary requirements effectively and efficiently (sound financial management)

✧ Developing a policies and procedures manual. This is a basic written guide for the occupational therapy department/unit that has many components. Some of these are:

  ▲ Philosophy (mission statement and objectives)

  ▲ Personnel (table of organization; description of the work environment; orientation procedure; performance evaluations; job descriptions; promotion procedures; vacation, personal, and sick leave; and career development)

  ▲ Programming (program descriptions and services offered, assignment of staff, client scheduling procedures, clinical conferences and team meeting, priority scheduling for client intervention, tardiness and missed appointments, family and client education)

  ▲ Documentation (initial evaluations, progress notes, re-evaluations, and discharge notes)

  ▲ Emergency and health safety (fire emergency procedure, bomb emergency procedure, electrical systems emergency procedure, hygiene and protection from infectious disease procedures)

  ▲ Equipment and billing (ordering supplies and equipment, and billing)

  ▲ Clinical specialty services (special group programs, home visits, positioning and wheelchair clinic, support groups, and follow-up)

  ▲ Student training program (student affiliation and contracts, students' objectives and goals, and scheduling student's fieldwork)

A policies and procedure manual is constantly updated. When a new procedure replaces an existing one, its date of adoption also needs to be added.

Much of the information presented on policies and procedures has been gleaned from an excellent resource:

✧ Burkhardt, A. & Gentile, P. A. (2001, January 1). Creating a policies and procedures manual that works. *OT Practice, 6*(1), 15-18.

These are some of the major responsibilities of management. There are a number of management styles (e.g., authoritarian, democratic, participative, laissez-faire, rules-oriented, and consultive). However, the manager can combine styles and invent new strategies and methods that are compatible with the needs of the organization and the manager's personality. Effectiveness and efficiency of occupational therapy service delivery are the primary outcomes to be achieved.

CULTURAL CONSIDERATIONS

CULTURAL COMPETENCY

Learning to be culturally competent has vast implications for practicing clinicians. Each client is an individual possessing a unique cultural background. In order to understand another person's culture, one must first understand his or her own cultural attitudes, values, and beliefs in relation to others. Learning more about other cultures permits one to become culturally competent and client-centered.

When conducting an appropriate occupational history interview, it is extremely important to identify the unique cultural beliefs and values of each client. Meaningful intervention and goals can be more readily established. It is also important to note that understanding another's culture is helpful in improving communication.[12]

For those who are beginning to understand the ramifications of cultural competency, Lyons suggests three interesting approaches that are helpful in broadening one's cultural level:[12]

✧ Know your own beliefs and understand how these compare with those of your clients.

✧ Learn more about other cultures (e.g., go to the library and read about the specific cultures of your clients). Look at the client's unique culture within the larger system.

✧ Listen to what your clients are telling you about themselves and their values. Be open to your clients' suggestions.

Cultural Communication and Occupational Therapy

Communication is a major key in being able to understand your client (and having your client understand you). Language proficiency is another aspect of culture and cultural competency.

"In communicating with consumers and their family members, words are the primary tools used in evaluation and intervention. Therefore, if language incongruity exists between practitioner and consumer, communication may be difficult and care may be compromised."[12, p. 3]

For instance, when evaluating persons with mental illness, both process of thought and content of thought become difficult when the consumer and the evaluator speak different languages. It might be difficult to judge if a client's language is slow due to poverty of ideas, because of depression, or because the client just doesn't understand the language well and needs time to translate the words back and forth in his or her own language. Again, it becomes difficult to evaluate whether a client's speech is fast because of cultural differences that occur in speech patterns or if it is a sign of flight of ideas. It might be problematical to discern if the logic of a person's speech is due to a schizophrenic thought disorder or due to an individual who is struggling with syntax sequencing in his or her secondary language.[13]

This writer witnessed a major miscommunication when a client told a physician (a newly arrived resident from Asia) that he was experiencing "butterflies in his stomach." It was an American idiom for saying that one's stomach was somewhat upset. The physician actually thought that the client truly thought he had butterflies in his stomach. Luckily, the physician spoke out loud about these thoughts and was surprised to learn from the client and others that this was an expression of feelings rather than a literal fact.

Taugher states that "Communication with caregivers remains one of the biggest problems for persons with limited English proficiency. This includes instrumental communication, in other words, strictly information exchange as well as linguistic and cultural communication."[12, p. 3]

Because the nature of occupational therapy involves a great deal of nonverbal and symbolic communication, therapists (through daily occupations and the personal interactions that surround them) may begin to break down some of these communication barriers by means of natural, everyday settings. Thus, a dialogue can begin and communication can improve as language skills increase for both the caregiver and the consumer. Occupational therapy practitioners have wonderful opportunities to find creative and meaningful ways to communicate by utilizing their unique skills to help family members and consumers address and resolve their conditions and problems.[13]

DOCUMENTATION

Documentation is the written record and the major way in which occupational therapy clinicians are able to communicate to others (the professional team, third party payers, accrediting agencies [e.g., Joint Commission on Accreditation of Healthcare Organizations; Commission on Accreditation of Rehabilitation Facilities; federal, state, and local governmental agencies], and the client) that services are being provided. It can also serve as a basis for measuring quality assurance and as legal evidence that services were rendered. It very importantly serves to justify reimbursement. Therefore, in order to be reimbursed, clinicians must constantly justify intervention through clearly stated documentation that is both necessary and reasonable for the condition being treated and that follows accepted guidelines for standards of care.

There are a variety of types of documentation needed in treating a client. The following represents a basic outline.

THE EVALUATION

First, there is the occupational therapy evaluation (which is preceded by a physician referral). This usually includes background and identification information, specific evaluation and assessment results, and recommended intervention. Recommended intervention involves the intervention plan (sometimes referred to as the plan of care).

THE INTERVENTION PLAN

In most instances the intervention plan is a part of the evaluation. Sometimes a separate intervention plan form is issued for both the therapist and the physician to sign. Whether the intervention plan is part of the occupational therapy evaluation or standing separately, specific information is needed. These essential elements include: a statement as to rehabilitation potential; rationale for occupational therapy intervention; a listing of specific modalities and methods recommended (including equipment and supplies as needed); time (e.g., 30 minutes, 1 hour, a visit or intervention session); frequency (e.g., three times weekly, five times weekly); duration (e.g., 6 weeks); prognosis assessment; and long- and short-term measurable goals.

Depending upon the work setting, there may be numerous variables involved in the intervention plan. The following serves as an example of a specific plan of care that is used in home health in the United States, known as the HCFA 485. The specific information needed includes:

◇ Certification and recertification
◇ Principal diagnoses
◇ Other diagnoses if appropriate
◇ Surgical procedure(s)
◇ ICD9 code
◇ Exact date of onset
◇ Start of care
◇ Medications
◇ Supplies and durable medical equipment
◇ Safety measures (e.g., bleeding precautions, remove environmental barriers, limited activity by pain or fatigue)
◇ Pain level
◇ Allergies
◇ Nutritional requirements (as appropriate)
◇ Functional limitations (e.g., legally blind, dyspnea, endurance, hearing, amputation)
◇ Activities permitted (e.g., complete bedrest, up as tolerated, no stairs, exercise prescribed)
◇ Mental status (e.g., oriented, comatose, forgetful, agitated, disoriented, depressed appearance, lethargic, confused at times)
◇ Prognosis

Some of the specific intervention modalities for occupational therapy services involve:

◇ D2—independent training/activities of daily living training
◇ D3—muscle re-education
◇ D5—perceptual motor training
◇ D6—fine motor coordination
◇ D7—neurodevelopmental treatment
◇ D8—sensory treatment
◇ D9—orthotics/splinting
◇ D10—adaptive equipment and training
◇ D11—other (could be another specific intervention that the therapist would deem reasonable and necessary)

✧ D20—home exercise program/therapeutic exercise

✧ D21—range of motion exercise

✧ D22—strengthening exercise

It should be noted that there is not to be any duplication of services with another discipline. The rehabilitation of the client needs to be assessed (e.g., good, fair, guarded, poor). Goals, both long- and short-term, need to be stated in functional terms (e.g., client will become independent in safe tub transfers and able to shower in the tub independently in a safe manner, client will be independent in dressing with the use of a stocking donner and dressing stick). Time, frequency, duration of intervention, and a statement as to expected discharge status (e.g., D/C to self-care, able to remain in the residence with supervisory assistance of a caregiver) are included in this part of the intervention plan of care.

The physician in charge of the case will review the occupational therapy recommendations (plan of care), discuss the case with the therapist or other team members (if needed), and then issue orders as related to the occupational therapy recommendations. Once this is done intervention can begin.

THE INITIAL CONTACT NOTE

In many instances an initial contact note stating that the occupational therapy evaluation was completed on a specific date with a brief summary of the findings, intervention recommendations, and goals (long-term and short-term) is required. Included are time, frequency, and duration of intervention. Subjective observations are also part of the initial note. For example, the information could include the fact that the client was cooperative and pleasant throughout the evaluation process, and the client's spouse was also present. Any statements that the client made during the evaluation would also be part of this note.

PROGRESS NOTES

Progress notes reflect the client's response to intervention. The most commonly accepted progress note form is the problem oriented medical record approach. Progress "SOAP" notes are directly used in this system. "S" stands for subjective. The clinician records information that is reported by the client, significant other, or family member. It is often a statement made by the client that is not measurable (e.g. "I feel much better today"). "O" is identified as objective. In this section the clinician records observable, measurable data, as well as a history or medical information. The emphasis is upon functional gains. "A" represents assessment. At this juncture the clinician records his or her professional opinion of limitation or functional expectations as related to the given objective data that was recorded in the previous section.

Here, again, it must be remembered that the emphasis is upon functional outcome. For instance, the client is making excellent progress in occupational therapy because he or she can now brush his or her teeth independently (including squeezing the toothpaste onto the toothbrush, rinsing it afterwards, and then putting it away). At the previous intervention session the client needed moderate (50%) assistance. "P" is identified as the "plan" part of the progress note. In this final section of the note the clinician records a plan of action to resolve problems. Information such as new short- or long-term goals, how long it is estimated that intervention should be provided, and how many times the client should receive intervention is recorded in the "P" section.[14]

Some agencies and institutions are now using checklist formats along with short answer sections (for such areas as subjective findings, objective findings, problems requiring service, client outcome interventions, objective findings, and new goals). Attention is now being paid as to whether the client has been informed of the benefits versus the risks of continuing therapy and if, in fact, that client wishes to continue therapy. Other aspects of the progress note may also involve documenting whether or not verbal or written instructions were issued to the consumer and whether that individual was able to understand the instructions.

Measurable functional goals are an important aspect of occupational therapy documentation. The following represent some examples of measurable goals that use a functional basis:

 ✧ Ms. Smith will participate in three social activities weekly with encouragement and support from the therapist for a minimum of 20 minutes at each activity session.

 ✧ Mrs. Jones will be able to button her blouse independently with the use of a button hook device within 3 minutes.

 ✧ Mr. James will be able to enter and exit the tub at a supervisory level in a safe manner with 15% verbal cues from the caregiver.

 ✧ Ms. Brown will be able to participate in the craft group (without taking all the available supplies in her section of the table) for at least 10 minutes, when verbally cued by the therapist at the beginning of each craft session.

It is important to note that goals are a collaborative effort. It is not the job of the clinician to think of goals in isolation. Rather, the client, the therapist, and the caregiver discuss goals that all feel are achievable and desirable.

In terms of writing goals, the following resource is very valuable:

 ✧   Allen, C. K., Earhart, C. A., & Blue, T. (1992). *Occupational therapy treatment goals for the physically and cognitively disabled*. Bethesda, MD: The American Occupational Therapy Association, Inc.

For most reimbursement purposes the therapy (intervention rendered) must be necessary and reasonable as related to the client's injury or illness and require the skills of an occupational therapist or a certified occupational therapy assistant (who is supervised by an occupational therapist). The intervention approach that is provided needs to be considered as that which follows accepted standards of practice.

RE-EVALUATION

During the course of intervention it may become necessary to re-evaluate the client (due to a variety of reasons such as a change in status or a request from the physician). The re-evaluation usually follows the same format as the evaluation.

THE DISCHARGE/DISCONTINUATION REPORT

The last piece of documentation is the discharge or discontinuation report. In this type of document the client's course of therapy is summarized (including such areas as modalities provided, the number of sessions/visits, if goals were met or not met). The condition/status and functional outcome of the client is carefully described. Recommendations and follow-up care suggestions are also important aspects of the discharge report. The discharge report must be signed and dated by the therapist. The physician in charge of the client's care needs to be apprised by the therapist of the client's status and in agreement with the rationale for discharge. Many agencies, facilities, and institutions also require a short discharge progress note that states that the client has been discharged and a brief summary of status at time of discharge.

In all documentation the occupational therapist and certified occupational therapy assistant must sign their full title (registered, licensed, degree) at the end of their names. The date and time are also part of the documentation process.

SPECIFIC OCCUPATIONAL THERAPY EVALUATION FORMATS AND CHECKLISTS

The evaluation of the client is one of the most important aspects of documentation because it lays the foundation for the intervention plan and program. The following evaluation, The General Occupational Therapy Evaluation for Geriatric Clients/Patients (Form 12-1) is a basic geriatric evaluation that can be useful in a number of therapeutic settings in which rehabilitation has taken place and the consumer is in his or her home or plans to return to his or her home.

GENERAL OCCUPATIONAL THERAPY EVALUATION FOR GERIATRIC CLIENTS

1. Name of client _____   Primary language _____

2. Name of caretaker and phone # _____   Primary language _____

3. Address and phone # of client _____

4. Case number _____ Date of birth _____ Sex _____

5. Physician (name and phone #) _____

6. Primary diagnosis/diagnoses _____

7. Medical history _____

8. Conditions/contraindications/general needs _____

9. Personal history (avocation, vocation, education, role relationships [married? single? significant other? mother? father?])

_____

_____

_____

10. Client goals at present time. The therapist asks: "At the present time what are the two most important goals you would like to see achieved?"

_____

_____

_____

11. Muscle/motor strength (upper body)

Areas		Right upper extremity	Left upper extremity	Comments
Shoulder				
Elbow				
Wrist				
Hand	Fingers			
	Thumb			
Neck strength				

Note upper body characteristics (e.g., blanched, cold, hot, edematous, handedness, muscle tone)

_____

_____

12. Range of motion (upper body)

Areas		Right upper extremity	Left upper extremity	Comments
Shoulder				
Elbow				
Wrist				
Hand	Fingers			
	Thumb			
Neck (ROM)				

(continued on next page)

Form 12-1. General Occupational Therapy Evaluation for Geriatric Clients.

13. Bilateral coordination (upper body) good_____ fair_____ poor_____
14. Trunk control   good_____ fair_____ poor_____
15. Fine motor coordination (include grip—prehension pattern, grasp, flexibility, dexterity)
    Comments:

Right upper extremity	Left upper extremity

16. Balance (for activities of daily living) good_____ fair_____ poor_____
    Comments:

    Any history of falls?____ How?_____ When?_____ Where?_____
17. Functional transfer (e.g., toileting)   good_____ fair_____ poor_____

18. Endurance   good_____ fair_____ poor_____
19. Ambulation (for activities of daily living) good_____ fair_____ poor_____
    Comments:

20. Use of device   yes _____   no _____
21. Use of wheelchair   yes _____   no _____
    Comments:

22. Visual/hearing/awareness

	Good	Fair	Poor	Comments
Visual				
Hearing				
Communication				
Mental status				
Mood				

    Comments:

(continued on next page)

Form 12-1. General Occupational Therapy Evaluation for Geriatric Clients, continued.

23. Perceptual status (comment regarding spatial relationships, stereognosis, body image, figure ground, L/R neglect, proprioception, visual field tracking, depth perception, color identification, and form constancy)

_____

_____

24. Sensation (comment as appropriate regarding hot/cold discrimination, dull touch, deep touch, paresthesias, light touch, two-point discrimination)

_____

_____

25. Activities of daily living (self-care and instrumental)

Activity/skill _Self-care_ (Include adaptive equipment in all categories)		Independent	Assistance (25%, 50%, 75%)	Dependent
Bathing/showering		Upper		
		Lower		
Dressing	Don	Upper		
		Lower		
	Doff	Upper		
		Lower		
Toileting		Hygiene		
		Management		
Grooming (hair, teeth, nails)				
Self-feeding				
Drinking				
Instrumental				
Meal preparation				
Meal planning				
Making bed				
Laundry				
Shopping				
Money management				
Cleaning				
Transportation				
Use of telephone				
Medical health management				
Other				

Comments (include safety in home environment as appropriate):

_____

(continued on next page)

Form 12-1. General Occupational Therapy Evaluation for Geriatric Clients, continued.

26.   Equipment on hand? _____
(include adaptive devices)
27.   Equipment needed? _____
(include adaptive devices)
28.   General statement/rationale for occupational therapy intervention
(include potential for rehabilitation)

_____

_____

29.   Modalities (intervention plan recommendations and use of specific
methods)

_____

_____

30.   Short-term goals (include time frame)

31.   Long-term goals (include time frame)

_____

_____

32.   Frequency _____ Duration _____
33.   Client/caretaker in agreement with intervention plan? Yes ___ No ____

         Therapist signature _____
         Date of evaluation _____

         (Reprinted with permission of Sandra C. Lewis, MFA,OTR/L, 2001)

Form 12.1. General Occupational Therapy Evaluation for Geriatric Clients, continued.

For those clinicians working with the older adult in the home setting or for those practitioners who have a potential to return home, specific checklists in home safety are recommended. Some therapists, as discussed in Unit 1, have branched out to become solely involved in safety management in the home setting.

Areas to evaluate include safe management of activities of daily living (cooking, dressing, bathing, shopping, transportation [e.g., driving/use of public transportation], cleaning, meal preparation), and actual safety within the physical aspects of the home.

Checklist questions concerning physical and hygiene safety in the home are helpful in determining potential and real safety hazards. The following basic questions help comprise a safety checklist:

✧ Electrical Equipment
  ▲ Are extension cords and outlets overloaded?
  ▲ Are there frayed electrical cords in the home?
  ▲ Are any electrical cords under rugs or under furniture?

✧ Fire Hazards
  ▲ Are smoke detectors readily available on each floor of the home, and are they in working order?
  ▲ Are flammable items (e.g., gasoline, solvents, rags, paint) stored away from heat sources?
  ▲ Are the correct fuses being used?
  ▲ Are there safety screens in front of or around fireplaces and kerosene heaters?
  ▲ Do independent heaters have automatic turn-off switches if they get turned over?
  ▲ Does the household have a fire escape plan?

✧ Rugs/Runners/Flooring
  ▲ Are throw rugs taped to the floor?
  ▲ Is the carpet pile low?
  ▲ Is flooring glossy and/or slippery?

✧ Bathroom
  ▲ Do the bathroom doors have safety release locks (able to open on both sides of the door)?
  ▲ Are there night lights in the bathroom?
  ▲ Do showers, bathtubs, and bathroom floors have nonskid surfaces?
  ▲ Are grab bars needed in the bathroom? If so, where?
  ▲ If grab bars are already present, are they attached in wall studs? Are grab bars appropriately and usefully placed?
  ▲ Is scalding prevention equipment needed? Does the client check the water temperature by hand before entering the shower/tub?
  ▲ Is a raised toilet seat with armrests needed?
  ▲ Is a bath bench or bath seat needed in tub/shower area?

✧ General
  ▲ Are pets underfoot?
  ▲ Is pet equipment (bowls, dog/cat play items, pet beds) in a safe area?

⋏ Can the client use a key to open the front/back door?

⋏ Can the client open locks on the windows?

⋏ Is dwelling clean (e.g., dust, dirt, litter)?

✧ Telephone/Communication System

⋏ Is the telephone accessible in case of accident?

⋏ Is the night light near the phone?

⋏ Does the phone have illuminated dial buttons?

⋏ Are emergency numbers clearly posted on or near the phone (e.g., 911, poison control, cardiologist, and other physician numbers as appropriate)?

⋏ Is another type of emergency call system needed?

✧ Kitchen

⋏ Are cupboards and shelves organized so that frequently used items are the most easily reached?

⋏ Is there a scalding prevention mechanism at the sink?

⋏ Is the sink accessible to the client? Can the client use the faucet with ease?

⋏ Does the client or caretaker wash hands before preparing food?

⋏ Are kitchen cloths and towels laundered frequently?

⋏ Does the client/caretaker wash fruits, vegetables, fish, and chicken before preparing a meal?

⋏ Is perishable food refrigerated?

⋏ Is frozen meat, poultry, fish taken out of the freezer and left to thaw in the refrigerator?

⋏ Are the tops of cans wiped clean before opening?

⋏ Are the knives appropriately used (and stored when not being used) when cutting/preparing food?

⋏ Is any special equipment needed in the kitchen (e.g., jar openers, doorknob turners)?

⋏ Can the client/caretaker hear a teakettle whistling?

⋏ Can the client/caretaker smell fire/smoke?

⋏ Are dials on the stove, oven, and microwave large enough to read with ease?

⋏ Is garbage contained in an appropriate manner?

✧ Bedroom

⋏ Is furniture protruding? Are walkways clear?

⋏ Is a night light available?

⋏ Is a bed appropriate height for client?

⋏ Is the mattress firm?

✧ Living Room

⋏ Are rugs appropriate (e.g., low pile; if runner or throw, are they secured by tape or tacked down)?

⋏ Is the chair or couch firm and high enough so it can support neck and back? Is the client able to touch floor while sitting?

⋏ Do chairs and couch have firm arm support for arising?

▲ Is lighting non-glare and luminous to meet the client's requirements?

▲ Can the client adjust room temperature?

▲ Are all tables stable with firm legs?

▲ Is furniture protruding?

▲ Are walkways clear?

▲ Are any electrical lines (e.g., from television, lights, clocks, computer) loose and not secure?

✧ Stair and Passageways

▲ Are stairways well lit (including night lights)?

▲ Are stairs clear of objects?

▲ Are handrails on both sides of stairway and securely fashioned?

▲ Are passageways clear of objects (e.g., are pet dishes, plants, newspapers, furniture placed so walkways are narrowed)?

▲ Are doorways clear of obstructions?

▲ Does the client wear textured and rubberized slippers/shoes (not stocking feet or socks) when relaxing in the home?

✧ Medications

▲ Are medications readily accessible?

▲ Is medication schedule listed and legible?

▲ Does the client understand his or her medication schedule?

▲ Are medications marked so that the client can easily read the label?

▲ Does the client know the side effects of each medicine?

▲ Does the client take medication as prescribed (e.g., with/without food; no grapefruit juice for some drugs)?

▲ Does the client wash hands before handling medication?

▲ Are medications stored as directed by label (e.g., reference to heat, light, moisture)?

SPECIFIC SAFETY CHECKLISTS

These checklists can be found in the following resources:

✧ Cook, A. & Miller, P. (1996). Prevention of falls in the elderly, Appendix B: Home Assessment and Check for Fall Hazards. In K. O. Larson, R. G. Stevens-Ratchford, L. Pedretti, J. L. Crabtree (Eds.), *The role of occupational therapy with the elderly* (2nd Ed., pp. 743-763). Bethesda, MD: The American Occupational Therapy Association, Inc.

✧ Mandel, D. R., Jacobson, J. M., Zeanke, R., Nelson, L., & Clark, F. (1999). *Home safety evaluation and home safety tips to prevent falls. Appendix 3: module handouts. Lifestyle redesign: Implementing the well elderly program.* Bethesda, MD: The American Occupational Therapy Association, Inc.

Resources Concerned With Evaluations and Assessments

There are many excellent resources that contain valuable information concerning evaluations, assessments, and tests that are useful to occupational therapists. The following represent a number of highly recommended resources:

✧ James, A. B. (1996). Evaluation and intervention for the performance components: Section 1—The sensorimotor component. In K. O. Larson, R. G. Stevens-Ratchford, L. Pedretti, & J. L. Crabtree (Eds.), *The role of occupational therapy with the elderly* (2nd Ed., pp. 548-572). Bethesda, MD: The American Occupational Therapy Association, Inc.

This resource section describes assessments of sensorimotor skills, sensory testing, stereognosis, perceptual and motor deficits, vestibular function, tests of motor function, and assessments of visual perceptual function:

✧ Levy, L. L. (1996). Cognitive integration and cognitive components. In K. O. Larson, R. G. Stevens-Ratchford, L. Pedretti, & J. L. Crabtree (Eds.), *The role of occupational therapy with the elderly* (2nd Ed., pp. 573-596). Bethesda, MD: The American Occupational Therapy Association, Inc.

Several tests and an inventory concerning cognitive functioning are amply discussed:

✧ Allen, K. A., Kehrberg, K., & Burns, T. (1992). Evaluation instruments. In K. A. Allen, C. A. Earhart, & T. Blue (Eds.), *Occupational therapy treatment goals for the physically and cognitively disabled* (pp. 31-84). Bethesda, MD: The American Occupational Therapy Association, Inc.

This chapter details the Allen Cognitive Level Test (a standardized leather lacing task). There are three versions. The enlarged or Large Allen Cognitive Level Test (LACL) is used specifically with geriatric clients who manifest cognitive disabilities and physical limitations. The Routine Task Inventory (RTI) is a pragmatic observational measure of performance (associated within Allen's framework of cognitive disabilities). It serves to identify qualitative differences in functional performance. The Cognitive Performance Test (CPT) was designed to provide a standardized ADL-based tool for assessing the client's functional level in Alzheimer's disease.

These tests and inventory are highly detailed throughout the chapter so that the practicing therapist can readily use them in the clinic:

✧ Trombly, C. A. (1995). *Occupational therapy for physical dysfunction* (4th Ed.). Baltimore, MD: Williams and Wilkins.

This resource is involved with a wide variety of evaluations and assessment tools useful in physical dysfunction. It includes a wealth of evaluations, assessments, and tests concerned with the biomechanical and physiological aspects of motor performance, and it also examines aspects of the human experience such as clients' roles and their importance in the performance of activities of daily living:

✧ Neistadt, M. E. & Crepeau, E. B. (1998). *Willard and Spackman's occupational therapy* (9th Ed., pp. 185-290). New York: Lippincott.

This comprehensive text examines a variety of evaluations that measure performance areas such as driving, sensory and neuromuscular performance, perception, cognition, psychological skills and psychological components, mental status, activities of daily living, and proprioception:

✧ Pedretti, L. W. (1996). *Occupational therapy practice skills for physical dysfunction* (4th Ed.). St. Louis, MO: Mosby-Year Book.

This is another excellent resource that includes a wide variety of assessments and evaluations. Some of these include evaluations of joint range of motion, muscle strength, motor control, cognitive dysfunction, physical dysfunction, dysphagia, visual deficits, sensation, and perceptual deficits:

✧ Laver, A. J. (1996). The Occupational Therapy Intervention Process, Section 1: Occupational therapy and evaluation of older adult clients. In K. O. Larson, R. G. Stevens-Ratchford, L. Pedretti, & J. L. Crabtree (Eds.), *The role of occupational therapy with the elderly* (2nd Ed., pp. 508-537). Bethesda, MD: The American Occupational Therapy Association, Inc.

This chapter is rich with descriptions of a variety of assessment tools that are appropriate for many areas of occupational therapy practice. The following is just a partial listing of some of the assessment resources:

✧ The Life Experiences Checklist
✧ The Role Checklist
✧ The Functional Assessment and Safety Tool
✧ The Safety Assessment of Function and the Environment for Rehabilitation Tool
✧ The Structured Observation Test of Function
✧ The Kitchen Task Assessment
✧ The Assessment of Motor and Process Skills
✧ The Mini-Mental State Examination
✧ The Home Occupation-Environment Assessment
✧ The Canadian Occupational Performance Measure

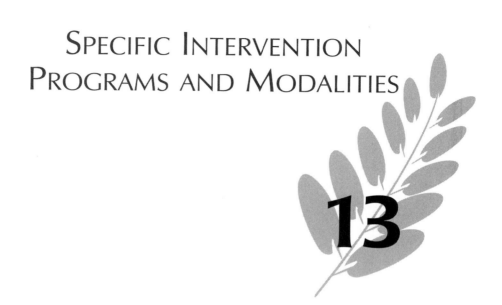

SPECIFIC INTERVENTION PROGRAMS AND MODALITIES

13

COGNITIVE PROGRAMMING IN DEMENTIA

Dementia, an acquired organic syndrome, is a condition in which there is a progressive deterioration in global cognitive functioning. It is of such severity that the individual's social and occupational performance is deeply affected. Alzheimer's disease (dementia of the Alzheimer's type) is the most common form of dementia in the United States. Other types of dementia include Parkinson's disease, normal pressure hydrocephalus, and an array of vascular diseases (e.g., multi-infarct dementia, now termed as vascular dementia, and mixed, multi-infarct/vascular dementia and Alzheimer's disease).[15,16] Dementia not only affects the older individual who is afflicted, but also it affects all those involved in the care of that individual.[16]

The first step toward intervention is to assess the cognitive level of the client. The Allen Cognitive Level test (ACL) or the enlarged Allen Cognitive Level test (LACL) are recommended.[16] These tools were described in the preceding section entitled, Specific Occupational Evaluation Formats. Warchol recommends implementing the ACL because it can readily identify cognitive deficits and abilities, it enhances the delivery of customized intervention plans and programs that emphasize the client's remaining abilities while compensating for deficits, it enables the therapist to write realistic intervention plans and goals, and finally it is helpful in demonstrating increases in safety and functional level.[15]

The Cognitive Disability Theory and Its Application to Dementia

Claudia Allen's Cognitive Disability Theory is highly useful and instrumental when one is designing an intervention program for dementia clients. This theory includes six cognitive levels and 26 performance modes. These modes are extremely sensitive to changes in the individual and are descriptive of that individual's abilities at every stage.[17] "By identifying what abilities still remain, we have a series of positives to build on and can present activities at a comprehensive level, enabling the client to maximize function and safety. The complexity of tasks can be graded to match the client's cognitive level and remaining abilities."[15, p. 17]

At each of the six cognitive levels Levy offers interventions that provide environmental stimulation and support so that the functional capabilities of the client can be maximized and confusion can be decreased. At the same time, the individual is enabled to retain a sense of mastery and competency despite impairments of a significant nature.[16]

This approach provides caregivers with guidelines so that they are educated in the best techniques to support the client diagnosed with dementia throughout the course of his or her illness.[16] In order to understand the management and intervention of this model, one must first review some basics of Allen's Cognitive Disability Theory. Allen proposed a hierarchy of six cognitive levels that involve the dimension of information processed while pursuing everyday normal life activity. Qualitative differences in functional capacity and limitations were also considered. Furthermore, Allen utilized three dimensions of sensorimotor information processing. These stages are part of each of the six cognitive hierarchical levels.[16] These dimensions include:

Attention to sensory cues. This involves the ability to attend to sensory input from the environment. Capabilities of this range involve: sensory cues that sustain attention from internal cues (proprioceptive and subliminal); sensory cues that are externally concrete (tactile, visual, and verbal); and complex abstract cues (symbols, ideas). In intervention, practitioners must learn to adapt activities in order to maximize the functional capabilities of the client. One needs to capitalize on cues that the client can attend to and limit exposure to activities that are beyond that person's comprehension.

The ability to translate cues into functional performance (goals). These include goals that are implicit in initiating a response to an action as well as goals that are explicit (that follow a conventional outcome). For example, at lower levels a client may be able to only comprehend the motions involved in a desired activity (such as pushing a vacuum back and forth). This same person would be unable to comprehend the more conventional goal of being able to clean a rug.[16]

Motor actions. These represent the final stage of Allen's information-processing model. They are composed of two parts. There are the spontaneous actions that are self-initiated from memory stores, and there are imitative actions that are cued by motor and visual channels via a demonstration by another person. As an example, a lower level cognitive individual might only be able to initiate and imitate motor actions that are near to reflexive (or are very familiar behavioral actions). A person with a more advanced cognitive level would be able to participate in planned actions that reflect attention to abstract cues (e.g., he or she would be able to utilize conceptual information to produce solutions to problems).[16]

Cognitive Disability Theory demonstrates the effectiveness of using activity analysis in determining the relative difficulty of an activity in terms of its information-processing demands. From this analysis one can deduce and identify environmental factors that can constrain or facilitate productivity of each cognitive dimension. Rehabilitation strategies are derived from the conceptualization of how best to use environmental elements (associated with each cognitive dimension) so that the environment can be modified within the structure of the desired activity to make use of remaining cognitive abilities to develop strategies that compensate for cognitive limitations. The emphasis, then, is to place desired activities in the grasp of the client's control and comprehension.[16]

Practitioners modify the structure of a desired activity (to compensate or capitalize upon) by adapting sensory cues that the individual can attend to, the quality of sensorimotor associations (or goals) that the client is able to conceptualize, and the degree of assistance that is needed to enable the client to complete a desired motor action.[16] Levy includes concepts for intervention with the discussion of Allen's six hierarchical cognitive levels.[16]

Cognitive Level 6—Planned Actions (Assistance Code: Independent). This level is characterized by the absence of disability. It involves normal functioning. A person in this category can make use of complex information to carry out desired activities with safety and accuracy. Errors are avoided, problems are anticipated, and consequences of actions are an integral part of problem solving. Sensory cues are rich and varied (e.g., diagrams, drawings, concepts involving gravity, speed, time, and three-dimensional space are well understood). Deductive reasoning can be used to confirm, validate, or refute a course of action. Abstract reasoning can be captured by symbolic and abstract cues. The goal, in this instance, is to use abstract reasoning to plan actions and to anticipate errors. Motor actions are planned in advance.[10,16]

Cognitive Level 5—Exploratory Actions (Assistance Code: Stand-by/Supervisory for Cognitive Assistance). The client is able to learn through visible, concrete, and meaningful stimuli. Attention is captured and then sustained through the use of external cues (especially interesting properties pertaining to concrete objects). The goal of action involves the exploration of the effects of self-initiated motor actions upon physical objects and then to investigate those effects utilizing overt trial and error problem solving. Motor actions are of an exploratory nature and extend through the use of visual memory. The client is able to follow through on concrete four- or five-step process and is able to learn new concrete activities through imitation. Avoid activities that involve abstract skills (e.g., reading comprehension, mathematics, writing skills, complex conversation, shopping, driving, and managing finances).

The client also experiences great difficulty with judgment, reasoning, planning ahead, *semantic memory* (involves general knowledge about the meanings of numbers, symbols, and words), and *episodic memory* (the ability to recall information and personally experienced events to a specific place and time). However, *procedural memory* (the recall of necessary procedures and skills to perform a task; it involves remembering how to perform familiar motor activities) is less affected at this level. The client is able to complete dressing, eating, and grooming activities without assistance. On the other hand, the client may need assistance in establishing safety procedures and in anticipating a hazardous situation, as these activities are of an abstract nature.[16]

Cognitive Level 5 corresponds to Stage 4 of the Predementia Stage of the Global Deterioration Scale for the Assessment of Primary Degenerative Dementia. It is termed Late Confusional. This is a frequently used medical scale that physicians use for staging the progression of primary degenerative dementia.[16,18]

Cognitive Level 4—Goal-Directed Activity (Assistance Code: Minimum Cognitive Assistance: Usually recognized as 25% assistance). At this level attention is directed to visible and tactile cues. Attention is sustained by means of the completion of short-term activities. In terms of goal selection regarding performing a motor action, the client perceives a concrete cause-and-effect relationship that exists between a visible cue and a desired outcome. Problem-solving abilities are lost, and the individual is not able to notice mistakes. Motor capacities are limited to being able to follow two- or three-step activities that are highly familiar motor processes (which can lead to the accomplishment of goals that are visibly predictive). Individuals utilize what they see in the environment for cues as to what they should do.[16]

Activities that can be accomplished are those that are adapted to capitalize on the client's ability to use two- or three-step familiar motor actions that possess predictable visible results. Activities that compensate for the client's inability to notice mistakes or comprehend unpredictable results are also essential to the completion of successful activity.[16]

At Level 4, the client should be provided with opportunities to engage in relatively error-proof activities that are simple, concrete, and supportive of desired social roles. These activities can be incorporated into a client's daily routine (e.g., straightening up the linen closet, folding laundry, waxing the car, and raking leaves). Instructions cannot be remembered, and clients are disoriented to time and/or place. Calendars and clocks with the date, day, and year are helpful. Labels and pictures may provide reminders of the location of objects and daily activities. Supervision is needed as individuals can forget daily care (e.g., to bathe, shave, let household chores pile up) and the placement of possessions. A system to organize and secure items that can ensure the safety of possessions (e.g., promotes that items have not been stolen or lost) is necessary by the supervisee. In terms of daily care, dressing and bathing can often be accomplished with a task set-up. Individuals can eat independently but need guidance regarding seasoning food and eating an appropriate amount of food. Areas in grooming (such as washing one's back, shaving under the chin) that are not visibly seen may be completely forgotten.[10,16]

Clients at this level need protection from potential safety hazards. Attention needs to be focused upon the following situations: removal of loose rugs or use of two-sided rug tape to hold rug down; removal of clutter; ensuring that the lighting is adequate; ensuring that electrical appliances, wiring, and hot water pipes are safely secured; securing of firearms, knives, power tools, medications, chemicals and any other potentially dangerous substances or objects; and supervising tub and shower activity. Persons at this level frequently wander and may get lost. Therefore, it is helpful to secure an identification bracelet for the client. In this respect, it is also advised to have identifying photographs of the client on hand should the occasion arise when this type of visual information would be needed. Twenty-four-hour supervision is recommend to ensure client safety.[16]

Many older adults at this stage can manifest anxiety and depression. Consistency of the environment is helpful and comforting. If the client becomes agitated, involving him or her in success-oriented manual activities is helpful.[16]

This level is comparable to Stage 5, the Early Dementia stage, of the Global Deterioration Scale.[16,18]

Cognitive Level 3—Manual Actions (Assistance Code: Moderate Cognitive Assistance: Generally interpreted as 50% assistance). Attention is directed toward tactile cues that can be acted upon and to familiar objects that the client can manipulate. Other objects and persons are scarcely noticed. The goal in performing motor actions is focused upon tactile exploration that relates to the effects of one's actions upon the environment. Goals are not related to outcome. Motor actions are limited to one-step very familiar, action-oriented direction that has been demonstrated. Individuals at this level cannot learn new behavior.

Behavior becomes confused at this stage (e.g., using keys indiscriminately in locks, pouring soup into a coffee maker, clicking dials on and off of a television set). Clients at this level should be provided with adapted activities that reinforce the relationship between predictable tactile effects on the environment and one's actions. Some of these activities include walking, washing cars, drying and washing dishes, cleaning countertops, and vacuuming. Sensory overload should be avoided. Decreasing unnecessary sources of stimulation can help the client cope more effectively. Because the individual will be drawn to any item that can be manipulated or touched, potentially dangerous appliances such as coffee makers, toasters, microwaves, and blenders should be hidden from view. Whenever possible, pushbuttons and knobs on the stove should be either covered or removed. The client's environment should be routine, comprehensible, and predictive.[16]

The client, at this level, is able to wash his or her hands and face and brush his or her teeth. When the individual is dressing or bathing, the caregiver needs to present items one at a time and supervise the client so that the appropriate order is followed (e.g., the client does not put underwear over slacks or wear a nightgown to go outside). At this level 24-hour supervision is required to ensure client safety.[10,16]

Level 3 correlates to Stage 6, the Middle Dementia Stage of the Global Deterioration Scale.[16,18]

Cognitive Level 2—Postural Action (Assistance Code: Maximum Cognitive Assistance: Generally interpreted to be 75% assistance). The client manifests highly disorganized thinking. Attention now involves internal cues. Objects and people in the environment are generally ignored. The goal in performing motor actions involves repeating a one-step motor action component of the activity purely for the pleasure of its effect on the body. The process and not the outcome becomes important. Motor actions are limited to the ability to imitate demonstrated one-step directions that are near reflexive, highly familiar, gross motor patterns. Demonstrated simple movement, modified sport activities, and calisthenics that can be imitated by the client are usually very successful at this level. Most activities need to be short-term (approximately 15 to 30 minutes). However, one-step activities (e.g., polishing furniture, folding laundry) can only be imitated if these actions were nearly habitual prior to the onset of the disorder. Many activities of daily living can be accomplished if the client is provided with a demonstration or model to follow. For example, the caregiver can demonstrate washing his or her own face with a washcloth in order to enable the client to wash his or her own face.[10,16]

When addressing the client, simple sentences (one simple statement at a time) are helpful. Routines need to be predictable. All self-maintenance activities need to be broken down with step-by-step processes that involve comprehensive one-step motor actions.[10,16]

At this level the client manifests spontaneous behaviors that are largely unproductive and appear bizarre (e.g., dressing and undressing, reapplying the same lipstick multiple times, sitting backward on the toilet and driving it as if it were an automobile, and aimless pacing).[16]

Caregivers and practitioners need to try to communicate on an emotional level and be sensitive to the emotionality of the tones. Emotional connection and building trust are essential elements in communicating at this level.[16]

Individuals may be able to eat finger foods (e.g., french fries, cut apples, hamburgers, or tortillas). However, any items such as artificial fruit and flowers should be removed as these individuals are unable to determine what they should and should not eat. Since aimless pacing is common at Level 2, it is helpful to structure the environment to provide a safe space for wandering (e.g., unobstructed walkways, combination locks on doors, nonslippery and nonglossy floors). Clients should be escorted to the lavatory every 2 hours when they are awake to avoid urinating in unacceptable locations. Receptacles and wastebaskets should be removed in order to prevent the client from mistaking these items for a toilet. Treasured possessions should be placed on furniture surfaces so that these items can be easily seen. This helps the client to feel secure that his or her favorite items are not "lost" or "stolen."[16]

Gentle stimulation of the senses involving familiar or favorite sensations are helpful (e.g., a house pet provides a "tender touch," gentle massage, favorite fabrics to touch, favorite musical CDs or tapes, and rocking chairs throughout the home or facility) and can be reassuring. Round-the-clock supervision is essential.[10,16]

Level 2 corresponds to Stage 6, Middle Dementia, of the Global Deterioration Scale.[18]

Cognitive Level 1—Automatic Actions (Assistance Code: Total Cognitive Assistance: This is generally regarded as being dependent or requiring close to 100% assistance). Attention at this level is limited to subliminal internal cues (e.g., taste, smell, hunger). Although the individual may be conscious, he or she will largely be unresponsive to external stimuli. Goal selection has no application. Motor actions are limited to, at times, being able to follow near reflexive one-word directions such as "sip." [10,16]

Clients at this stage need to be assured of adequate nourishment. The individual may need to be fed or, if still able, be allowed to eat finger foods. Assisted ambulation and assistance with transfers from bed to wheelchair are indicated in the earlier part of this level. Later, regular turning in bed and passive, active, and/or assistive range of motion may be needed in order to prevent bed sores, osteoporosis, infections, and contractures. Dressing and bathing activities are provided by the caregiver. The environment should be consistent, familiar, and modified to elicit orienting experiences. Favorite foods, hand lotion, gentle touch, massage, and fragrant plants are helpful in providing pleasant and familiar orienting experiences. At the same time providing a loving touch and relaying messages of concern and care are exceedingly important.[10,16]

Clients at this level are profoundly impaired and need constant 24-hour supervision.[16]

Although this level marks the terminal phase of this disease, death usually occurs prior to the last stage of this level. Secondary complications of dementia and comorbidities (e.g., infection, trauma, aspiration, malnutrition, and pneumonia) are usually responsible for the cessation of life.[16]

Level 1 corresponds to Stage 7, the Late Dementia Stage, of the Global Deterioration Scale.[18]

Levy has demonstrated, through the use and adaptation of the Cognitive Disability Theory, how functional performance can be maximized throughout the deteriorating course of this disease. Practitioners can provide caregivers (be they family, significant others, or aides) with guidance on ways in which cognitive capabilities of the client can be capitalized upon and how compensation for specific cognitive limitations can be carried out by modification of the structure and demands of desired life activities and occupations.[16]

Behavior Management of Dementia

Clients diagnosed with dementia often manifest bizarre or inappropriate behavior. With all types of dementia one of the most frustrating aspects of caring for these individuals is inconsistency of affect and mood. Another major problem is their inability to make necessary associations without the appropriate stimulus of an object before them (e.g., a client may void in an inappropriate place because the stimulus of "toilet" has not been seen). The person with dementia is frequently confused with memories of the past that keep intruding upon the present. Current memories (such as having moved to an assisted care or nursing home facility) are, for the most part, not being stored for future application.[19] Thus, many persons afflicted with dementia may often state that they need to "go home," or "go to work," or "go to school." They will attempt to find an exit so that they can leave to perform these tasks.[19]

There are a number of ways to communicate and modify unwanted behavior. The following are recommendations that deal with improving communication and behavior of the dementia client:

⬦ Avoid situations where reasoning is required. Reasoning with dementia clients places those persons in an adversary role as they have little in the way of resources to defend their position.[19]

⬦ Listen to the client. Every forgetful person deserves the dignity of being heard. Active listening in a concerned and caring manner can often help that individual respond in a positive way.[19]

⬦ Maintain a trusting relationship. Avoid giving false promises or false information (so that one can calm a person temporarily). Maintain courtesy at all times. Avoid merely issuing orders.[19]

⬦ Offer choices whenever possible. The feeling of having some sense of control can be supported by offering choices (usually no more than two options to avoid confusion).[19]

⬦ Communicate effectively. Provide relevant (not abstract) information that is needed to facilitate care in the present moment (e.g., "It is cool out today; you will need a jacket"). The client is usually unaware of rules of a new facility and the fact that he or she now needs 24-hour supervised care. Intervention should include possible needs. For example, if a client has wandered away from a supervised area, communication should be designed to alleviate the confusion. The client should be redirected back to a safe area without causing an embarrassing moment. Using phrases such as "I was just going for a walk; would you keep me company" can be helpful in preventing accusations, questions, or commands that the dementia client cannot answer.[19]

⬦ Decrease demanding social situations. If a client has become reclusive, it may be due to the fact that the client's memory and cognitive skills have declined, and the individual's ability to engage in conversation has become greatly diminished. It is important to achieve a less demanding social situation. Caregivers and therapists should provide emotional support and remove the client from high-stress social situations (e.g., a large party) when the client manifests signs of agitation.[20]

✧ Simplify approaches and the environment during "sundowning." It has been noticed that from mid-to-late afternoon and into early evening many elders with dementia can become disoriented, agitated (often yelling), restless, combative, and manifest increased confusion and wandering. Because many of these behavioral changes occur at the time of sunset, the terms sundown syndrome or sundowning are used to describe this phenomenon. The increased rates of falls and elopements from facilities during this time period is testimony to the hazards of this behavior.[10]

Possible causes of these behaviors may be fatigue, limited tolerance of others and the environment, failure to continue coping, dehydration, a need for simplification of requests or participation expectations, circadian rhythm disruption, and biochemical factors.[10,21] It is interesting to note that in many facilities the "change of shift" occurs during sundown time and that this behavior might be directly linked to sundowning (clients sensing that one group of employees is leaving and that a new group has "come aboard," that daily reports are being given, and that discussion about these events is taking place).

Intervention helpful with sundowning behaviors involves simplifying the environment and approaches toward the sundowner. The following area specific strategies useful in decreasing sundowning behavior:[20]

✧ Use adequate lighting.

✧ Provide a safe area for physical activity.

✧ Give reassurance in a calm and caring manner.

✧ Urge the client to drink fluids during the day.

✧ Reduce noise and clutter.

✧ Avoid, if possible, restraining the client at this time.

At three Life Care Centers in eastern Tennessee, a "wandering room" was developed to monitor specific residents with dementia when the afternoon change of shift occurred.[20]

Provide effective strategies for coping with anger. There are numerous reasons why an older adult with dementia might strike out in anger. The individual may not be able to convey feelings of frustration and helplessness in a rational manner. This older adult might also be angered because he or she believes that more help is being offered for a task than is required.[19] He or she may be experiencing fear, a variety of misinterpretations, and challenges to understanding personal survival.[21] Specific strategies for dealing with anger include:

✧ Assess the situation (one's role and the effect of the client's outburst on others).

✧ Respond, distract, and make needed changes as soon as possible in order to avoid escalation of the aggressive behavior.

✧ Move slowly, speak slowly—and with determination.

✧ Try to maintain eye contact.

✧ When approaching a stressful situation, adopt a casual tone of voice. Address the individual as a peer and offer distracting conversation.

✧ If the client objects to a particular procedure, reduce the amount of assistance offered.

✧ Express regrets and understanding regarding the client's frustration. These individuals need this type of acknowledgment.[19,21]

✧ Promote meaningful intervention when dealing with catastrophic reactions. *Catastrophic reactions* (such as sudden changes of mood, where the individual without an apparent reason resorts to: anger; combativeness; restlessness; repetitive foot and hand motions like the stamping of feet, clapping of hands, crying, or throwing items) are responses of distress that demonstrate the inability to interpret, understand, or cope with an imagined or real situation, environment, person, or self. These changes may be due to unrealistic demands, being rushed, too difficult a task, feelings of being manipulated, inability to express one's fears and needs, caffeine, unfamiliar environment, too much confusion or noise, strangers, reflections, disliked persons present, an onset of illness, misunderstanding a television program, or an inability to perform a purposeful movement.[21]

Ways to intervene include:

✧ Anticipate or perceive problems or stressors.

✧ Rephrase negatives such as "no" or "don't" to positive statements such as "we can do it this way" or "come with me."

✧ Distract the client/resident with food or by asking for assistance.

✧ Use familiar routines.

✧ Simplify tasks.

✧ Allow time to respond.

✧ Allow physical movement to defuse agitation.

✧ Reduce environmental stimuli.[21]

Cope effectively when a client displays inappropriate sexual behavior. Occasionally the client with dementing illness might make offensive invitations or remarks, fondle others inappropriately, masturbate in public, or expose him- or herself. For most of these individuals, their ability to control inappropriate or impulsive behavior is severely impaired. When these types or behaviors are displayed, reminders that these actions are inappropriate and subsequent involvement in some type of constructive activity is helpful in defusing the situation. At no time should the impaired elder be subjected to ridicule, emotional lectures, or threats. If this individual persists in continued inappropriate sexual behavior, he or she should then be directed to the privacy of his or her own room to avoid any public consequences.[10,19]

Deal appropriately with pacing and wandering behavior. Many late life impaired adults wander or pace. This may be due to: a method of expressing needs (such as exercise, urination, or hunger and thirst), an expression of medication reactions, looking for something that they cannot describe or name to others, not being able to recognize signs of fatigue or how to stop and sit down, the inability to realize when they have become lost, increased stress and anxiety, or responses to feelings of tension, insecurity, fear of being manipulated, and not being able to understand what is expected of them.

Intervention in this area of management includes:[21,22]

✧ Assessing what the wandering might be manifesting (e.g., illness, response to medication, or hunger).

✧ Using a calm approach, keep arms at the side, and maintain eye contact.

✧ Providing signs for cueing (e.g., client's name on bedroom, bathroom).

✧ Using distraction techniques to break the pacing pattern (e.g., look at pictures or view a scene from the window; as both the caregiver and client walk, offer to sit with the client or provide a drink of juice).

◇ Providing other opportunities for activity and movement (e.g., relaxation sessions, exercise sessions, recreational activities, and adapted sports).

◇ Simplifying requests and tasks.

◇ Providing rocking chairs as a source to ease tension.

◇ Using appropriate lighting.

◇ Providing uncluttered and safe areas in which to pace (both outdoor and indoor).

◇ Providing areas and nooks that promote a chance for exploration and discovery as well as privacy.

◇ Monitoring fatigue.

◇ Maintaining fluid intake.

◇ Monitoring client's feet (watch for blisters or calluses).

◇ Using "medic-alert" bracelet with wristband identifying client.

◇ Providing reassurance, attentiveness, and acceptance.

◇ Walking with the client, converse and build up trust. Then redirect in a clear voice, "Let's go this way."

Cope effectively with pillaging and rummaging behaviors. Pillaging and rummaging are behaviors that involve searching, holding, touching, looking at, and moving items from one place to another. These behaviors can lead to accusations that others are taking or stealing beloved objects, increased anxiety (not knowing what one is looking for), safety dangers (e.g., hoarding spoiled food, sharp items or toxic substances found in kitchens or bathrooms), increased confusion, taking others' belongings, and feeling lost.

Assistance to these individuals involves:

◇ Providing a sense of security that the client's needs will be met.

◇ Learning favorite "hiding places" (e.g., tissue boxes, underneath the mattress, underneath the bed, and behind the drapes).

◇ Ensuring that the client has familiar items from the past that he or she can carry and hold.

◇ Utilizing "straightening up" as an activity.

◇ Fabricating cloth scrapbooks (sew on straps and attach to the individual's chair) that have familiar and meaningful items.

◇ Providing activities that use sorting as a strategy (e.g., tiles, poker chips).

◇ Marking items with the resident's name.

◇ Monitoring surroundings for unsafe items.

◇ Providing special areas such as closets or drawers for rummaging.

◇ Accompanying the client and make the activity "fun" (thereby changing it from a fear-driven activity).

◇ Not scolding, teasing, punishing, or responding with anger; instead being gentle and speaking softly.

◇ Fabricating busy boxes with safe items that can be handled (e.g., balls of yarn, ribbons, work-related safe items such as large erasers).

✧ Using distraction (such as "Let's get a glass of juice" or "Come, let's walk together") as a way to direct the client away from another person's possessions or space.[21]

✧ Promoting discretionary assistance with activities of daily living routines. Many late life clients with dementing illness are not able to recall a series of instructions and activities that relate to daily routines (e.g., dressing, getting ready to go to bed, washing). Often these individuals, if sent to the bathroom to toilet, wash, and undress, will emerge with only one of these tasks completed. Therefore, these persons need assistance in daily care in which activities are "broken down" into simple routines. It is important for caregivers to be able to casually assist clients with routine activities and anticipate any needs these individuals might have (e.g., have necessities such as a toothbrush, a comb, and denture materials when grooming in clear view so as to provide visual cues).[19]

Meaningful activities are an essential part of life. The impaired older adult with dementia is in need of a satisfactory, varied, and productive day. Not only is this helpful in enabling these individuals to feel worthy, but it also ensures that they will be sufficiently tired to fall asleep at an appropriate time. In this way sleepless nights can be avoided. Inclusion in small group activities such as tea and coffee klatches, simple crafts, walks, simple games, exercise sessions, and helping with simple chores are examples of activities that many impaired late life adults can benefit from.[19]

The following are recommended behavior management resources useful when coping with a variety of dementia and neurological disorders:

✧ Cleland, M. (1988). *Prevention and management of aggressive behavior in the elderly*. Portland, OR: Good Samaritan Hospital and Medical Center.

✧ Matthies, B. K., Kreutzer, J. S., & West, D. D. *The behavior management handbook: A practical approach to patients with neurological disability*. Available from Therapy Skill Builders (a Harcourt Health Science Company), 555 Academic Court, San Antonio, TX 78204-2498.

✧ Robinson, A., Spencer, B., & White, L. (1988). *Understanding difficult behaviors: Caregiving suggestions for coping with Alzheimer's disease and related illness*. Ypsilanti, MI: GECM/Eastern Michigan University.

These behavior techniques and recommendations are exceedingly helpful to therapists who are consultants, company directors, and employees working in dementia care as well as to families and facilities.

Specific Activities/Occupations Useful for Older Adults With Dementing Illness

It is important to remember that any program designed for clients with dementing illness must match the specific level at which that individual is currently functioning. This means that activities and occupations must be carefully monitored and adapted as changes occur.

Carly R. Hellen, OTR/L suggests a variety of activities that she has found to be helpful in promoting meaningful occupations among those clients diagnosed with dementia of the Alzheimer's type-DAT. Hellen proposes that objectives of an activity should focus on abilities, not limitations; be purposeful in the use of time; provide a sense of belonging; promote positive behavior; be a tool to diminish unwanted to negative behavior; and finally become a vehicle for appropriate verbal and nonverbal communication.[21]

Successful activity criteria include the following characteristics: First, it must be safe (not a hazard to staff, family, or the client or any residents living in the same area as the client). Second, it must be modifiable (simplified, able to be "broken down" into small tasks and adapted for success). Third, it needs to be repetitive, familiar, and routine. It should also be adaptable (e.g., small group, individual, seated, or lying down if needed). It needs to be pleasurable (e.g., enabling the client or resident to use past skills and interests in an enjoyable manner). Finally, and most importantly, it must be dignified (ensuring the client's sense of worth and self-respect).[21]

Some examples of successful activities in the cognitive arena that Hellen has used are: who's who (pictures of famous persons familiar to the client) and going shopping (using catalog pictures or advertisements in which one can guess the cost of an item, this game can be altered by using old catalogs to see the changes in what items cost 20 years ago and what they cost today); reminiscing kits (reminiscing kits can be made of familiar items that are meant to be seen, touched, or smelled. For example, a kitchen kit can contain a ladle, a vegetable brush, measuring spoons, an eggbeater, measuring cups, and a sponge to spark discussion. Likewise, a toolbox kit can consist of a ruler, a screwdriver, a hammer, sandpaper, and a c-clamp to initiate conversation. Sports boxes or sewing kits are other items that can be used in promoting communication and reminiscence); personalized memory boxes (with this type of a project the client keeps a box filled with familiar photographs and other personal memorabilia. These boxes can serve as a point of communication as well as a way to enhance one's identity); and sorting activities (poker chips, wash cloths, tiles, and sensory games [sea shells, pine cones—participants listen to the sounds in the sea shell or smell the pine cones and then discuss these sensations. Other items that have any type of sensory connection can be used]).[21]

In the area of physical activity, Hellen suggests beginning exercise and movement groups with head-to-tail directions, going from the midline of the body to the sides, and using bilateral movement before unilateral movements. Other activities that promote physical movement are tossing games (balloons, soft balls, bean bags); movement to music; circle dancing; and tour of the facility as an opportunity to walk and greet staff).[21]

Activities and occupations that encourage positive psychosocial participation are also effective. These can include involvement in service projects (in which the participants fabricate pictures and scrapbooks for children in a hospital or individuals can become involved in caring for pets or plants).[21] Most of the above activities that Hellen has recommended are useful in facility settings. However, clients residing with their families may also benefit from some of these recommendations.

Intervention Approaches Useful in Combatting Dementia

Barbara Szekais offers a number of intervention approaches for those older adults with dementing illness. She identifies intervention, in dementia, as essentially the management of problems that are produced by the illness and finding solutions or ways to meet the challenges that face both the client and caregivers (be they staff or family).[22]

Szekais recommends that before initiating intervention, the occupational therapist evaluate physical, sensory-perceptual, cognitive, psychosocial, and activities of daily living components as well as include pertinent information from family and significant others to determine the client's functional level.[22]

To enhance cognitive functioning Szekais suggests counseling (in the early stages), cognitive facilitation and stimulation (e.g., modified reminiscing groups, completion of partial song lyrics); relaxation (e.g., quiet music, rocking chairs, and tapes of soothing environmental sounds); structured communication; environmental structuring (compensating for functional deficits by changing or rearranging the client's physical environment); sensorimotor therapy (may include spontaneous and automatic movement or multi-sensory stimulation); intergenerational activities; structured activities; and self-care (structured as needed) activities.[22] A number of these intervention options will overlap into other functional areas.

To improve affective functioning, Szekais recommends the following: counseling (in the early stages); relaxation activities; appropriate medication intake; structured socialization; structured activities; movement and exercise; intergenerational activities; activities that allow for spiritual expression, and milieu therapy. This involves identifying a range of tasks in which clients can be involved. These tasks can address a number of skill areas such as affective, social, perceptual, sensory, cognitive, and physical.

These tasks are then matched with the client's skills, interests, and needs as much as is possible. The client is given responsibility for chosen tasks that reflect his or her interests and is given assistance as needed. The client's tasks match needs that should be reviewed and adjusted regularly to meet changes in the client's condition as the disease progresses. In an adult day care center the client can become part of a group that makes new members feel welcome. In a skilled nursing care facility a client/resident may have the responsibility of providing plant care.[22]

To enhance sensory-perceptual functioning, Szekais suggests that the first priority should be the provision of appropriate physical aids (e.g., hearing aids, corrective lenses, or non-glare lenses). Other modalities and methods include: environmental structuring; the use of adaptive techniques and equipment; sensorimotor therapy; structured activities; and adjunctive therapies (e.g., pet therapy, dance therapy, and horticultural therapy).[22]

Social functioning is another important aspect of meaningful occupations. Szekais recommends the following to promote improving the client's social skills: counselling (in the early stages), milieu therapy, adjunctive therapies, structured socialization, and intergenerational activities.[22]

Language and communication are two very important aspects of human activity. There are a variety of modalities and techniques useful in supporting appropriate communication. These include structured verbal and nonverbal communication techniques, cognitive facilitation and stimulation, behavior modification (some examples are operant and respondent conditioning, positive and negative reinforcement, reinforcement schedules, shaping, and extinction), and environmental structuring.[22]

In the area of self-care activities there are a number of modalities and techniques that are useful. Adaptive techniques and equipment enable the client/resident to perform these vital skills as much as he or she possibly can. It is also important to explain to the caregiver the rationale involved in activities of daily living so that the caregiver will comprehend their importance and not try to "do for" the client what he or she can do for him- or herself. Performance of activities of daily living promotes gross and fine motor coordination; sensory stimulation; reinforcement of old learning; reinforcement of self-image; and pride in self as well as an improved sense of reality.[22] It is suggested that exercise and sensorimotor therapy, environmental structuring, behavior modification programming, and milieu therapy are helpful modalities in enhancing self-care skills.[22]

In the area of promoting sound physical health and appropriate sleep patterns, relaxation activities, sensorimotor and exercise therapy, structured activities, environmental structuring, the monitoring of medications, and the use of natural sleep inducers (such as herbal teas and warm milk) are helpful.[22]

Nutrition and elimination can best be enhanced by positioning equipment and appropriate chair and table heights to promote physical function when eating, using adaptive equipment as needed (e.g., non-skid mats, enlarged two-handled cups, covered glasses and cups, enlarged handles on utensils, and divided plates); providing a conducive eating environment such as a quiet area that is home-like and separated from visual distraction; and establishing formal eating programs.[22] Behavior modification, exercise and movement therapy, and the monitoring of medication all aid in improving nutrition and elimination.[22]

Motor function is an important aspect of human activity. Except with immobilized very impaired elders, movement (in a variety of forms) provides an activity or occupation in which most clients can participate. Simple movement can help work off excess non-directed energy that might otherwise become pacing or agitated behavior. Exercise and sensorimotor therapy, the use of adaptive techniques and equipment, environmental structuring, and the monitoring of medication are all important activities that promote improved motor function.[22]

It is important to note in any comprehensive dementia intervention program, such as that described by Szekais, the caregiver involved must be given "time out" and an opportunity to attend to his or her own needs. Within the home, volunteers, friends, other family members, hired caretakers, or church members can provide respite care. Outside the home setting, adult day health and day care centers, nursing homes, assisted living facilities, adult family homes, or hospitals can provide short-term supervision and care. Respite should be part of the weekly schedule of the caregiver and client.[22]

Environmental Structuring in Dementia

The environment is always the silent partner in any intervention effort, and although it may appear passive, it is a powerful tool in shaping behavior and functional ability. The use of environmental structuring and adaptation includes not only physical functioning but also perceptual functioning, sensation, memory, social interaction, and communication.[22] It is an exciting avenue of occupational therapy practice that can be used in a number of settings.

Compensating for sensory-perceptual loss by means of "response facilitators" can include the use of improved and appropriate lighting (e.g., non-glare fluorescents versus indirect lighting); the promotion of high-contrast coloring or textured surfaces and the use of objects for stimulation and demarcation of geographical contours; the provision of tactilely safe and varied objects that can be handled; visual blocks; and the use of soundproofing to eliminate distraction.[22,23]

In facility settings there are a number of ways to enhance memory. Large-print wall calendars, daily schedules, name plates, photographs of significant events and others, favorite memorabilia, seasonal decorations, familiar furniture, photographs of a favorite pet (facsimiles of stuffed cloth animals may also be helpful if no photograph or picture is available), favorite music, and notices of current events are all examples of restructured environments that are helpful with memory-impaired older adults. In terms of improving social interaction, common areas that are structured so that residents/clients can face each other serve to enable these individuals to communicate more freely. Also, these settings can be furnished with soft pillows, meaningful photographs or pictures, areas for personal memorabilia and knickknacks, and scrapbooks of familiar happenings.[22]

The environment for late life persons with dementia must be as consistent and calm as possible (e.g., the reduction of loud and objectionable noises). Items need to be placed so that they can readily be seen. For example, in the bathroom open shelving can be used (items such as soap, a toothbrush, toothpaste, a washcloth, and an electric razor can be displayed) and can serve as a visual cue to promote good grooming.[23]

Dressing tasks can be simplified by structuring the way clothing items are stored. A task can be visually sequenced by putting an outfit (e.g., a blouse and a skirt) on the same hanger. Adjustable closet rods and hangers should be stored at eye level. Drawers and cupboards need to be placed at the appropriate height for the individual. One type of item should be placed in a drawer. For instance, all socks should be placed together in a drawer.[23]

Persons with dementia often become upset with locked closets or cupboards. This may lead to anger and frustration as the individual may think something is stuck and repeatedly try to open it. Magnetic closures that are inconspicuous are helpful.[23]

A safe indoor walking space or a secure enclosed garden area are helpful for those individuals who need to pace.[23]

When there is a security concern about an individual leaving a house, a monitoring system can be utilized (e.g., a bell can be installed to signal that a door has been opened; an individual monitoring device is another method).[23]

Painter discusses a variety of environmental strategies that she has found helpful in enhancing or maintaining functional performance among those diagnosed with *dementia of the Alzheimer's type* (DAT).[24]

In the United States, 70% of people with DAT live at home. Three out of every four caregivers are women. The average cost of caring for a person with DAT throughout the course of the disease is $174,000.[25]

Painter contends that the environmental context has a major impact in maintaining function and monitoring behavior. The home needs to be modified throughout the progression of the disease. It is imperative that practitioners develop an understanding of how environmental cues, in conjunction with normal aging, can influence behaviors and performance.[24]

Painter has developed an Alzheimer Home Evaluation that encompasses cognitive, psychological, physical, and social needs of persons with DAT. Specific information relating to this evaluation can be found in:

❖   Painter, J. (1996). Home environmental considerations for people with
     Alzheimer's disease. *Occupational Therapy in Health Care, 10*(3), 45-63.

Before the initial home visit, Painter also makes use of an environmental checklist (for the caregiver to fill out) and/or a telephone interview may also be used with the caregiver. Suggestions for a telephone discussion with the caregiver include the following questions:

❖ Does the individual appear to have increased behavioral problems in certain rooms or during certain times of the day?

❖ Does the person live in more than one residential setting? Is there a time of the day when there are more people in the home? If so, when?

✧ Is the impaired elder left alone at any time of the day?

✧ Did the individual ever get lost in the neighborhood?

✧ What are the sleeping hours of the impaired older adult?

✧ Are there any pets in the home?

✧ What is the impaired elder's age?

✧ Provide a judgment as to the individual's cognitive level.

✧ What are the person's present and past hobbies?

✧ What were the impaired older adult's volunteer and work experiences?

✧ What is the educational level of the individual as well as the caregiver?

Answers to these questions will assist the therapist in (1) making the home evaluation appointment during a time when the individual with DAT will be most alert and aware; (2) researching and analyzing the caregiver's questions; and (3) bringing adaptive equipment, catalogs, and any other materials deemed appropriate based on the client's cognitive level.[24]

The person-environment fit model was used in the Alzheimer Home Evaluation. This model is based upon the legibility of the environment (quality and quantity of particular cues and their stability). Cues relate to the information that is provided by the environment. Stability is related to the constancy of environmental stimuli and the constancy of furnishings in relation to the behavioral patterns and functional capabilities of the individual with DAT. Stability and environmental cues have psychological, social, and physical aspects. For example, predictability and orientation are considered to be part of the physical component. The psychological aspect relates to the emotional tone of a situation, and relationship and roles with others are part of the social components.[24] When environmental cues become more than an individual can manage, functional performance and behaviors may become unmanageable. Changes in the environment such as remodeling a bathroom to make it more accessible (e.g., widened door, new paint on door for color contrast, new shower installed instead of a bathtub) may cause the client to appear agitated, confused, and unable to independently perform grooming and hygiene tasks.[24]

In order to avoid negative behavior, caregivers must consistently continue to modify the environment of a client with DAT as the disease progresses. Physical cues that relate to rooms, furniture, and objects should be readily visible, meaningful, comprehended, and adapted to normal sensory changes that occur with the aging process. These physical cues must match physical and cognitive changes that occur with the progress of the disease.

An example can be seen in the fact that initially the client with DAT may not have difficulty finding his or her bedroom, but as the disease advances, the caregiver will need to make a number of environmental changes that are directly related to physical cues. Painting the bedroom door a color that is the client's favorite may temporarily aid the individual with DAT in independently being able to locate his or her bedroom. As abstract thinking declines, the client with DAT may no longer be able to comprehend the meaning of the colored door. Next, the caregiver may need to place a sign on the door that indicates, "This is Mary's Room."

As the disease continues to progress, the caregiver can then place a picture of the person and the bed (at eye level) on the door so that these visual cues can indicate that this is the client's bedroom. With further advancement of the disease, even greater concrete physical cues will be needed. A favorite item may be placed by the door, and the bedroom door can be opened, allowing the individual with DAT to see the contents from a short distance. In the bedroom pictures may need to be placed on closet doors, drawers, and other items so that the client may be guided to the items that are needed for daily living tasks.[24]

The client with DAT may not be able to recognize normal sensory changes that occur with aging. An example of this can be seen when the person with DAT is able to locate the closet (with various physical cues), but he or she is unable to locate the appropriate clothing, because this individual does not know that there is a need to wait for visual accommodation to darkness, or he or she forgot to turn on the closet light. An automatic light that turns with movement is helpful in alleviating the problem.[24]

Environmental social cues enhance communication by promoting an understanding of what others mean as well as promoting interactions with other individuals. When an older adult with DAT moves into a new environment (such as a retirement community, a relative's home, or a nursing home), it is important to provide a rich social environment that personalizes the individual's living space with familiar objects and prized possessions, as the person with DAT may feel that his or her self-identity has been lost (if these important social cues are not part of the new living environment).[24]

The manner in which information is communicated to the client with DAT is another aspect of the social environment that needs attention. There are a number of ways in which caregivers can promote activity and social engagement:[26]

⋄ Give directions succinctly and clearly.
⋄ Speak slowly and directly to the client so that this individual is allowed time to process the information.
⋄ Use body appropriate gestures and body language that demonstrate what is being discussed or what is expected.

Social cues also are crucial in enhancing positive behaviors and functional performance by preparing both the client and the environment prior to actual tasks. This involves eliminating distraction in the following manner:[10,24,26]

⋄ Remove all items from the table except the task at hand.
⋄ Close the blinds to decrease outside activities and glare.
⋄ Turn off the television, tape, radio, or CD player. Turn down the telephone ringer.
⋄ Make certain that the light in the room is appropriate (non-glare, appropriate lumination).
⋄ Guide the client, prior to and during the task, through each step of the activity as needed.

Psychological cues aid in establishing the emotional tone of the client's home environment. This includes the general environmental ambiance as well as those persons who visit and live in the home. Environmental psychological cues involve a variety of strategies: (1) provide an appropriate color scheme in the rooms of the home that the client is most likely to use (e.g., neutral and pastel colors produce a relaxed atmosphere as compared to extremely bright colors that may be "too busy" for the client to manage); (2) organize the daily schedule of the client (provide a large print calendar for orientation to person, place, time, and the daily schedule); and (3) avoid distractions (the family may need to limit the number of persons in the same room with the client or eliminate extraneous noises). Only one person should speak at a time.[24]

Environmental stability is a major component that guides the client with DAT in terms of behavioral and functional performance. Therefore, it is important to utilize environmental strategies that negate continual change and, instead, stress constancy. A stable environment is necessary to assist the client with DAT in orientation and activity engagement.[24]

In terms of physical stability it is important to avoid changes that involve the client with DAT's living space (including furniture and its arrangement, interior decorations, and structural alterations). If changes must occur, it is important to suggest to the family that these be implemented on a gradual basis (or during the early stage of the disease). If a piece of furniture has become worn or in need of reupholstering, the family should try to find similar material and keep the item in the same previous arrangement. If the family needs to rearrange other rooms, it should be done one room at a time (only after the client becomes comfortable to the first room's rearrangement should another room be considered for rearrangement).

If the client moves to a nursing home or assisted living arrangement, personal objects and prized possessions (including furniture) should be arranged in the new living area in a similar and familiar fashion as the individual had previously experienced. No matter where the client with DAT lives, it is of utmost importance for practitioners to suggest strategies that encourage maintaining the stability of physical cues. In this way, these physical cues can serve as aids in guiding the client in activities.[24]

Social and psychological stability are essential in ensuring that the client with DAT can participate appropriately in daily activities. The constancy of the moods of the people who are in contact (on a daily basis) with the client with DAT, the consistency of the client's daily schedule, and the stability of "how" information is transmitted are all important factors in assisting the client through each day's activities. Ideally the promotion of social and psychological stability can be accomplished by:[24]

◇ Maintaining the same people (in small numbers) who deal with the client with DAT.

◇ Using the same method to communicate (whether the client lives in an assisted living situation, a nursing home, his or her own home, or any other type of living arrangement). Encourage all persons to use similar phrases and gestures (e.g., "Please put on your shoes"). Keep the phrases brief and basic.

◇ Developing daily schedules that describe specifically when various activities will occur. This schedule should be kept in the same location and indicate who is to help the client with DAT with each activity.

Painter offers some excellent recommendations that help the client with DAT deal with the temporary change of a caregiver. For instance, if the caregiver plans a vacation or needs to be away for a period of time, it is wise (prior to the leaving of the caregiver) to have both the replacement and the caregiver who regularly cares for the client to be together for a brief period of time. This allows for the temporary caregiver to understand the client's daily routine and the communication methods the primary caregiver uses when caring for the client. It also permits the client to know the temporary caregiver in a secure situation. To enhance the continuity of transition, it is of the utmost significance that the primary caregiver write out the daily schedule, write explicit directions, and complete any other household tasks for the temporary careperson during the primary caregiver's absence.[24]

Environmental instability may also occur during holiday events. Practitioners should recommend that family members not make any changes in the primary rooms that the client with DAT uses (especially the bedroom). However, if this is not possible, then the client's favorite holiday decorations, plates, or other holiday items can be utilized. This will promote some stability and encourage facility employees or family members to help the client reminisce.[24]

Painter describes a number of ways of combatting inappropriate or dangerous behaviors to prevent the client with DAT from harming him- or herself. First, to prevent the client from eating unsafe items (such as seashells, candles, potpourri, or other similar types of objects), Painter recommends that these articles be placed in a secure area that is out of sight and out of reach of the client. All types of equipment that might be hazardous (space heaters, accessibility to detergents, hair dryers, cleaners, medicines, knives, matches, lighters, scissors, house plants, sewing machines, and power tools) should also be kept in secure and out of sight places. The water heater setting should be securely set not higher than 120°F. Safety plugs should be placed in any outlets not being used.[24]

There are also other safety hazards in the immediate outdoor environment and neighborhood. The locations and availability of poisonous plants, lawn mowers, tools, hot tubs, swimming pools, bicycles, electric outlets, garbage cans, types of driveways and road surfaces, neighborhood animals, and street traffic should be carefully noted. All potentially dangerous items should be disposed of or stored in a secure area that avoids the scrutiny of the client. Hot tubs and swimming pools should be covered. It is essential that the family provide a safe environment in which the client can pace or wander but one that does not allow for the client to be placed in a dangerous situation or get lost. Therefore, it is important for the client to wear a medical alert bracelet and to inform neighbors about the client's condition.[24] If the family lives near water hazards (e.g., the ocean, a lake, a pond, or a creek), the use of an alarm system that identifies the opening and closing of the outside door may be needed.[24]

In many home situations, caregivers have many needs that are centered on their stress levels, responsibilities, and fatigue levels. These, in turn, influence the ability of the caregiver to concentrate on the level and quality of care that can be rendered. These factors also affect the careperson's ability to care for other family members and themselves as well. Painter suggests that the occupational therapist also provide information regarding addresses and phone numbers of local adult day care centers; nursing homes and/or assisted living facilities that provide weekend respite care for those with DAT; the phone numbers and addresses for support groups; contacts for services such as meals-on-wheels; and phone numbers and addresses of state and national DAT groups and associations. These services could provide some respite and worry-free periods of time to the careperson. This, in turn, would have a positive effect on the quality of care that the client with DAT receives.[24]

Occupational Therapy and Dementia Care: An Evolving Specialty

Although strategies and techniques that deal with the intervention and management of the dementia client have been discussed, it is important to note that a number of entrepreneurially oriented occupational therapists have banded together to form companies that specialize in dementia care. For example, Kim Warchol, OTR/L is the owner of Five Star Health Care Seminars and is president of Dementia Care Specialists, Inc. As a lecturer she provides dementia consultation and workshops concerning Alzheimer's disease interventions. Two other colleagues, Chris Ebell, OTR/L and Caroline Copeland, OTR/L are equally involved in Dementia Care Specialists, Inc.[15,17]

Dementia Care Specialists have established a community-based occupational therapy practice that evaluates and treats the person with dementia in the home environment and provides caregivers with training and education in order to maintain the individual's best functioning ability so that he or she can remain at home for as long as possible.[15,17]

Besides this community based focus, the training and education of caregivers in nursing homes is another major avenue of occupational therapy service. Maintenance planning, instruction, and training are essential to good care (as is documenting the competency of caregivers in carrying out the plan prior to discharge from therapy services). Maintenance plans are a highly necessary and critical aspect of care when working with the client diagnosed as having dementia. It is a good maintenance program that allows the individual with dementing illness to utilize his or her highest possible physical and cognitive abilities in the areas of self-care, instrumental activities of daily living and recreational pursuits. In the United States, occupational therapy services can be reimbursed (by Medicare, for instance) for grading the cognitive complexity of tasks and then designing maintenance programs that match the cognitive demand of the task with the cognitive capabilities of the individual. As professionals we need to document the amount of cognitive assistance the individual requires as well as the type of cognitive cueing that is necessary to perform meaningful activities and occupations.[17]

Warchol points out that documenting modified approaches and outcomes has been increasingly important in seeking reimbursement. The following information provides some approaches to increasing opportunities for reimbursement when working with the client with DAT:[15]

✧ Follow the Medicare guidelines for skilled service:
1. Must relate to the plan of care.
2. Must be reasonable and necessary for the intervention of the client's condition.
3. Must require the judgment, knowledge, and skills of the occupational therapist. The therapist should include how the cognitive approaches and the environment of the caregivers were altered, and how new learning deficits were compensated for.

✧ Meet the requirement of *medical necessity*. This means answering the question, "Why are occupational therapy services needed now?" It should be clearly delineated what would happen if occupational therapy did not intervene and why occupational therapy interventions are necessary to improve the client's safety, function, and quality of life. Practitioners need to elicit remaining abilities in order to facilitate significant improvements in function and safety by identifying and utilizing those abilities that remain while at the same time compensating for deficits.

✧ Use accurate ICD9 and Current Procedural Terminology (CPT) codes. In using the ICD9 codes, always try to add an intervention diagnostic code and any other additional medical diagnosis codes that reflect the conditions being treated. Because a number of intermediaries will not reimburse DAT or related dementias as a "stand alone" diagnosis, it is very important to add other diagnoses, if appropriate, when using the CPT codes. It is essential to utilize the CPT code that most accurately describes the outcomes of the services provided during the intervention session.

The need for meaningful therapeutic programs for dementia clients is expanding. Large numbers of assisted living facilities and long-term care facilities are opening up dedicated wings that are devoted solely to dementia care. There presently are numerous specialized dementia services and environments exploding around us. Occupational therapy can "have a big influence on their placement criteria, specialized therapy and activity programs, and environment designs."[15, p. 18] "Perhaps the greatest reward is the satisfaction derived from using our unique expertise to improve the quality of life of a very underserved, challenging group of persons who desperately need our help."[15, p. 19]

The need for occupational therapy services has never been greater, and it will become even more so as our population continues to age. This is an exciting service opportunity for practitioners.

COGNITIVE PROGRAMS AND MODALITIES USEFUL WITH BRAIN TRAUMA AND NEUROLOGICAL DISORDERS

An Overview of Cerebrovascular Accident and other Disorders

A *cerebrovascular accident* (CVA) is an insult to the brain that is caused by an insufficiency in the brain's vascular supply (may be due to an embolus, a thrombus, a hemorrhage, an aneurysm, or anoxia). A CVA is most often caused by the atherosclerosis, hypertension, or a congenital weakness in the artery wall.[27]

Cognitive deficits may be severe, and devastating residual problems following a CVA, traumatic brain injury, or acquired disease can result in brain injury.[28] Cognition involves abilities and skills in the following areas: orientation, attention, ability to follow directions or commands, numerical concepts, memory, problem solving and reasoning, concentration, sequencing, ability to initiate, decision making, judgment, categorization, organization, awareness, mental tracking, understanding, knowing, abstraction, and insight.[27-31]

Evaluations and Assessments Useful to Determine Cognitive Deficits in Brain Injury

In evaluating the client's cognitive abilities it is important to observe the client in a number of activities and settings at different times of the day; use standardized tests and functional activities to establish baseline measures; and identify the components of a specific skill that is to be evaluated (that are relatively intact versus those skills that are impaired).[28,29]

The following are several tests that screen and evaluate a range of cognitive skills:

MINI-MENTAL STATE

(First appeared in):

❖ Folstein, M. F., Folstein, S. E., & McHugh, P. R. (1975). Mini-Mental State: A practical method for grading the cognitive state of patients for the clinician. *J Psychiatr Res, 12*(3), 189-198.

This test screens orientation (time and place), registration, attention, calculation, recall, and language skills.[27] However, the mini-mental state is heavily laden with language, and therefore may misclassify clients with aphasia.

THE GALVESTON ORIENTATION AND AMNESIA TEST (GOAT)

Courtesy of Harvey S. Levin, Division of Neurosurgery, Department of Surgery, University of Texas Medical Branch, Galveston, Texas (Levin, O'Donnell, and Grossman, 1979)

This is a brief memory and orientation test which has 10 questions. It was originally designed for amnesia clients. However, it is useful with CVA clients.

  ✧   Daniel, M. S. & Strickland, L. R. (1992). *Occupational therapy protocol management in adult physical dysfunction* (pp 62-63). Gaithersberg, MD: Aspen.

THE COGNITIVE ASSESSMENT OF MINNESOTA

This measure assesses cognitive abilities and consists of 17 subtests (some examples—attention span, memory, orientation, mathematics, visual neglect, following directions, object identification, judgment, reasoning, and safety). These subtests were designed to test the manipulation of knowledge, the fund of knowledge, social awareness, and abstract thinking.

Rustad, R. A. and Associates: The Cognitive Assessment of Minnesota. Available from:

  ✧   Therapy Skill Builders
      555 Academic Court
      San Antonio, TX 78204
      1-800-211-8378
      www.tpcweb.com

THE CONTEXTUAL MEMORY TEST

Developed by Joan P. Toglia, MA, OTR

This test assesses memory capacity, strategy of use, and recall in adult clients with memory dysfunction.

Also available from Therapy Skill Builders (see above).

THE ARNADOTTIR OT-ADL NEUROBEHAVIORAL EVALUATION (A-ONE)

Provides an analysis of functional activities to identify cognitive skill deficit areas. Found in:

  ✧   Arnadottir, G. (1990). *The brain and behavior: Assessing cortical dysfunction through activities of daily living*. St. Louis: CV Mosby.

Because problem solving, memory, and other higher intellectual functions all have an attentional component to their skills, the client's attentional ability should always be evaluated at the very beginning of a functional cognitive assessment.[29,30] A variety of cognitive evaluations and test references can be found in:

  ✧ *The Adult Stroke Patient: A Manual for Evaluation and Treatment of Perceptual and Cognitive Dysfunction*[29]

  ✧ *Vision, Perception, and Cognition: A Manual for the Evaluation and Treatment of the Neurologically Impaired Adult*[30]

  ✧ Chapter 17 of Willard and Spackman's *Occupational Therapy* (9th Ed.)[31]

  ✧ Chapter 15 of *Occupational Therapy: Practice Skills for Physical Dysfunction* (Revised 4th Ed.)[28]

Cognitive abilities should always be considered in relation to other potential deficits. The quality of a person's cognitive skills and processes depends on the integrity of the individual's perceptual, visual, language, and sensory abilities. Therefore, it is paramount that occupational therapists administer visual, perceptual, and sensory evaluations before evaluating cognitive testing. Also, during these precognitive tests it is important to gain information and insight regarding the client's language abilities.[28] It is equally important to have definitive information regarding the client's premorbid cognitive functioning before initiating testing. This information can usually be provided by the client's family, friends, or significant others.[28]

In terms of intervention, limiting environment, extraneous information, and distractions is critical. Enough time should be allowed for the client to respond, and the utilization of sensory cueing, whenever possible, is highly recommended.[25,28]

Attention and Orientation Intervention Strategies

ATTENTION

Attention has three components: (1) alertness—preparing the individual to mobilize to attention, (2) selectivity, and (3) effort. This includes the ability to sustain attention over a period of time—known as *concentration-vigilance-effort*.[29,30] Attention involves two types of information processing—automatic and controlled. *Automatic processing* is utilized at a subcortical level. *Controlled processing* involves processing that is used when new information is being considered. An example of an automatic processing deficit (focused attention deficit—occurs when an automatic response is replaced by a controlled response) is seen when a client diagnosed with a CVA is concentrating on walking. A controlled processing deficit (divided attention deficit—occurs when the function of controlled processing is inadequate for the client to process all the information that is required for task completion) is manifested by the client becoming slow in behavioral processing and experiencing "overload" when dealing with several alternatives. The client may respond by reverting to focused attention. Thus, the client diagnosed with a CVA, when asked a question while ambulating, may frequently stop walking and engage in the conversation.[28-30]

In treating attention deficits the following are recommended:

✧ The environment can affect performance. Therefore, initiate training by utilizing a nondistracting environment with structure. As the client progresses, provide a more normal environment while gradually lessening the structure.

✧ Provide external feedback to modify behavior, and praise the client in proportion to the length of time that he or she attends to the task.

✧ Increase the duration of intervention and the complexity of the task as the client's tolerance improves.

✧ As appropriate, utilize external cueing.

✧ Teach the client to screen out distractions, use environmental cues, and identify them.

✧ Enable the client to develop internal attentional strategies (e.g., teach the client to prepare to attend by stating to him- or herself, "I must really concentrate and look at the person speaking to me").

✧ Ask the client to vocalize each step of the task as he or she is in the process of performing it. Once this is mastered, ask the impaired elder to subvocalize (silent vocalizing so that the technique is internalized).

Sensory input (auditory, tactile, visual) can be effective in relation to *motor output* (participation and attention to the task). Initially, provide sensory cueing (one at a time). Once the client can respond to a single sensory cue, multi-systems can progressively be applied.

Transfer to training is another strategy that can be utilized. For instance, if a client can appropriately use sequencing cards in the area of donning clothing, he or she should then be able to transfer this to actively being able to put on clothing.

Utilization of cognitive remediation modalities that include ADL tasks, board games, and computerized cognitive remediation programs are other strategies useful in promoting improved attention.[27,29]

ORIENTATION

Orientation is an understanding of the self and the relationship between the self and the present and past environment. Orientation to person, place, and time are essential to functioning in everyday activities in an appropriate manner. *Orientation to person* involves the self and others. *Orientation to place* is manifested by the client's ability to understand where he or she is (being able to report the name and location of the place as well as integrating and understanding direction and distance). *Topographical orientation*, considered a component of orientation to place, involves the ability to follow a route (the ability to describe the relationship between one place and another), to use visuo-spatial skills, and to incorporate memory components.[31] *Orientation to time* refers to knowing the date, the season, and the time of day.[31]

Improvement of orientation can involve external aids (calendars, orientation boards, and bulletin boards that contain information such as the name of the facility, the season, the date, and major current events). Some facilities schedule an orientation group at the beginning of each day to review the previous day's happening and to receive information concerning the day's upcoming events.

MEMORY

Memory is an important component in cognitive functioning and has been described in Unit 2. The "breakdown" in the memory process can occur at any level. For instance, a client may be able to store information but not be able to retrieve it.

Memory strategies can be divided into two groups—external and internal. *External strategy* methods are those used by the therapist in the environment to improve a person's recall. Examples may include: adapting the external environment (e.g., color coding, chaining, breaking tasks down into steps [links] and then adding additional steps [one at a time—once each step has been learned], signs, cue cards, written instructions, notebooks, pictures, timetables, diaries, computer data storage units, and alarm watches or timers). *Internal strategies* are those that are conducted by the mental effort of the client. Internal strategies may include: visual imagery, association, mnemonics (some examples involve: the utilization of first letters of a word within a phrase to represent the first letters of information be recalled; "rhyming-a-word"—the use of rhymes with the information to be recalled "fun-sun") and rehearsal (the client silently repeats information to be recalled).[28,29]

REASONING AND PROBLEM SOLVING

Reasoning and problem solving are other aspects of cognition. It is abstract thinking that enables a person to discriminate relevant from irrelevant detail, and it allows an individual to understand relationships between objects, ideas, and events (permitting problem solving and reasoning to occur). Problem solving involves a number of cognitive skills such as attention, memory, planning, organization, and the ability to reason and to make appropriate judgments. In the problem-solving process there are two major types of reasoning—*deductive reasoning* (the ability to arrive at conclusions) and *inductive reasoning* (the ability to make generalizations from specific experiences).[28]

In terms of intervention, five major steps comprise the problem-solving process. They consist of: defining the problem, developing possible solutions, choosing the best solution, executing or acting on the solution, and evaluating the outcome. The sequence can be taught to the client, with instructions to use the steps when a problem occurs. This technique can be transferred to a number of different situations.[28]

EXECUTIVE FUNCTIONS

The ability to perform executive functions is another component involved in cognition. *Executive functioning* consists of goal formation, planning, carrying out the plan, and appropriate performance. Being able to initiate a plan is also a part of this type of functioning. In terms of intervention, a client who can appreciate the implications of inactivity may be able to respond to environmental cues or self-monitoring strategies. An individual who is unable to comprehend inactivity or is unable to initiate an activity may need a significant other to set up a daily routine and provide verbal prompts and a system of environmental cues as needed.[28]

INSIGHT

Another major issue in cognitive functioning involves the ability to have insight and awareness into one's functioning. Many persons with brain injury have decreased insight and awareness of their functioning capacities. A consequence of this is impaired or compromised safety. Strategies in dealing with improving insight and awareness focus upon: asking the client questions concerning his or her prediction of performance of a specific task and discussing the outcome, self-questioning during an activity and then following with a self-evaluation upon the completion of the task, and role reversal between the client and the therapist. In terms of gaining insight into behavior that may be inappropriate, direct feedback should be presented to the client. Internal strategies such as "time out" (where the individual leaves the situation) can be taught if the client's level of insight and control warrants it.[28]

COMPUTER-ASSISTED PROGRAMMING

Computer programs have been used in cognitive remediation. This is a high-growth industry. Games, puzzles, and specific tasks involving a number of cognitive strategies are available in program format. As therapists review these resources, the following guidelines are helpful:

◇ Games and programs should be uncluttered and simple.
◇ The keyboard input should be simple (alternatives to a classic keyboard can include a joystick, space bar, light pen, track ball, and voice recognition).
◇ Games should contain a low basic performance level as well as a high ceiling.
◇ Large print numbers and letters are recommended.
◇ Programs should continually adjust to the client's performance.
◇ Select simple-to-use tools (modules, cartridges).
◇ Software (program) instructions should be concise and easy to follow.
◇ The content of the programs should be accurate. No parts of the program should be displayed in a demeaning manner.

✧ Programs that allow one to control the variables (e.g., the length of time a stimulus is displayed, the level of difficulty, the ability to enter one's own items into the program in addition to being able to use only the preprogrammed items, the time that is needed for the client to respond, the speed of task performance, the type and time of reinforcement, and the size of letters or words) are the most flexible and useful.

✧ The format should be consistent so that the client does not become confused.

✧ The feedback should be age appropriate.[29]

Other literary resources that are helpful in promoting cognitive rehabilitation include:

✧ Carter, L. T., Caruso, J. L., & Languirand, M. A. (1984). *The thinking skills workbook: A cognitive skills remediation manual for adults.* (2nd Ed.). Sprigfield, IL: Charles C. Thomas.

✧ Harrell, M., et al. (1992). *Cognitive rehabilitation of memory: A practical guide.* Gaithersburg, MD: Aspen.

✧ Katz, N. (Ed.). (1998). *Cognition and occupation in rehabilitation: Cognitive model for intervention in occupational therapy.* Bethesda, MD: The American Occupational Therapy Association, Inc.

✧ Levin, W. (1991). Computer applications in cognitive rehabilitation. In J. S. Kreutzer, & P. H. Wehman (Eds.), *Cognitive rehabilitation for persons with traumatic brain injury.* Baltimore, MD: Paul H Brooks.

✧ Mathews, C. G., Harley J. B., & Maler, J. F. (1991). Guidelines for computer-assisted neuropsychological rehabilitation and cognitive remediation. *Clinical Neuropsychology, 5*(3).

The following represent suppliers of computer cognitive rehabilitation materials:

✧ Brain Train
727 Twin Ridge Lane
Richmond, VA 23233
1-800-822-0538
www.braintrain.com

✧ Critical Thinking Books and Software
P.O. Box 448
Pacific Grove, CA 93950
1-800-458-4849
www.criticalthinking.com

✧ Page Minder
3623 South Ave.
Springfield, MD 65807
1-888-882-7787
www.pageminder.com
(sends customized reminders to text pager for medication, appointments, daily living skills)

◇ Computer Input
  Interactive Therapeutic, Inc.
  P.O. Box 1805
  Stow, OH 44224-0805
  1-800-253-5111
  www.interactivetherapy.com
◇ Big Keys Co.
  P.O. Box 1888
  Huntersville, NC 28078
  1-800-249-5397
◇ Equal Access Computer Technology, Inc.
  222 Grant Way
  Lancaster, MA 01523
  978-466-9199
  eact@world.std.com
◇ Keyboard Alternatives and Vision Solutions, Inc.
  537 College Ave.
  Santa Rosa, CA 95404-4102
  1-800-953-9262
  www.keyalt.com

Mental Health and the Older Adult

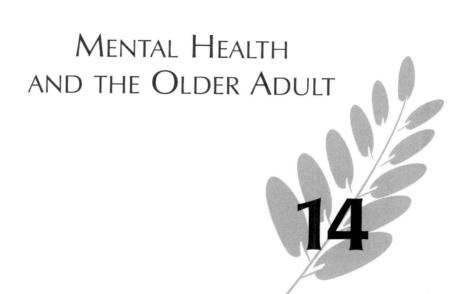

14

Depression

A significant number of late life adults experience loss of self-esteem and depression. Many elderly persons experience losses in the course of aging (loss of family members, loss of a spouse, decline in physical abilities, loss of a home that one has lived in for a long period of time, loss of health—most older adults experience at least one chronic health problem, loss of employment resulting in a decrease of financial assets; sensory losses—especially hearing and vision, loss of mobility—difficulty driving at night, and feelings of isolation and helplessness/loss of control).[32] The suicide rate for persons over 65 is three times higher than the general population. The highest suicide rate worldwide is for white males over the age of 80.[10,32]

For the purpose of this remediation component a brief review of some of the most commonly seen symptoms involved in late life depression will be explored. Somatic complaints are frequent. The individual experiences fatigue; poor concentration; a decline in the ability to solve problems or make decisions; devaluation of the self (these individuals often think of themselves as worthless, helpless, and burdensome); a decline in the ability to enjoy any pleasure (*anhedonia*); and these persons receive no satisfaction from completing a task or a project.[32] Depressed late life adults often complain that they do not feel like doing anything. They experience difficulty sustaining the interest, energy, and attention to perform daily activities (dressing, bathing, eating) and can become irritable and critical of others.[32]

Dysthymia (known as *dysthymic disorder*) is related to depression in that many of the symptoms are similar. However, dysthymia (also described as a state of unpleasant mood) involves symptoms that are generally not as disabling as major depression. Persons with dysthymia can also experience a superimposed major depression.

Despite this list of symptoms it is essential to note that depression and dysthymia are amenable to intervention and can be expected to remit.[32]

Generalized Intervention Approaches in Depression

When providing intervention to the depressed late life adult, the practitioner should note that short-term success-oriented activities are indicated. Tasks should be graded in a hierarchy of difficulty. Successful experiences are helpful in increasing a depressed person's performance and a positive attitude toward him- or herself. Initially, it is best to start with shorter work periods and tasks that have a low level of energy expenditure. These individuals require a lot of encouragement from the clinician. If a client is complaining and ruminating, redirection to a concrete task is indicated, and more constructive adequate time needs to be allotted to these depressed older adults, as it takes them longer to organize their thoughts.

Decisions regarding a project need to be limited to just a few options (e.g., "Would you like to paint this pink or green?"). In this way the client is allowed some autonomy while he or she engages in exerting some control and decision making. The clinician needs to provide feedback to the client so that he or she can appraise his or her accomplishments accurately and identify and establish realistic goals.[32]

Social encouragement and engagement need to be emphasized. Providing simple, small essential tasks can be helpful in this respect. For instance, putting colored sugar on cookies that a group is making provides immediately visible results, and the task is a "true" contribution to the group's effort.[32]

At any time a client expresses suicidal intention or ideation, it is imperative that this information be given to the staff and physician in charge, verbally and documented, as soon as possible.[32]

Involvement in daily living tasks needs to be encouraged. Programs that deal with hygiene and behavior modification can assist in engaging the depressed person to participate in self-care activities. In this respect, an arranged visit to the beauty salon or barber shop for hair care and a manicure can be quite beneficial.[32]

Day Intervention and Depression

Day intervention can be divided into three separate models—the social model, the health maintenance model, and the rehabilitation model. The *social model* offers recreation and socialization in a protective environment and provides respite care for caregivers. Most often health care professionals are not involved. At times, depending on individual circumstances, health care providers may be "called in" on a case-by-case contractual basis. The *health maintenance model* emphasizes the maintenance of health and the prevention of further functional loss. Day care clients in this arena are those individuals who have deficits that are not expected to improve such as chronic schizophrenia, dementia, and stroke. Occupational therapy personnel are often found in these settings.

The *rehabilitation* or *restorative model* provides therapeutic programming to clients who have mental health and/or physical problems in which there is a good prognosis for improvement. Therefore, progress goal attainment and active intervention are stressed. Health professionals such as those in nursing, occupational therapy, physical therapy, speech and language therapy, social work, psychology, and psychiatry are usually employed on either a full- or part-time basis.[10,33,34] Besides providing direct client care, occupational therapy personnel have also served as coordinators, administrators, consultants, and program supervisors in this type of day intervention setting.[10,33,34]

Day intervention in geriatric mental health care is important in breaking the downward spiral of isolation, withdrawal, and depression. Day intervention is a form of intensive psychiatric outpatient intervention. Often described as partial hospitalization, it is reimbursed under Medicare. The intervention services are prescribed by a psychiatrist. There is a plan of care that is periodically reviewed by the staff and the psychiatrist. The client's condition must be treatable, and the primary diagnosis cannot be dementia. In order to continue with the program, the client must make progress during the course of intervention, and this must be documented in the client's medical record.[34]

The role of occupational therapy in this setting is to foster the development of competence in coping skills through planning, participation, and evaluation of purposeful goal-directed occupations. These occupations may include crafts, arts, hobbies, group games, exercise sessions, training in activities of daily living, insight groups, and individual client assignments to research community support systems and resources.[35]

Wolfe and Paulson aptly describe their successful geriatric day intervention program's objectives. These include providing experiences that promote:

- Increased feelings of mastery
- Management of transitions (dealing with grief and loss)
- Accessing community resources
- Exploration of leisure skills
- Identification and validation of feelings
- Improvement of communication skills
- Providing education concerning the aging process, depression, chronic illness, and relapse prevention
- Improvement of self-esteem
- Development of coping skills for daily living with significant others and family members
- Reduction of negative self-talk

Occupational therapists, in this setting, address all these areas through the application of purposeful occupations.

Wolfe and Paulson provide a number of intervention approaches. The specific group experience described here represents just one example. It is focused upon improving the client's self-esteem. Many older adult clients come to day intervention with feelings of low self-esteem. This may be a result of life's events or they may have experienced a lifetime of low self-esteem. Feelings of guilt or unworthiness are components of depression that can contribute to a poor image of the self.[35]

In promoting increased self-esteem, poker chips were used to indicate to members the amount of negativity that their thought processes and conversations contain. During an activity group, the clinician hands each member of the group a red or white poker chip every 15 minutes. No explanation is given. Red is used for negative comments and white is used for positive comments.

At the end of the activity, each group member can see and begin to understand how positive or negative their behavior was. An example, such as this one, can help give members insight and awareness of their negativity and aid them in beginning to try to improve their attitude, manner, and feelings.[35]

In their chapter, "Day Treatment for Behavioral Health Needs," Wolfe and Paulson include three excellent examples of assessment materials that they use to gain initial information on a client's status. First, there is the Hope Day Treatment Program Psychosocial Intake Assessment.[35] This includes questions concerning information about: the client's age; referral source; current situation (such as living arrangements, social problems, legal problems, and employment); presenting problem and history of presenting problem; substance use/abuse; assaultive and/or suicidal ideation/behavior; past psychiatric history; medication of both the past and present; personal development and family history; health and medical conditions; mental status examination (that also includes a physical description); interests and leisure activities; impressions and/or significant findings; therapy goals; and rationale for recommended intervention modalities.[35]

A second document is the Problem Checklist.[35] In this tool, 12 items are listed (such as loneliness, isolation, anxiety, grief, feeling overwhelmed, difficulties with one's family, depression, feeling helpless and hopeless). The client is asked to put an "X" in front of any problems he or she would like to work on that are part of the checklist. In addition, there is also space for at least four more problems that the client can identify that were not specified on the list. The last part of the checklist ends with the question, "What would you like to change about your life?"[35]

The last document is entitled Occupational Therapy Assessment Domains.[35] This includes identifying specific information (problems/strengths/abilities) in the following areas:[35]

- ✦ Physical systems (past medical history, range of motion, strength, coordination, sensation)
- ✦ Mobility/ambulation
- ✦ Hearing/vision restrictions/precautions
- ✦ Cognitive systems (short- and long-term memory, attention span, task organization, and problem solving)
- ✦ Psychosocial systems (support systems such as those found with family and friends, coping mechanisms, interaction styles)
- ✦ Social and work history (attitudes toward aging, attitudes towards disease/disability, relationship history, work history, retirement history)
- ✦ Activities and leisure interests (past, current, and future considerations)

Day intervention offers occupational therapists who are interested in the gerontological mental health field varied interventional approaches from which to remediate depressive symptoms.

The Use of Occupational Therapy (as Applied to Beck's Cognitive Therapy in Combatting Depression)

Butin has clearly been influenced by the work of Dr. A. Beck and occupational therapists Cynkin and Robinson. In order to develop programming and to establish a baseline, Butin suggests a number of assessment tools that are helpful with the recognition of depressive syndromes. These assessments (both standardized and validated) are as follows:[33]

The Geriatric Depressive Scale. This scale provides the rater with a valid and reliable measure of depression. It contains 30 "yes" or "no" questions. The higher score is seen as being indicative of depression. This tool is sensitive to the somatic presentation that is often seen with older adults. Found in:

❖   Gallo, J., Reichel, W., & Anderson, L. (1988). *Handbook of geriatric assessment*. Rockville, MD: Aspen.

The Beck Depression Inventory. This tool is well validated and sensitive to psychosomatic presentation that many late life adults exhibit. The higher score in this inventory is indicative of depression. Found in:

❖   Gallagher, D. (1986). The Beck Depression Inventory and older adults: Review of its development and utility. In: T. L. Brink (Ed.), *Clinical gerontology: A guide to assessment and intervention* (pp. 149-163). New York: Haworth Press.

The Short-Care. This is a multidimensional assessment (validated and reliable) for use with older adults. It is a 45-minute interview that assesses dementia, functional disability, and depression. The focus is on six areas: sleep disorders, depression, subjective memory impairment, somatic symptoms, activity limitations, and dementia. This assessment is available through Columbia University and requires training. This tool can also be found in:

❖   Gurland, B. & Wilder, D. (1984). The Care Interview Revisited: Development of an efficient system of clinical assessment. *J Gerontol, 39*, 129-37.

The plan of care is important in that it enables the depressed older adult to examine the relationship between perceptions, feelings, and his or her current involvement in activities. Activities health can be described as the ability of the older person to participate in directed socioculturally delineated activities with the feeling of satisfaction.[33] An activities health assessment (similar to a time configuration) is helpful in examining and comparing past and present activity patterns and interests. In this way a person can determine how his or her time is spent. Butin recommends the following six questions (to act as a guide) when examining a client's activities health assessment.[33]

❖ What is most striking about your activities health assessment?

❖ From your observations, how would you say your current health impacts on the way you use your time?

❖ Are there major differences that you notice with this configuration as compared to the way you would like to spend your time?

❖ Is there anything you enjoy in this configuration?

❖ Is there anything you do because you feel you must?

❖ Is there anything you would like to change?

This tool aids in (1) beginning the problem-solving process by identifying the way that depression has impacted upon the involvement of daily activities, and (2) assisting in defining intervention goals and the means by which these goals can be achieved.[33]

Butin recommends the following book to explore the concept of activities health:

❖   Cynkin, S. & Robinson, A. M. (1990). *Occupational therapy and activities health; Toward health through activities*. Boston: Little Brown.

As a frame of reference for treating the depressed elderly, Butin recommends cognitive therapy as espoused by Dr. A. Beck. Its basic assumption is that an individual's thoughts can influence behavior. Actions are based on perceptions and thoughts. According to cognitive therapy principle, a "triad" develops when an individual becomes depressed. For example, a man of 78 who has suffered a stroke and can no longer move his left arm might say, "I'm not good because I can't move my arm any longer." He then might see that there is little in the way of activities that he can perform in his environment. This may lead to a thought process that says, "I can't do anything." Next, he might generalize the belief that the future is hopeless.[33]

In terms of intervention, the depressed older adult needs assistance in understanding how his or her belief system is interacting and influencing his or her ability to function.[33] In this manner, the individual can learn about the relationship of depression to symptoms. It is important to discuss the inactivity cycle with the client. Butin summarizes this process as follows: "The less you do, the less you feel like doing until you're doing little that you can feel good about. This cycle can lead to depression."[33] A therapeutic partnership can be forged by stating, "Let's break this inactivity cycle together."[33, p. 617]

Activities must be within the client's abilities. Tasks should be analyzed and broken down into manageable, success-oriented steps so that feelings of satisfaction and self-worth can be generated. This is how the possibility of shifting mindset and altering perceptions concerning one's capabilities can begin.[33]

Through the therapeutic relationship between the clinician and the client, a safe place to practice skills that are necessary for recovery can be developed. Groups are capable of providing a powerful mechanism for discovering the commonality needs among late life adults. Once group planning is initiated, the clinician should continually assess and analyze the client's goals so that there is an understanding as to how the activity will foster the skills that are necessary to accomplish these objectives.[33]

Butin postulates that groups (within the mental health care setting) can be classified into four areas of occupation (self-management, leisure, family, and work). In this instance work is defined as paid employment and/or meaningful volunteer job placement.[33] Some of the therapeutic groups (both inpatient and in-community intervention) that Butin describes include budget and resources group, fit and fabulous group (choosing and buying clothing, grooming, and establishing an exercise routine), tai chi, video group, fitness walk, intergenerational programming, and family activity group.[33]

Occupational therapy involvement in restoring the quality of life and function in late life depressed older adults is an essential service that is both meaningful and cost effective. Therapists need to make clear to insurers, the elderly, and their families of its value.

Mental Health Home Care

In 1979 Medicare expanded its home care benefit to include psychiatric home care (must be ordered by a psychiatrist) as a reimbursable service. In October 1997, Medicare's requirement that only a psychiatrist could order mental health home care changed to permit any physician to order these services (under the condition that the physician was willing to oversee psychotropic medications and approve and sign the care plan that would include mental health home services). Medicaid and managed care companies have followed the criteria that Medicare has set forth for home care. These criteria include:[36]

◇ The client must be homebound. This criterion is described as the client not having the normal ability to leave home or that his or her illness is manifested in part by a refusal to leave home or the client's disability is of such magnitude that it would be considered unsafe for him or her to leave home unattended. Diagnoses that support this homebound definition are:

⮝ Paranoia

⮝ Panic disorder

⮝ Agoraphobia

⮝ Thought process disorders (e.g., delusions, agitation, hallucinations, or impairments of cognitive thought that compromise the client's decision making and judgment and ultimately affect the client's safety)

⮝ Acute depression

⮝ Mental health problems that are associated with medical conditions that render the client to be homebound

✧ Services must be provided under a home health plan of care (in the United States, HCFA 485). This must be approved and signed by the physician.

✧ Services must be reasonable and medically necessary for treating the client's psychiatric symptoms or condition.

✧ A skilled psychiatric nurse must be involved to provide care.

The most prevalent conditions, as seen by the home health team, are depressive disorders.[36] However, clinicians are trained to treat the whole person. As such we have a wonderful opportunity to provide services to an aging population that is complex. For instance, even though an older adult's major diagnoses might be psychiatric, there are often a number of concomitant physical conditions (e.g., COPD, diabetes, cardiac conditions, hip fracture) that also need to be treated.

Home mental health care occupational therapists provide skilled services that involve evaluation (the Allen Cognition Level Test is recommended[36,37]), planning (the development of the plan of care), and implementing therapeutic programs. Occupational therapy's specific interventions in mental health home care include activities of daily living, life management, and safety in the home. In terms of activities of daily living, occupational therapy is responsible for teaching task-oriented therapeutic activities that are designed to increase and restore cognitive abilities and functional participation in activities of daily living. Clinicians address the planning and implementing of individualized therapeutic activity programs as well as adapting the environment as part of an overall active intervention program. Lastly, the clinician is responsible for assessing and planning for improving home safety issues.[36]

Whether a mental health clinician is working in a hospital, a day intervention center, or a home health setting, he or she is given the opportunity to improve the depressed older client's functioning capacity by means of a variety of intervention techniques and modalities. It is a challenging and rewarding area of occupational therapy practice that can promote a new or renewed positive self-image among late life adults.

THERAPEUTIC GROUP PROGRAMS FOR THE CHRONICALLY ILL

Promoting and providing meaningful and effective communication and an awareness of the self as it acts in the environment are important basic skills needed for "everyday living." Awareness and social interaction programs need to center around the abilities, interests, skills, capabilities, and functioning levels of the participating clients.[10]

Sensory Stimulation

Leona Richman developed a program to help late life adults who manifested severe psychomotor retardation and experienced deficits in discriminating between and responding appropriately to environmental stimuli. The clients in her sensory training program suffered from sensory deprivation that was based upon disuse, malfunction, and psychological retreat from the environment. Most of these individuals assumed the role of being a nonparticipant. It is Richman's contention that sensory discrimination can be trained and greatly developed through practice. The main objective of sensory training is to increase tactile discrimination and sensitivity though the stimulation of all sense receptors. In this way, the regressed older adult's ability to interact in the environment is greatly increased. In sensory stimulation training, the sensory receptors are stimulated in isolation and simultaneously in a multisensory approach.[10,38]

The following are areas of stimulation that are emphasized with each sense being stimulated separately.

Olfactory. This involves the identification and discrimination of odors. Different odors bring different responses. For instance, the use of cloves and garlic can be very alerting. On the other hand, if one wants to introduce scents that evoke various aspects of pleasant past life experiences, mint, vanilla, and oranges may be used. These scents should be presented in a manner in which the identification of the item is not visible (e.g., a small opaque container). Thus, the client has to concentrate more fully on the task at hand (identifying the odor).

Tactile. Discrimination of various textures and contact (hand shaking, hand touching, hand holding) between group members is encouraged. The use of varied textures (a sponge, a piece of wood, a ball, a piece of fabric) is presented to each participant to feel and describe to the group. Discrimination between objects helps to make a person feel that the environment is real and more manageable.

Auditory. This involves the ability to attend to vibrations and sounds. The participant closes his or her eyes and names the sound that is being demonstrated (e.g., ball bouncing, hand clapping, coffee brewing, whistles being played). The actual sounds can be initiated by the trainer or a tape/CD can be played.

Kinesthetic and proprioceptive. This includes awareness of one's movements in relation to body parts and joints. Each participant is asked to identify and move various body parts.

Vision. This involves the development of the ability to see and control eye movements. Pictures of bygone days, bright colored scarves, clothing of the past, visual pursuit activities, slides, movies, or videos of historical events can be helpful in improving the late life adult's visual sense as well as providing a format for meaningful discussion topics.

Gustatory. This includes the awareness of various tastes by means of using taste receptors. Participants can be asked to identify different gelatin or ice cream flavors (with vision occluded). Another way to stimulate the gustatory sense is to involve group members in assisting the making of fruit punch by having him or her decide what ingredients might need to be added.

Self and body awareness. This is promoted through the use of self-identification with the use of breathing over a handheld mirror or by blowing soap bubbles (this enables the individual to become more aware of his or her body processes). In this way, breathing takes on a more concrete form.

Cognitive, social, and verbal stimulation. This involves the promotion of social stimulation, interaction, and awareness of verbal responses.[10,38]

The program format consists of a group seated in a circle. Each participant is given individual attention. The clinician/trainer introduces each participant by his or her name. Tactile stimulation in the form of hand shaking (greeting) is encouraged. Each individual in the group is then asked to identify various sensory components.[38]

Sensory training can be divided into two groups: a *primary group* (contains the most regressed individuals and requires concrete and structured activities) and a *secondary group* (tasks are more challenging). For instance, the more functional client might be asked to compare more than one stimulus.[10,38]

Paire and Karney demonstrated in a controlled study that sensory stimulation therapy was effective because it enabled long-term psychiatric clients to improve their self-care skills (eating, grooming, toilet usage, and hygiene were used as criteria). Improvement was also noted in interpersonal skills as clients who had participated in sensory stimulation programming demonstrated and manifested an improvement in overall word group participation even after therapy was discontinued. Thus, a major achievement from sensory stimulation therapy was that it was helpful in rekindling interest in the environment.[10,39]

Interactive Group Therapy: Five Stages

In her book, *Integrative Group Therapy: Mobilizing Coping Abilities With the Five-Stage Group*, Mildred Ross expands upon the benefits of this type of therapy with chronically regressed and/or neurologically impaired late life adults.[40] Benefits of client participation include: the client being able to reflect in a prevailing mood of alert calmness, demonstrating acceptable behavior, and being able to participate in at least one of the activities that comprise the five-stage group.[40] Improvement in motor behavior is also noted in that the client's ability to copy demonstrated or verbally directed movement in balance, endurance, object handling, and posture improves relative to each participant's initial performance within the group session. Social behavior such as respecting each other's spaces, sharing time and use of items, and being able to observe each other with more awareness becomes increasingly appropriate within the therapy session. Those older adults who are nonverbal because their expressive language is limited or because they cannot vocalize expand their ability to communicate by actions or signing. Those who do use language to express themselves become more articulate, initiate communication, and improve word knowledge.[40]

Ross makes the following assumptions regarding neurophysiological characteristics that underlie the five-stage program. Some of these are listed below:[40]

◇ Selective proprioception, tactile, vestibular, or other sensory stimuli promote the brain's ability to register, organize, and respond adaptively. An organized sequence of inputs enhances responses as well as the probability of a response.

◇ Stimulation and activity can be heightened, motivated, and improved by activities that are presented in a systematic and sequential matter.

◇ Routine organized sequences enhance the likelihood of an automatic habitual response.

◇ Activities and stimulation have properties that affect central nervous system functioning.

◇ Neurologically impaired older adults who are able to register tastes, auditory, visual, and tactile senses in their environmental system find them pleasurable, are motivated to interact, and habituate the experience.

✧ The five-stage group process appears to restore or improve a participant's ability to interact with others.[40]

In terms of logistics the easiest way to manage seating is to utilize a circle format. Activity is used to organize the individual. When presenting an activity to the group, the group leader must help the participants to become ready to receive the activity and act on it responsibly. The selected activity needs to also be designed to have the "just right" amount of challenge.[40]

Following are the five stages of integrative group therapy:

STAGE 1: ORIENTATION

All actions and activities are designed to welcome group members, promote continuity of intervention of the previous day or previous sessions, and aid in enabling group members to focus their attention. The acknowledgment and welcoming of each group member is the initial phase of Stage 1. Each member is encouraged to state his or her name and members can hold wrists or hands with one another. "Hello," can be said in a whisper, in a foreign language, in sign language, or by traditional hand shaking. The therapist or a group member can approach each participant and shake his or her hand. These suggestions are some of the ways to acknowledge each group member and to focus awareness and attention of each participant. It is also a time to briefly state the purpose of the session (e.g., "We are here to learn from one another and stretch a bit").

Besides the introductory part of this stage, which is used to arouse the participants' alerting centers, there are a number of other 1-minute activities that can be used to evoke pleasurable and appropriate responses. Some of these may have a calming and relaxing effect:

✧ With the individual's permission, the use of a vibrator on one's hand in a slow and light manner by the therapist

✧ Proprioceptive input, as in passing a 2- to 3-lb bag and demonstrating how each member can hold it high and pass it along

✧ A 12-inch Nerf ball (Hasbro, Providence, RI) can be used to provide isometric exercise to the chest and arms of each member.

✧ Passing and applying hand lotion has a pleasant tactile and soothing effect. Passing items (candle collection, rhythm instruments, music boxes, a bell) around forces continuous interaction and focuses the attention of group members to watch one another while each one awaits his or her turn. This stimulates the tactile and touch tracts.

In addition, the therapist or assistant can present a brief prelude to discussing emotions. An example of this would be to present feeling words (e.g., sleepy, joyful, energetic) on cards cut into different shapes and ask participants to choose a feeling. A brief period for serving light refreshments (e.g., tiny pieces of oranges or lemons) can be utilized at the conclusion of this stage.

In summary, these familiar and routine activities that make little demand but provide significant satisfaction signal the limbic, thalamus, and reticular activity systems of the central nervous system that those initial conditions are physically comfortable, interesting, and emotionally safe. In this manner, Stage 1 promotes sensory registration.[40]

The entire therapy program can take anywhere from 30 to 50 minutes or to a full hour. Stage 1 can last from 5 minutes to one-fifth of the time that is allotted for the entire group.[40]

STAGE 2: MOVEMENT

This stage emphasizes movement and bodily responses. Movement theories and activities are used to increase endurance, muscle tone, and postural alignment as well as to facilitate adequate balance and to promote a positive self-concept. By reducing movement to basic first steps, therapists are able to facilitate a balanced combination of novel and routine movements. These in turn stimulate the cerebellum, the brain stem, the thalamus, the cortical areas, the basal ganglia, and the touch tracts.

During Stage 2 sensory processing takes place.[40] In general, movement aids in retraining, increasing, and sustaining arousal and a sense of connection with other group members. Movement is a method for practicing motor planning as the movement flows from one posture to another. Movement assists in connecting group members to each other as everyone is doing approximately the same thing in the same manner at the same time. The therapist can encourage this by using phrases such as "we are working together to keep the ball moving." Stage 2 uses the senses to develop body scheme, center of gravity awareness, reflex maturation, postural balance, motor planning, the ability to balance between the protective and the discriminatory when using the sensory system, and an awareness of the two sides of the body.[40]

A series of movements or exercise should always be introduced at the simplest level and gradually more complex movement can be demonstrated as slowly as needed so that group members can process the movement and its changes. Exercise and movement need to be self-directed. Members must be allowed to copy the exercises in their own manner.[40]

Ease in response to movement can be encouraged by providing an object for each member to use during movement activities. These items can include bells with a variety of tones; chiffon scarves; cones; flowers (paper, plastic, or real); fans (paper or light wood); hoops; individual balloons to bounce from hand to hand; thin newsprint (approximately 5 by 8 inches to be used for wadding and then to be bounced on heavy plastic plates); Nerf balls (3 to 7 inches in diameter); and musical instruments of any kind.[40]

Other movement activities that help the group to feel connected are parachute movements (materials used can include stretchy cloth, king-size sheets, "see-through" lightweight drop cloths, and pantyhose that is made into a circle by cutting it at the top of the leg and knotting it together with another pair so that there is enough for a circle that is 6 feet in diameter) in which group members pull together to form a cohesive movement.[40]

Ross makes use of Range of Motion (ROM) Dance as established by Harlow and Yu. This total program includes a variety of dance movements. It also provides a comprehensive approach to understanding different kinds of relaxation exercises and pain management techniques. This dance program is an excellent resource for planning and conducting a series of group sessions. Helpful cassette tapes, videotapes, and a book are available from ROM Dance:

❖   Harlow, D. & Yu, P. H. ROM Dance: A Range of Motion Exercise and
       Relaxation Program. Madison, WI: The ROM Institute.
       ROM Dance Network
       P. O. Box 3332
       Madison, WI 53704-0332

Breathing exercises are a dynamic part of Stage 2. During this segment, the therapist and assistant can ask the group members to hold up their index finger and blow
on them so that they can feel the movement. Pinwheels, party blowers, plastic kazoos,
whistles, and blowing up balloons are all activities that promote blowing and help the
participants to realize the strength of their breathing process.[40]

Relaxation exercises can also be utilized at this time. One of the relaxation exercises that Ross recommends is the Benson Relaxation Response:

❖   Benson, H. (1989). *The relaxation response*. New York: Avon Books.
❖   Benson, H. & Proctor, W. (1989). *Your maximum mind*. New York: Avon Books.

There are other motor activities that can be utilized in this stage. First, there are the
brief primary motor activities. These consist of asking other group members (whether
seated or standing) to raise their feet one at a time to march in place. Then the therapist or assistant can focus upon upper extremities by instructing members to hug themselves. Throughout this routine the therapist or assistant should alternate between
lower (ankles, feet, legs) body activities and upper (arm, hands) body activities.[40]

Large swings, rocking chairs, and rocking boards are other types of motor activities
that many group members enjoy. Slow vestibular stimulation appears to lead to relaxation and has a calming effect on the participants.[40]

Moderately advanced motor activities are yet another component of Stage 2.
Participants are encouraged to receive more information concerning their bodies while
they move body parts in a progressive manner.[40] Motor activities in this part of Stage 2
can include: ball activities (a selected group member is the leader and should stand in
the center of the circle throwing the ball to each member, one at a time; each group
member throws the ball back to the designated leader); mat activities (members can be
creative by finding different ways to get across a long mat); members pass an object
from one to another with their feet or their hands; touching and identifying body parts
through movement—each participant is asked to touch as many body parts as possible
with a selected body part (e.g., "use the right elbow to touch the knees, hip, right ankle,
left wrist, etc.); and movement activities that promote balance (for instance, members
are asked to hold hands in a group circle and stand on one foot at a time, circle left
and circle right, jump, or hop).[40]

Stage 2 can be one-fifth or more of the time that is spent in the entire group process.
This portion of integrative group therapy generally provides the benefits of generating
interest and energy among the participants.[40]

Stage 3: Visual-Motor Perceptual Activities

New challenges are promoted at this stage. Group members need to reflect on their
performance in order to respond in a more studied manner to activities that increase
demand and that provide features to stimulate the thalamus, the cortex, and the brain
stem. This stage promotes adaptive responses and the display of sensory integration
responses.[40]

Perception is the interpretation and awareness of the physical world as each individual relates to it. It is influenced by stimuli from sensory systems and feedback from
movement that evokes emotional associations and memory processes.[40]

In Stage 3 sensorimotor abilities are used to help the individual develop ocular motor control, postural adjustments, eye-hand coordination, auditory skills, visual-spatial skills, and the development of feelings of adequacy, emotional stability, and mastery of the environment.[40]

Suggested activities for this stage include:

✧ Games that use a common object (e.g., shine a flashlight around the room to locate objects or make designs).

✧ Guessing games that use a pointing movement (e.g., the leader states, "I see something that goes on and off" [light switch], "that goes up and down"[window shade]). Members may take turns being the leader.

✧ Games that utilize skills of directionality, matching, and hand-eye coordination (e.g., construct 3- to 5-foot puzzles on the floor or a table by drawing the human figure on two large poster boards. Cut the second drawing into parts that can then be placed on top of the first. Ask the participants to identify body parts, direction, importance, and planes).

✧ Games that use the skills of constancy of form (e.g., introduce the game in this manner: "I am thinking of something in this room that is red," "…square").

✧ Games that estimate weights and distances (e.g., with the group, estimate the number of steps a group member or the group leader needs to reach a predetermined place, measure items that are distant and close to the group's members; weigh different items on a scale and ask the group beforehand which item looks heavier).[40]

✧ Activities that promote figure-ground skills and concepts (e.g., games and activities that involve following a pattern and finding the sequence; hanging photographs and pictures around the room—asking group members to search for the one with the dog or the one with trees; asking group members to identify sounds on tape [many tapes that have a variety of sounds such as musical instruments, animal, atmospheric, and industrial sounds may be found in public libraries]).[40]

✧ Activities that provide tactile stimulation and touch discrimination (e.g., place items in a paper or plastic bag in which participants are asked to "fish around" for smooth, rough, soft, light, or heavy items; construct two sets of sample textures [e.g., leather, corduroy, a feather] by gluing them to small pieces of board, one set is distributed while the other is laid upon a table. Ask members to close their eyes and see if they can match the texture they received to those that are on the table.)[40]

✧ Bilateral body scheme reinforcement activities that focus upon the body as a means of relaxation (e.g., ask group members to imitate movements of the therapist such as "close your eyes," "clap your hands," "shrug your shoulders"; the therapist can state the use of a body part as a way of cuing the group members to supply the name of that part as associated with the action of that part [e.g., "I walk with my _____"]; "I hear with my _____"; and using rhythm instruments to tap out the syllable to each name with a clap).[40]

✧ Exercises that promote body image (e.g., draw a person on the blackboard with an incomplete line or a body part missing and ask members to complete the image).[40]

✧ Games that reinforce the concept of body parts (e.g., "Looby Loo," "Red Light," "Simon Says," "Hokey Pokey").[40]

◇ A moderately weighted mirror that is passed around to promote proprioceptive input when it is held up to the face (e.g., ask members to verbalize what feature on their face they like the most).[40]

◇ Action poems that encourage movement responses. These can be chanted as members respond to the movement (e.g., "Hands on your hips, hands on your knees, put them behind you if you please...").[40]

◇ Pantomime drama that utilizes imagination and motor planning (e.g., elicit a theme like making a garden; group members describe, in sequence, what needs to be done to make a garden. Then, related garden activities are acted out).[40]

◇ Computers and robots emphasize visual-motor perception and cognitive social objectives (e.g., in regard to computers, members in small groups can take turns creating a design or running an image).[40]

◇ Challenges to improve coordination and physical skills (e.g., use the "Forward Pass" [available from Developmental Learning Materials' Teaching Resources, 1-800-527-4747], which is a football with two ropes that pass through it. Two or four players can play by moving the football back and forth on the ropes. Coordinated bilateral shoulder abduction and adduction are utilized with these types of movements).[40]

◇ Common objects can be used to initiate discussions (e.g., two pictures of similar subject matter such as animals or babies are used to discuss differences and similarities).[40]

In all five stages, the emphasis is upon lowering emotional levels while at the same time increasing the members' ability to attend to new interests, positive feelings, and healthful thoughts. These, in turn, can cushion responses to stressful conditions.

The third stage is especially appropriate for providing meditation, guided imaging, aromatherapy, and mood music. All of these are relaxing and calming techniques, and most group members will feel rested and relaxed at this point. However, the next two stages (in order for the participants to be empowered to function and appropriately handle the rest of the day, Stages 4 and 5 [which include activities that will arouse the participants and prepare them in feeling alert]) need to be included to complete the program.[40]

Stage 3 involves more judging, risk taking, and decision making than the previous stages. Stage 3 can be very flexible timewise as it can merge into Stage 4 as a natural continuation of a discussion regarding an activity.[40]

STAGE 4: COGNITIVE STIMULATION AND FUNCTION

This stage acts as a high point of sharing and cohesion within the group.

Additional activities to be included in this stage can be the use of poetry or other types of literature (e.g., short verses of limericks or published poetry, short stores, riddles, or jokes).[40]

Many kinds of memory games are useful (e.g., hide something that has been previously reviewed with the group and then ask the group members to remember what has been hidden). Memory games should be played with sensitivity. For instance, in learning group members' names, the members can participate in training to remember names by creating an association with the name (e.g., Paul is tall; Joan is wearing a red dress).[40]

Concentration is another important aspect of this section.

Pictures presented in pairs (e.g., two flowers, two cards, two types of tools, two animals) can be used mounted on 8- by 5-inch cards. One group of cards is placed on a table or the floor, and the participants are asked to match the items.[40]

Prepare two sets of items (e.g., sponges, cubes, empty spools, tiny plastic flowers, an eraser) and place one complete set into a container. One item is chosen to be hidden from the group by a group member whose actions are not to be seen by the group. The hidden item is placed in another container. Pass both containers around and have the participants guess which one of the displaced items is hidden.[40]

Pictures or photographs of nature (either seasonal or unseasonal) can be used to express a wide range of emotions. Feelings such as sadness, happiness, joyfulness, and innocence can be represented in these pictures or photos. Members are then encouraged to discuss their feelings about each "nature image."[40]

Show-and-tell can be used as a modality. Members and the clinician can present collections of souvenirs, hobbies, or photographs to discuss with the group.

Blackboard activities can be utilized at this time. Some of these include: (1) write "I wish" on the blackboard and encourage each member to add to the list—until everyone has had the opportunity to write; (2) a blackboard can be filled with at least five rows of single-digit numbers. Each participant can be given a different task (e.g., one is asked to put a circle around all 3's, another can be asked to circle all 4's); and (3) letters can be placed in a sequential format on various parts of the blackboard. Members are then asked to draw a connecting line that follows the correct sequence (colored chalk is helpful in denoting this).[40]

Music can also be presented. Tambourines and drums can be offered to group members so that they can keep the beat of the music that is played on a tape or CD; music presentations can also encourage participants to hum, clap, or assume postures.

Felt board activities are another modality that is useful. A felt board (about 3 by 2 feet) can be constructed, and felt cutouts can be used to dramatize an impromptu poem or story. Felt shapes, colors, and categories of food can be produced and used as decorations.[40]

During this stage it is expected that group members will be able to demonstrate a high level of impulse control, awareness of each other, attentiveness, and group cohesion. The time allotment for this section is approximately one-fifth of the total time.[40]

STAGE 5: CLOSING THE SESSION

This stage represents the ending or closing of the group program. Familiar relaxing and routine activities that promote the closing of the session on an affirmative note are utilized. Internal control is strengthened by appropriate leave taking, reminders, and hand clasps. To promote a tone of calm, stimulation is directed to the limbic systems and the reticular formation. This stage evokes an environment of trust. The focus of the program has been one of preparing the group participants to feel organized and affirmative about their abilities so that they will increasingly seek to take responsibility for their own welfare.[40]

Activities useful for Stage 5 include: using upbeat activities with group participants that require increased arousal (e.g., provide a beverage, sing a goodbye song and clap along, hold hands and move them in various directions); using routine activities to maintain an alert and calm state (e.g., pass a caring touch, participants can hold hands—then elbows and shoulders—swaying together before pulling apart); using relaxing activities when the group displays high spirits (e.g., serve a snack or a bever-

age, encourage group members to recite a poem, ask members to encourage participants to state an interest); and as the group is in the circle, close eyes and hold hands
for as long as possible. Someone in the group, without being prompted, will usually
announce that the session should close, and cleaning up and clearing up as well as
announcing the next meeting time are other ways to signal closure.[40]

Sensory Integration and Sensory Processing Theory as Related to Integrative Group Therapy

It should be noted that integrative group therapy is very much related to sensory
integration and sensory processing theory. In this theoretical approach, specific structures within the central nervous system provide an organized approach to conceptual-
izing the central nervous system.[40]

Ayres postulates that vestibular and tactile input performs a critical role in integrating and organizing sensory stimuli (primarily at the brain stem level).[41] Sensory input
and integration are essential in developing appropriate size and visual form constancy
and reliable localization of auditory stimuli. All of these are important features that
enable the late life adult to utilize his or her environment effectively and appropriately.[10]

Sensory integration is an important model for understanding the relationship
between the sensory centers (including the tactile, proprioceptive and vestibular systems). Normal development promotes the acquisition of physical skills for motor performance. It is these physical skills that underlie the mastery and competence that is
required by all individuals to grow toward responsibility and independence.[40]

Integrative Group Therapy: Mobilizing Coping Abilities With the Five-Stage Group
also contains an assessment, the Smaga and Ross Integrative Battery (SARIB).[40] This
tool assesses range of motion; posture and gait; balance; general strength (shoulder and
hand grasp); proprioception; visual performance (eye-tracking ability, field of vision,
depth perception); moving two-point discrimination; stereognosis; motor planning and
coordination; L-R fine motor control test; auditory figure-ground perception; memory
(short-term/long-term); unilateral neglect; judgment; and behaviors that influence performance (coping behaviors, motivation, performance time). It is best suited to a population that manifests chronic illness and is used to predict any individual's degree of
functional independence. It also judges the amount of supervision and support a person may need for living within the community. It has been used with adults who have
histories of developmental disabilities, mental retardation, mental illness, and late life
adults with physical disability.[40]

SOCIALLY ORIENTED PROGRAMS

Social Skills Training Program

Social skills training focuses upon conversational skills and general "getting along
with others." Social skills can be defined as a person's ability to obtain and give information and to exchange and express emotions, opinions, and attitudes.[42] For older
adults who have experienced a series of psychiatric commitments or institutionalization, this type of programming can be helpful.

Although medication can address the psychiatric client's positive symptoms (e.g., loose associations, hallucinations, and delusions); negative symptoms (e.g., low voice volume, avoidance of eye contact, and isolation) can be treated best through social skills, training, and development. Those clients with a diagnosis of depression are also able to benefit from this type of intervention.[42]

Some of the abilities needed in order to perform effective social skills include: recognition of nonverbal cues, resolving nonverbal and verbal conflicts, predicting the consequences of a social situation, comprehending a sequence of social events, generating possible verbal and nonverbal sending modes, generating possible responses, and choosing an appropriate response.[42]

The social skills training group is initiated with an "ice breaker" or warm-up activity. A conversation topic is then presented. This is followed by a role-play situation. In the role-playing component, the key to success is practice and repetition. The group then concludes with some type of light refreshment and an informal socialization time. Whenever possible, it is helpful to have female and male co-therapists as they can serve not only as instructors but also as role models.[42]

The following illustrates one specific aspect of the program—the warmup. There are a wide variety of warmup activities (such as socially oriented games). The one discussed here is entitled, "What is different?" In this activity the participants are paired up to study each other's appearance. Next, they are told to turn away from each other and change one item or thing about their appearance. The next step includes turning back to one another and trying to identify what is different about the other individual. After three rounds with the same partner, the participants are asked to switch with another person and play three more rounds (with a new partner). The participants continue to change until each player has had an opportunity to pair up with all possible partners. The clinician then closes the group and asks all the participants how they felt about the activity. The skill areas addressed in this activity include attention, concentration, recall, attention to details, socialization with all who are in the group, expressing feelings, using eye contact, and learning to give constructive criticism.[42] Other useful topics can include discussing a season or holiday event and giving each member an opportunity to talk about it with cues or prods from the clinician, such as asking each participant to list the signs of a particular season.[42,43]

A major component of social skills training involves role playing. In this example the participants of the group are asked to role play giving directions to one another on how to get from one part of a building to another section (for instance, the individual is sitting in the lobby and a visitor comes in the front door and asks how to get to the "office area"). The dysfunctional areas addressed are disorientation and perception. The skill areas include awareness of surroundings, directionality, space visualization, and clear informational communication.[43]

In general, social skills training programs address the following long-term goals: participants will demonstrate decreased anxiety in social situations, increased eye contact with others, improved fluency, increased control of anger, and improved conversational skills.[42,43]

Discussion Groups

For those older adults who display little confusion, there are other types of group interaction programs that serve to stimulate greater cognitive awareness and social awareness. These socially oriented programs can include groups that focus upon special subject areas such as world news, literary reviews, sports, travel, history, the arts (art, photography, music, dance, the theater, the cinema, fashion), and community events. In all these groups the clinician can act as a guide and resource person. As each group matures, individual group members can "take turns" in assuming the leadership role.[10]

In these types of groups there are goals that involve both cognitive and social development. These include improvement in:[10]

- ◇ The ability to understand what is being said and to put the important issues in an order of priority
- ◇ The capacity to respect and understand another person's point of view
- ◇ The ability to express one's own point of view so that others are able to comprehend the speaker's intent
- ◇ The ability to engage in cognitive pursuits (conversation, discussion, thinking, organizing one's thought process, the ability to give and retain information)
- ◇ The ability to develop positive relationships within the group

Intergenerational Programming

Grandparenting has long been a natural role for older adults. In this situation a wise elder assumes an interest in the development and well-being of a younger person. In the case of a grandparent, it is one who is a family member; however, there are many instances when an elderly neighbor may take on a similar role with a young neighbor.

In psychiatric hospitals that serve the elderly and in nursing homes, most late life adults rarely have the opportunity to interact with or even see children.

Butin describes several situations where positive interaction can occur between the very old and the young. First, there is the concept of an intergenerational cooking group. Depressed late life adults and hospitalized adolescents can be provided with an opportunity to practice and transfer the interpersonal skills that are needed for relationships with family members in the home setting.[33]

Butin also suggests utilizing the Reader's Digest Foundation Intergenerational Program to permit older adults (who are in community psychiatric intervention) to practice and model communicating with young children in order to improve relationships with their own grandchildren.[33] The program's members were trained in play therapy and child development. They purchased books and toys for this activity.

The program consists of three specified activity models. First, there is the Grandparent Story Hour. In this segment the late life adult chooses and reads books to preschoolers at the local library. Prior to reading before the children, the older adults practice reading and receive feedback from peers. Secondly, there is the Adopt-a-Tot component. This part of the program lasts approximately 1 hour. It involves crafts and finger play and gross motor activities with 3- and 4-year-olds at a local day care center. The last component is entitled Heal-the-Children. In this activity late life adults attend the family health clinic (which is upstairs from the psychiatric day treatment center) so that they can play with the children in the waiting room.[33] The Reader's Digest Foundation Intergenerational Program can also be used with the well-elderly population.

There are other types of intergenerational giving and sharing activities that promote intergenerational relationships between chronically ill elderly psychiatric clients and brain-damaged children.[10] In one instance, six elderly female psychiatric inpatients, during occupational therapy sessions, fashioned hand puppets (out of papier mache and hand sewn costumes) to give to six physically and emotionally disabled children (students at a nearby center for handicapped children). Arrangements were made between the center and the occupational therapist (who worked with the women) for the clients to visit the children and personally hand deliver the gifts. At the center, the women were greeted with "Thanks you's" from the children and all enjoyed light refreshments together.[10] Another group of inpatients (five late life males) constructed a toy train set out of wood (again during occupational therapy sessions). They, too, visited the center and personally presented their gifts. This time the children entertained the clients with a gymnastic program as their way of saying, "Thank you."[10]

Another group of older adults in a nursing home were interested in the community surrounding them and, indeed, the world community. The group became involved in knitting baby blankets for AIDS babies.

"Providing opportunities whereby disabled late life adults are involved in productive activity… and where they are placed in the role of 'providers' instead of receivers add to enhancement of the self."[10] These were indeed meaningful experiences. One client told this author, "I felt useful again." Another client remarked, "I never had children of my own—it's good to know that I made a difference in someone else's life."[10] These statements are testimony to the importance not only of these types of activities but to the fact that these activities promote a new or renewed positive self-image among late life adults.

THE LIFE REVIEW AND REMINISCENCE

The Life Review: A Definition

According to Butler, "The life review is conceived of as a naturally occurring universal mental process characterized by the progressive return to consciousness of past experience, and particularly, the unresolved conflicts surveyed and reintegrated. It is assumed that this process is prompted by the realization of approaching dissolution and death."[44]

The life review is a progressive, usually spontaneous, and unselected return to past experiences. Older adults need the opportunity to allow for the reduction of past conflicts. If this does not happen, the late life adult might become depressed, filled with anxiety and guilt, or panic stricken. Contrarily, the successful reintegration of former conflicts can lead to the righting of old wrongs, a sense of serenity, a feeling of accomplishment and pride, and an acceptance of life's mortality.[10]

There are many ways that older adults accomplish the life review. Some late life individuals will tell stories about their past, others will reminisce and/or participate in mild nostalgia. Many older adults will tell their life story to anyone who is willing to listen, while others may conduct monologues without an audience.[10]

The late life individual's sharing of his or her life story is an important part of the developmental process.[7]

Reminiscence is manifested by recollections of past experiences and events, nostalgia, and storytelling.[7] The integration of various past experiences into one's present living situation helps to enable the older individual to achieve an acceptable and positive view of his or her life's worth. Reminiscence may also be responsible for promoting successful adaptation in late life by maintaining self-esteem;[7] "reminiscence can have therapeutic benefits, especially in helping older adults who are depressed or need to integrate past experiences with present losses or challenges."[7]

Stevens-Ratchford recommends that clinicians develop interview schedules that tap stories of the milestones from situations and events of the elderly person's life.[7] It is also important for the clinician to encourage storytelling or reminiscing about past experiences that indicated successful coping with adjusting to life's changes and other challenges.[7]

Programs Involving the Life Review and Reminiscence

There are many ways to therapeutically encourage the life review process. Some of these include: discussion groups (e.g., discussion of early childhood events—the Great Depression, education in a one-room school, the roaring 20s, World War II; later experiences—The Big Band period, being a teenager, seasonal celebrations, family experiences, recalling positive elements in past experiences, using common references to a life setting [such as photographs of parks, a city, or a farm to spark recall and conversation]). The clinician can enhance these experiences by bringing in tapes and videos of music (of past times). Frequently, public television offers programs that depict past events. "Jazz," a series which aired in January 2001, represents one of these offerings. This type of programming can be taped or purchased so that video libraries can be developed.

Other therapeutic groups and activities that utilize reminiscence include:

1. A collage group in which participants are asked to make a collage of an important positive experience in their past and describe it in the group setting.
2. A quilting group in which members can make a quilted square of their life's experiences in a combined group quilt or each member can produce a quilt of his or her own which can be presented to a family member or significant other as a memento.
3. The development of life story photograph albums in which one arranges his or her photographs into a life story and discusses it with other group members; it can later serve as a gift to family and friends.
4. Drawing or painting of an important moment in one's life.
5. Writing or taping one's life story and discussing these projects within a group can also serve as a gift to family and friends. These activities can be carried out as part of a group process or on an individual basis.

The life review process has been used by the well elderly in the community setting, by those in a facility setting, and by hospice participants. It is an opportunity for clinicians to assist the older adult in a normative process that has a number of therapeutic benefits.

DEVELOPMENTALLY DELAYED OLDER ADULTS

Developmentally Delayed Older Adults: A Definition

In general, a *developmental disability*, as defined by the Developmental Disabilities Assistance and Bill of Rights Act amendments of 1987, is a chronic and severe condition that:[45]

✧ Is manifested before the age of 22

✧ Is attributable to a mental impairment, a physical impairment, and/or both

✧ Results in substantial functional limitations in at least three or more areas of major life activity

✧ Is likely to continue indefinitely

✧ Reflects a need for a combination and sequence of specialized interdisciplinary, generic care, intervention, or services that are lifelong and are individually coordinated or planned

Typical diagnoses include mental retardation (at all levels of severity), neural tube deficits, cerebral palsy, autism, and pervasive developmental delay. It is estimated that between 1% and 3% of the total population has a diagnosis of developmental delay (DD).[45,46]

It is important to note that DD older adults are a growing segment of our population due to decreased early mortality rates and improved health care. Many of these adults had previously resided in large institutional facilities. However, from 1982 though 1988, it is estimated that the number of persons with profound levels of mental retardation (living in smaller community residences of fewer than 15 individuals) increased by 150%.[47]

Occupational therapists are in an excellent position to enable adults with DD to live in the community as successfully as possible. With our training in physical and cognitive dysfunction, task and activity analysis, and environmental adaptations, occupational therapists can readily evaluate and address the physical, vocational, self-care, and leisure needs of late life adults with DD who are living in the community.[48]

Besides having developmental disabilities, these late life individuals also experience similar health care needs as other older adults (e.g., cardiovascular problems, arthritis, hypertension, cancer, Alzheimer's disease, bipolar disorders, and depression). Therefore, there are shifts in the kinds of health care services that are needed by older DD clients. This encompasses increased health care access within the community setting (such as acute and rehabilitation hospitals, community clinics and home health care).[49,50] There will, most likely, be numerous opportunities for clinicians to offer occupational therapy intervention strategies that can enable these individuals to function at their optimal level.[48]

Evaluation and Assessment for Older Adults With Developmental Delay

First, it is important to begin with an evaluation. A number of factors need to be considered before this can occur. These include receiving information regarding the referring acute medical diagnosis; the interests and needs of the client; the priorities as expressed by the family, administrators, or agency workers; and the frame of reference as utilized by the facility, agency, or therapist.[48]

An interview (to the extent that is possible) with the client is the first step in the evaluation process as it will serve to guide the therapist on how to proceed. It is important to identify the client's communication patterns before conducting the interview (e.g., the client may be nonverbal or use an assistive device). Family, guardians, and staff members should also be part of the interview process as they provide important background information.[48]

Knowing the client's hearing, vision, cognitive and/or mental retardation level, communication, posture, and ambulation status as well as a quick screen of the client's needs and strengths will suggest areas upon which to concentrate.[48] Therapists also need to be aware of the evidence of changing functional status. There is a high incidence of concomitant disorders among individuals with DD. For instance, individuals with Down syndrome are at increased risk for early onset of deafness, eye disease, congenital heart disease, psychiatric disorders, and Alzheimer's disease.[50] Herge and Campbell caution that therapists should be ever diligent to detect changes that could be explained or missed by caregivers as part of the client's behavior. Changes that occur on a slow steady basis (such as a change in endurance level) may not be noticed in the same manner as dramatic changes. Therefore, therapists should include questions regarding the client's previous functional level that have occurred within the past 6 months.[48]

Herge and Campbell recommend the following assessment tools for determining the needs and the strengths of older adults with DD.

THE SENSORY INTEGRATION INVENTORY

This is a tool that is helpful in screening possible sensory integrative (SI) dysfunction. This tool is meant to identify possible patterns of SI dysfunction (not diagnose). With this inventory, the therapist usually interviews a caregiver who is familiar with the client, independently. If the screening indicates there may be SI dysfunction, a further specialized assessment may be required.

This tool can be found in:

✧ Reisman, J. & Hanschu, B. (1992). *Sensory integrative inventory—Revised for individuals with developmental disabilities*. Hugo, MN: PDP.

ALLEN'S COGNITIVE SCREENING/ALLEN DIAGNOSTIC MODULE

The Allen test batteries can be helpful in identifying a client's cognitive level. Intervention plans and environmental modifications can be developed from information obtained from this tool.

This screening tool can be found in:

✧ Allen, C. K., Earhart, C. A., & Blue, T. (1992). *Occupational therapy treatment goals for the physically and cognitively disabled*. Bethesda, MD: American Occupational Therapy Association, Inc.

THE KITCHEN TASK ASSESSMENT

This assessment is an objective, practical measure of cognitive functioning using a demonstrated common task (making cooked pudding). This tool is useful in helping the therapist determine the specific level of assistance a client may need to perform tasks safely. This assessment is very useful when contemplating discharge planning.

This assessment can be found in:

✧ Baum, C. & Edward, D. F. (1993). Cognitive performance in senile dementia of the Alzheimer's type: The Kitchen Task Assessment. *Am J Occup Ther, 47,* 431-435.

RUOCCO GERIATRIC ASSESSMENT

This assessment, designed specifically for older adults with DD, focuses upon identifying individuals who may be experiencing dementia. This tool includes the assessment of records of the client's medical history, the client's performance of activities of daily living, use of unstructured time, behaviors, and mobility. It is designed to be repeated at regular intervals. This assessment monitors and compares any changes in the client's routines and/or behaviors.

The Ruocco Geriatric Assessment can be found in:

✧ Ruocco, L. E. (2000, February). *Geriatric assessment of individuals with intellectual disabilities—A four part rating scale.* Paper presented at the Office of Mental Retardation, "Everyday Lives Conference," Hershey, PA.

ENVIRONMENTAL ASSESSMENT

The fifth area is an environmental assessment. Many facilities and agencies develop their own home environmental checklists and assessments. Typically, the evaluation involves: the kitchen, the entryway, the bathroom, the bedroom, and any other living areas.

This type of evaluation can be found in:

✧ Pedretti, L. W. (1996). *Occupational therapy: Practice skills for physical dysfunction* (4th Ed.). St. Louis, MO: Mosby-Year Books.

For other suggestions of environmental checklists and assessments, please refer to Chapter 12 of this unit.

Herge and Campbell recommend a number of strategies that are useful with the older adult:

✧ Present information in manageable steps. Present only one or two steps of a task at a time, and avoid using a patronizing tone.

✧ Develop alternative strategies/methods to elicit data (e.g., when testing for muscle strength on a client who can only follow one-step directions—ask the client to reach for something [manual strength grade of 3/5], to determine if the client has a higher grade of manual strength, ask him or her to lift something with a wrist weight [manual strength grade of 4/5]).

✧ Allow adequate time for the client to process cues. Keep instructions simple (avoid wordy instructions, avoid rephrasing the cue or repeating too frequently).

✧ Pair physical, verbal, or gestural cues (notice which type of cue elicits the best client response).[48]

Therapists will often need to adapt the evaluation process that is traditionally used in their setting so that the client's specific capabilities and needs can be addressed. For instance, a 6- to 8-inch Nerf ball can be thrown to the client to catch. By assessing the client's capacity to catch the ball and feeling it on the body, the therapist can evaluate awareness of the environment, reach, bilateral hand use, and grasp.[48]

Intervention Planning With the Older Adult Diagnosed With Developmental Delay

Intervention planning encompasses a number of considerations: the interests and needs of the client, family, and caregivers; agency priorities; funding priorities; environmental factors; the client's ability to process information, attend therapy, and learn new skills; and the caregiver's ability, capacity, and willingness to provide and promote follow-up care. The plan should actively involve participation of the client, family, service providers, and caregivers in an appropriate team process. All goals and objectives need to be achievable and measurable, and at the same time take into consideration the client's previous independence level and cognitive disability level. This, then, needs to be related to the rehabilitation process or the acute diagnosis.[48]

Any assessment findings regarding the client's cognitive functioning and specific cues, prompts, or adaptations need to be communicated to the team and recorded so that the client can receive the best possible care.[48]

Occupational Therapy Intervention Involving Rehabilitation of a Late Life Client With Developmental Delay

Often it is the occupational therapist who shares information regarding the client's ability to participate in his or her health care process. The therapist needs to always consider the client's cognitive limitations when making intervention and environmental decisions and considerations.

This author worked with a late life male with DD. The client had previously lived in an assisted living facility where he was independent for dressing and bathing. He was transferred to an associated skilled nursing facility when he broke his right hip. He needed to be brought through the process of using long-handled equipment (such as a reacher, a dressing stick, a sock donner, a long-handled shoe horn, and elastic shoe laces) slowly by the therapist. This was later reinforced by the aides (instructed by the therapist) in a.m. and p.m. care.

The client also needed to learn to wait for assistance (initially from maximum assistance, to moderate assistance, to minimum assistance, and finally to supervision/independent). Instruction on carry-over in safe entry and exit in the shower as well as washing oneself while in the shower was performed in the same manner. All shifts were educated in proper self-care techniques. When the client reached the supervisory/independent level, he was ready for discharge back to the assisted living facility. The therapist then instructed all morning and evening shifts in the assisted living facility as to the client's functional level. The follow-up by the aides was excellent and within 3 weeks the client was back to functioning independently.

In general, the therapist or assistant (instructing care providers) needs to be very specific as to the level of care that is necessary. Many performance repetitions are usually needed to ensure generalization and learning.[48] When establishing an intervention plan or home program, the therapist or assistant needs to consider the particular caregiver's (whether staff, family, or significant others) needs and strengths (capacities in carrying out and follow-up of the intervention program). Most families have a service provider or a case manager from their local county department who provides service to individuals with mental retardation. This person is responsible for coordinating all services for adults with DD or mental retardation. He or she can help in locating respite care and in-home support. At times the therapist or assistant may need to collaborate with this individual to ensure appropriate family support.[48]

Therapists and assistants working with this population segment have much to offer in enhancing the "client's ability to function independently and improve his or her quality of life in the community."[48, p. 23]

An excellent resource for adults with DD is a book by Mildred Ross and Susan Bachner (1988) entitled, *Adults With Developmental Disabilities: Current Approaches in Occupational Therapy*. The book includes activities, strategies, and case studies that focus upon service delivery to adults with DD. Some of its highlights involve providing a holistic intervention perspective regardless of primary diagnosis; demonstrating intervention effectiveness and accountability; reviewing the client's human and legal rights; offering strategies that focus upon the needs, applications, and potential outcomes for functional performance; promoting ways that the therapist and assistant can serve as advocates for adults with DD; and describing how the clinician can play a major role in providing team-based services that promote positive work and community outcomes for this group of individuals. This volume is available from the American Occupational Therapy Association (Bethesda, MD), 1 877 404-AOTA, www.aota.org.

PHYSICAL DISABILITIES AND OCCUPATIONAL THERAPY INTERVENTION APPROACHES

15

VISUAL DYSFUNCTION AND INTERVENTION FOR OLDER ADULTS

Visual perception is a process that integrates vision with other sensory input so that an individual can adapt and survive. Sensory input into the central nervous system is ever changing. Likewise, a person's decision as to how he or she could respond to a situation can change on a momentary notice (depending upon the alterations in the sensory context that the individual experiences). Vision, our most far-reaching sensory system, takes us out into our environment. It alerts us to danger (e.g., seeing a severe storm approaching) and to pleasure (e.g., seeing one's children playing in the school-yard as one drives up or viewing an art show in a museum). Vision is used to analyze situations, and it plays a key role in the decision-making process. There are numerous phrases that attest to the importance of vision in everyday life situations. For example, "I'll believe it when I see it" or "I can see what you mean" are phrases that literally reflect vision's powerful role. Vision is paramount in aiding us in the anticipatory process of problem solving as well as enabling us to adapt to the environment.[51] "It is how we 'see' a situation that triggers the planning and decision-making process."[51, p. 194]

The visual process begins as light enters the eye, passes through the cornea and the lens, and focuses upon the retina. The visual information is then passed from the retina to the optic nerve and tract to the lateral geniculate nucleus of the thalamus where it synapses (with information from the retinal hemifields of both eyes to provide binocular vision) and carries visual information over the geniculocal carine tracts to the visual cortex.[51]

There are two parallel routes that carry visual information from the occipital cortex to the prefrontal lobe and the frontal eye field. The *northern* or *superior* route carries information involving the parietal association cortex (where visual-spatial maps and orientation that includes movement detection take place). This information, in turn, is carried to the prefrontal lobe and frontal eye field. Decision making, planning ahead, and emotional tone are conducted at this juncture. The *southern* or *inferior* route carries visual information via the posterior temporal association cortex (visual object recognition that includes form and color are conducted here). This information is then carried to the prefrontal lobe and frontal eye field.[51]

Besides these pathways the brain stem contains several important neural structures that involve processing—particularly in the peripheral visual fields and eye movements. The subcortical areas of the brain aid in monitoring the peripheral visual field and help to keep the individual upright in space.[51] The hemispheres divide responsibility for some aspects of visual processing and differ in strategy that each employs to focus attention. Some examples of these differences can be seen as follows:[51]

1. In the left hemisphere: there is more detail orientation in relation to persons, places, and/or things; minute details are taken in and comparisons and contrasts to details are employed; visual information is processed sequentially in a systematic item-by-item, serial strategy search; and only right visual fields are able to attend.

2. In the right hemisphere: a more holistic and global approach is employed; a general view of the environment is taken in; multiple visual inputs are processed simultaneously and grouped into meaningful categories; and both left and right visual fields are able to attend on a global basis.

Visual perceptual function is based upon an organized hierarchy of skill levels that are interdependent upon each other within a unified system. *Visual cognition* is defined as, "the ability to manipulate visual information mentally and integrate it with other sensory information to gain knowledge and to solve problems, formulate plans and make decisions."[51, p. 198] Visual cognition serves as a foundation for academic pursuits (e.g., areas such as mathematics, writing, reading, and professions in art, engineering, architecture, science, and surgery). However, in order to perform intact visual cognition, a host of other skills need to be integrated. On the basic level are oculomotor control, intact visual fields, and intact visual acuity. On the next level is attention (involving the ability to be alert and to be able to attend); intact scanning is the next level; this is followed by intact pattern recognition, which is then followed by the ability to hold a visual memory. There are a minimum of seven visual skills that are needed to perform visual cognition appropriately.[51]

The following discussion represents those visual disabilities that are found in late life adults.

Deficits in Visual Acuity

Photoreceptors in the retinal field, lining the inside of the eye, are programmed to respond to discrete visual stimuli. Any deficit in the optical system such as the lens, the cornea, or the length of the eyeball can cause images to be poorly focused. *Myopia* (nearsightedness) can be corrected by a concave lens in the front of the eye, *hyperopia* (farsightedness) can be corrected by placing a convex lens in front of the eye, and astigmatism can be corrected by placing a cylindrical lens in front of the eye. Cataracts, cloudy media, and corneal opacities are the most common causes of decreased visual acuity in the elderly.[51-53] Other disorders that affect the integrity and health of the retina (such as macular degeneration, glaucoma, hypertension and diabetic retinopathy) also are responsible for the decreased ability for one to clearly identify visual detail.[51]

Refractive problems such as found on the physician's evaluation of the optical system can generally be corrected with the use of medication, surgery, or lenses. For other aspects of visual acuity in which there is a reduced ability to see color or contrast, an adaptive approach toward changing the environment is the most beneficial.[51]

The three most effective factors that can be used to adapt the visual environment are appropriate illumination, decreased use of pattern backgrounds, and the use of contrast.[51]

Illumination involves increasing the intensity of available light. Light needs to be provided that does not involve increasing glare. Fluorescent and halogen lighting are recommended over standard incandescent lighting. It is also important to minimize shadows. This is particularly useful when trying to identify a person's face. Fifty-watt halogen desk lamps provide the best illumination for reading (with a minimum of shadow).

Patterned backgrounds should be avoided as they have an effect of camouflaging objects lying on them. Instead, solid colors for background surfaces (e.g., bedspreads, dishes, countertops, rugs, placemats, furniture coverings, and towels) should be utilized. Pattern represents clutter in the environment. In this respect clients with difficulty identifying objects perform better with kitchen shelves (as well as countertops, bookshelves, closets, baskets, and clinic areas) that have a few orderly items rather than those that are filled with dozens of items.

The use of contrast is another way to improve the environment for those individuals who experience decreased visual acuity. To be effective the clinician must first determine what critical items in the environment are needed for identification and orientation. Once this has been done, contrast should be added to surrounding features (e.g., placing a carrot on a white cutting board rather than a tan cutting board, putting bright tape at the end of each step, using a black cup for drinking milk, using a white cup for coffee or tea, and marking the wheelchair brakes with red tape so that they will be easier to distinguish from the wheel).[51] Optical aids that are enlarged and that use contrast (such as enlarged clocks, timers, phones, and calculators) can also be helpful.[52] Meal preparation is particularly difficult due to the involvement of many low contrast details (e.g., stove dials, reading recipes, measuring, and pouring liquids).[53] Here again the use of contrast is helpful (e.g., painting the stove dials a different color and contrast from the stove, using large print with contrasting measuring devices).

Golisz and Toglia contend that visual-processing dysfunction includes a variety of components such as difficulty in detecting gross differences in size, direction, position, rotations, and angles; difficulty in visual discrimination between pictures of objects, basic shapes, and colors; difficulty in visually locating simple visual targets in space or judging gross distances between two objects; difficulty in drawing simple objects or shapes (e.g., a flower or a geometric shape); and decreased ability to detect simple part-whole relations in basic shapes or objects.[31]

Deficits in the Visual Field

Homonymous hemianopsia, the loss of the visual field in the corresponding left or right half of each eye, is one of the most common visual impairments following a CVA. Many of these individuals experience a narrowed scope of scanning as well as reduced speed of scanning in activities in which monitoring of the full visual field is needed (such as driving a car or moving about in a very active and busy environment). This narrowed scope of scanning creates safety hazards. Reading and performing mathematical calculations are also difficult. For example, a client with a left visual field deficit might read the number 10 as a zero. Many clients with these types of difficulties can lose confidence in their ability to manage a checkbook or pay bills.[51]

In terms of evaluation, the use of computerized, automated perimetry is the most exact way to measure field deficits. If this tool is not available then a confrontation test (examiner sits in front of the client and asks the client to fixate on a centrally placed target—often the examiner's nose. Then, the examiner holds up one, two, or five fingers or a clenched fist separately in each of the four visual quadrants. The client indicates how many fingers are seen during each trial) can be administered. This type of test must be done in combination with careful observation of the client's performance in activities of daily living. Client behaviors that often indicate visual field deficits include consistently bumping into objects on one side; changing head positions when asked to view objects that are placed on a certain plane; consistent reading errors; and misplacing objects in one field.[51]

Intervention involves a combination of strategies. First, the focus should be upon increasing the scope and speed of the scanning pattern. In this respect, the client must learn to turn his or her head as quickly as possible in order to compensate for the limited visual field. The Dynavision 2000 (Performance Enterprises, Ontario, Canada) is an excellent device that provides clients with practice in scope and speed of scanning skills. Balloon patting and ball toss (in which balls are tossed quickly from player to player) are activities that offer other helpful strategies.[51]

Driving, reading, and writing are three activities that rely completely on the visual process. Many clients with visual field cuts experience difficulty merging on and off of the roadways, changing car lanes and monitoring traffic in multilane situations. Training in the area of driving should focus upon increasing the speed and scope of scanning as well as providing specific strategies to handle the above mentioned traffic conditions.[51] Specific programming in driving remediation will be considered separately in a later section of this unit.

In reading, most clients' complaints focus upon their difficulties locating and maintaining the correct line of print and being able to accurately identify numbers and words. Often these individuals experience difficulty returning to the margin (of the affected side) of the reading material so that they can begin the next line of text. Drawing a bold red line down the side of the margin provides a visual cue to the client. For those individuals who experience difficulty staying on line or moving down the correct line, a plain card or a ruler may be used under the line of the print to promote enabling the client to keep his or her place.[51]

Other adults with deficits in the visual field may also experience problems with writing skills. Most of these individuals experience difficulty staying on line when writing. Intervention centers upon teaching the client to monitor the pen tip while maintaining visual fixation as the hand moves across the page into the affected side. The following information represents two approaches in dealing with this situation. First, the client can be asked to trace lines toward the side of the field loss (helpful in re-establishing eye-hand lock). Secondly, devices such as the talking pen (Wayne Engineering, Northfield, IL) offer feedback. These tools work well in training the client to monitor the tip of the pen while he or she is handwriting.[51]

Contrast, reduction of patterns, and appropriate illumination play an important part in enhancing daily living activities for those who experience visual field deficits. The following represent a few ways one can modify the environment:[51]

1. Use contrast in writing materials by providing black felt-tip pens on boldly lined paper.
2. Add color and contrast to key environmental structures (e.g., furniture, door frames, threshold).
3. Reduce pattern in the environment by using solid colored objects and cleaning out clutter.
4. Increase illumination (often this can positively affect reading speed and reduce errors).

Deficits in Oculomotor Control

Deficits in oculomotor control are most commonly the results of specific cranial nerve lesions that cause paresis or paralysis of one or more of the extraocular muscles that control eye movement. They can also be the result of the disruption of central neural control of the extraocular muscles that affect the coordination of the eye's movements. The functional result is decreased speed, coordination, and control of eye movements. During some types of traumatic brain injury, diffuse damage can take place throughout the brain stem. This, then, can affect the neural control centers that coordinate oculomotor actions (without affecting the cranial nerves).

Clients who experience *diplopia* (double images), due to a paretic muscle, can often be found assuming a head position that avoids the action of the paretic muscle. These individuals often tilt their head as a form of functional adaptation to stabilize their vision. Because many factors are involved with oculomotor control, clinicians involved in treating these clients should do so under the guidance and monitoring of an ophthalmologist or optometrist specializing in visual impairment from a neurological basis.[51]

Deficits in Visual Attention

Visual attention is accomplished through visual scanning. Deficits that affect visual attention can be observed by changes in the way the client scans for visual information. There are both focal (selective) visual attention and ambient (peripheral) visual attention. *Focal attention* allows for one to accurately distinguish visual details in such differences as those that exist between numbers and letters. Therefore, it highly contributes to academic excellence. *Ambient attention*, on the other hand, is involved with the detection of events in the environment as well as their location in space and in proximity to the person. The contributions of each of these areas of visual attention are equally important to perceptual processing. Normal brain scanning varies as to the task. When reading (in the case of the English and Romance languages), a left-to-right and top-to-bottom reticular strategy is utilized. When one is scanning a room (open array) a circular left-to-right strategy is generally used. The eye will usually follow a clockwise or counterclockwise pattern.[51]

Visual inattention is most often associated with right brain injury (usually after a CVA). Clients typically avoid viewing objects and the environment on the left side. Visual inattention has also been identified as visual neglect, hemi-inattention, or unilateral inattention. However, the term neglect is a misnomer as it implies that the client has some volitional part in this condition. In actuality the client is unaware of the incompleteness of his or her perception and responses to the environment.[31]

It is essential that the occupational therapist first distinguish between hemianopsia (visual field cuts or deficits) and unilateral inattention. Visual field cuts are hemiretinal, while visual inattention is hemispatial. Clients with visual field deficits are usually aware of their loss and make compensatory head turns and movements. Unilateral inattention can exist with or without visual field cuts.[31]

Traditional evaluation of hemi-inattention involves tasks of extinction and confrontation, line bisection, drawing tests, and cancellation.[31]

Warren suggests several tests for hemi-inattention:

A Simple Test of Visual Neglect

✧   Albert, M. L. (1973). A simple test of visual neglect. *Neurology, 23,* 658-664.

This is a scanning task with an instructional array. Numerous short diagonal lines are scattered over a page. The client is asked to place a line through each line that is seen. It is important to note as the client performs the test, the type of strategy that he or she uses to impose a structure while scanning the random display of lines.[51]

Behavioral Inattention Test

This test was developed by Wilson, Cockburn, and Halligan. It is composed of a number of parts and involves a variety of functional tasks that require scanning (e.g., setting a clock, reading a menu); paper and pencil scanning tests, letter cancellation, line bisection, and slash-the-line tests. The star cancellation test involves a series of large and small stars, intermixed with random letters that are scattered over the page. The client is asked to cancel out the small stars.

This test is available from:[51]

✧   Behavioral Inattention Test
    National Rehabilitation Services
    117 North Elm St.
    P.O. Box 1247
    Gaylord, MI 49735
    517-732-3866

The Scanboard Test (by M. Warren)

This test determines how the client applies scanning strategy to a broad space. Found in:

✧   Warren, M. (1990). Identification of visual scanning deficits in adults after cerebrovascular accident. *Am J Occup Ther, 44,* 391-399.

Intervention in hemi-inattention as recommended by Warren is as follows:[51]

✧   With right brain injury: These persons demonstrate asymmetry in scanning. The first step is to teach the client to recognize his or her scanning patterns by initiating scanning in the impaired area first. Two scanning strategies need to be taught—first there is a left-to-right rectilinear pattern for reading; next, there is a left-to-right circular pattern that should be used to scan an unstructured array. Activities such as checkers, solitaire, double solitaire, and dominoes can be used to help establish an appropriate scanning strategy.[51]

✧   With left brain injury: These individuals omit scanning for details in visual arrays.

    ➤ Provide activities that emphasize careful inspection and comparison of objects as well as activities that emphasize conscious attention to detail (e.g., matching or sorting activities, puzzles, dominoes, and formboards).[51]

▲ Provide activities that require the client to physically manipulate the objects scanned (e.g., ball games, enlarged tic-tac-toe games).[51]

To increase insight, teach the client how to monitor and control performance by learning to recognize and correct errors in performance. The client will need immediate feedback. Deficiencies should be pointed out. The client can also be taught to use self-monitoring techniques (e.g., activity prediction as to how the client predicts the successful performance of an activity as well as identifies where errors are most likely to occur).

Practice the skill within the context to ensure carryover of application to everyday activities (e.g., selecting clothes from a closet, searching for items on a shelf or in a refrigerator).[51-53]

The Use of the Discovery Process With Unilateral Inattention

Thamb, Borell, and Anders discuss their study in which the "discovery process" was utilized to enhance the participants' ability to fully use compensatory strategies and incorporate them for everyday use. The subjects were four female inpatients with right cerebrovascular lesions of less than 10 weeks' duration at a neurological rehabilitation clinic in Sweden. The subjects who also exhibited severe left extrapersonal unilateral neglect were interviewed during various phases of the process.[54]

The findings demonstrated how the discovery process (the process in which the participants experienced, discovered, and later learned to handle their disabilities) aided the clients in the study to improve everyday functioning skills. The discovery process included the following steps:

1. Experiencing the new and unfamiliar (e.g., not being able to utilize the left side of one's body as had formerly been done, not being able to understand what had happened)
2. Comparing the new world with the old
3. Searching for explanations
4. Becoming more familiar with the new
5. Understanding the disabilities
6. Learning to handle the disabilities in daily life
7. Incorporating new strategies

In the beginning, it seemed as though the left half of these clients' "world" did not exist for them. After interviews of these clients, it was learned that they experienced their surrounding world as if it were complete (unaware that they were missing the left side of their environment). However, they felt that their perceptions of time and space were strange and new.[54]

These clients, early in the discovery process, felt as though the left half of their body was unfamiliar to them—as one client remarked, "I feel like my left hand and foot are objects. I have to go up to my shoulder like this, to understand that it really is my hand that my arm is attached to."[54, p. 401]

Perceptual experiences in which the participants had a diffuse feeling of not being able to orient in their worlds contributed to their feelings of insecurity and disorganization.[54]

While staff or relatives would perpetually remind the clients to look to the left, these individuals (at this stage of the discovery process) could not understand why others were giving them these instructions. Often the subjects thought the reminders were reprimands.[54]

Next, as the discovery process progressed, the clients experienced different occupational situations. They could then begin to compare their new experiences with the old. They were able to describe and discover their limitations as they encountered them in everyday tasks. In essence they were experiencing the consequences of not being able to view their left side (e.g., they could no longer read or understand what they were reading—but at this phase they did not understand why). Although feelings of failure or anger arose from the participants, difficulties in performance of certain tasks (e.g., crashing into a door on the left side) seemed to lead to discovery of the disability. The participants, during this phase, began searching for reasons as to why their worlds were now different. The explanations they found were based upon their own experiences of only living in half of a world.[54]

As time passed (6 to 10 weeks into the study) the participants indicated that they were becoming more familiar with their new world. Although cognitively they became aware that they had orientation and interaction problems with the left half of their surrounding world, they were still not able to consciously use any strategies to compensate for their disabilities. Slowly, the participants began to incorporate left body parts into their daily activities, and they became more familiar with their left body parts in daily life.[54]

In the next phase, the clients began to understand that they had a limited ability to interact with the left part of the environment in everyday situations. "Understanding of the disabilities seemed to be an important prerequisite for being able to consciously search for new strategies to handle the disabilities in daily life."[54, p. 402] This understanding enabled the participants to begin to consciously use compensatory strategies. It was also easier to learn the use of compensatory strategies in occupations that had importance to the individual. In other words, it was easier to find an object to the left if they were interested in finding it. It was easier to handle walking and other known occupational activities that the participants had already learned through practicing frequently. Likewise, it was easier to learn compensatory strategies in activities if the objects involved were well known.[54]

Video feedback was also a highly effective way to demonstrate to the participants their actual performance (as most of the subjects said they often experienced difficulty perceiving their own performance).[54]

Some of the strategies that were generated from this study included: (1) conscious reflection during performance (concentrating on remembering to look to the left when starting to become involved in an occupation) and (2) search for an anchor on the left side (to enable the individual as to where to start or stop screening the environment on the left side). It is of the utmost importance that the strategies need to be based on the client's own understanding and occupational experiences.[54]

At the end of the discovery process (16 weeks) the participants had gained much experience in the conscious use of compensatory strategies. Their awareness and understanding appeared to have become deeper, and they had slowly begun to incorporate these new strategies into their daily routines.[54]

In summary, during this study, occupational therapy intervention had focused upon improving the participants' awareness of disabilities in everyday living. This included (on a daily basis) the therapist's empowering the subjects to gain experiences from task performances that confronted them with their difficulties. This, in turn, encouraged them to solve and describe the difficulties they encountered during task performance. Video feedback also played a supportive role in allowing the participants to become more aware of their problems during the performance of a task. During the rest of this time period the subjects received occupational therapy intervention that focused upon training in self-care activities (by adapting task contexts and demands as well as using the subjects' available abilities). The participants also received other individualized services (such as daily physical therapy). The basis for the specific awareness-training program was "to use meaningful everyday occupations as the therapeutic media to improve awareness of disabilities"[54, p. 399] The subjects were also supported in developing and using their own strategies. The findings in this study "demonstrated the importance of the awareness of disability before a person can consciously use compensatory strategies and incorporate them in daily life."[54, p. 404]

Deficits in Pattern Recognition, Visual Memory, and Visual Agnosia

Deficits in pattern recognition occur when the client does not efficiently and thoroughly scan objects. Persons with right brain injury are usually not able to become generally aware of objects that surround them. This leads to the individual failing to recognize a pattern or an object (because he or she does not notice it). Clients with left brain injury experience difficulty identifying objects because this is the hemisphere that directs focalized item-by-item attentional strategy. These individuals experience difficulty in being able to distinguish one letter from another (even though they may realize they are seeing a letter). Failure in the ability to recognize objects and patterns will decrease one's ability to establish an accurate understanding of his or her environment.[51]

In terms of evaluation for this deficit the star cancellation test of the Behavioral Inattention Test (discussed earlier in this unit) provides an excellent opportunity to observe the client's ability to recognize patterns and attend to visual detail. Other types of matching activities (matching a deck of cards, sorting items with similar features such as different sized bolts and screws) are also helpful when evaluating for deficits in pattern recognition. Attention to detail can also be evaluated through the computerized evaluation, MATCH.

This computerized test is available from:[51]

✧　Life Science Associates
　　1 Fenimore Rd.
　　Bayport, NY 11705
　　516-472-2111

Because complex visual processing depends upon the initiation of the stimulus through the means of a stimulus search strategy of selective visual attention, the clinician should select scanning activities that require careful inspection of detail in visual arrays. Intervention, then, should involve activities that require discrimination of subtle details. Matching and sorting activities as well as games of solitaire, double solitaire, Connect Four (Milton Bradley, East Longmeadow, MA), Scrabble (Hasbro, Providence, RI), and Dominoes (Pressman, New Brunswick, NJ) are helpful. Number and word searches, crossword puzzles, latchhook needle crafts, and large 300- to 500-piece puzzles provide opportunities for clients to develop and practice the skills that are needed for stimulus-by-stimulus search strategies. Throughout the performance of these tasks, clients should be encouraged to check their work (several times) to make certain that critical details are not missed. In order to ensure success in regaining selective attention skills, the client needs to employ a conscious strategy to compensate for the deficits created by inattention and the inability to recognize visual detail and patterns.[51] Insight on the part of the client into the nature of the visual deficit and how it has affected functional performance is critical to making learning compensation successful.[51]

Visual memory is dependent upon accuracy in pattern recognition. In order to establish a visual memory, one must first construct an accurate sensory image of the object as established within the mind's eye. Lower level skill deficits (in areas such as oculomotor control, acuity, visual field, attention, and scanning) may cause a critical part of an object to be overlooked and inaccurate construction of the visual model may result.[51] This inaccuracy of the visual model may result in the central nervous system's inability to comprehend and remember the object.[51]

Visual agnosia represents a condition where the individual is unable to identify an object. An effective evaluation involves a deficit-specific approach to object identification. The client is presented with actual objects (or pictures of objects) and asked to identify each object. To establish more specific information regarding object identification, the evaluation can conceptualize object recognition as a continuum of difficulty in which a variety of task conditions (e.g., amount, spatial arrangement, and environment) are presented in a conventional context, in an associated context, and finally, out of context.[31]

The Dynamic Assessment of Object Identification is detailed on page 269 of *Willard and Spackman's Occupational Therapy* (9th Ed.).[31]

In the intervention of visual agnosia, cues can be used to facilitate object recognition. First, the clinician can ask the client to "Look again, Mr. Green" (which provides the client with general feedback that his or her response was not correct). Next, the clinician can provide the client with specific perceptual cues to focus his or her attention on (such as a critical detail of the object—"Look, here, Mr. Green"). Any additional items that overlap the target item can be removed to allow the client to "see" the target item as a continuous whole. Specific cues that provide a choice array of possible groups that the object may belong to (e.g., "Mr. Green, does this item belong to the group of jewelry, tools, or clothing?") serve to narrow the range of possible objects (when combined with aid in identification and visual cues).[31]

Deficits in Visual Cognition

Visual cognition is the application of all the preceding skills (oculomotor control, visual field, visual acuity, attention, scanning, pattern recognition, and visual memory). It represents the highest level of visual skill integration. Deficits in these lower skill levels will decrease the client's ability to apply these skills so that they can adapt cognitively.[51] "Deficits in visual cognition result in difficulties in identifying the spatial properties of objects and mentally manipulating these properties in thought."[51, p. 207]

Selective attention is a major difficulty in being able to perform appropriate and accurate visual cognition. Most individuals who experience deficits in selective attention have difficulty in three major client performance areas:

1. They are unable to attend to the variables between objects and identify any critical features of an object or objects.

2. Scanning is often restricted to objects on the ipsilateral (sound) side.

3. They are not able to superimpose a structure in scanning an unstructured array.

In terms of evaluation, scanning tests that have a structured array are a good way to begin. Letter cancellation and line bisection are two scanning tests that are particularly sensitive to identifying visual inattention.[51]

Intervention of visual inattention and scanning deficits have previously been discussed in this section and should be applied where visual cognition deficits are indicated. As Warren aptly states, intervention should "focus on increasing the accuracy and organization of the sensory input to the system through manipulation of the environment and by providing the client with strategies to compensate for or minimize the effect of the deficit in daily living activities."[51, p. 210]

Most of the previously described conditions are due to visual dysfunction that has been caused by a CVA (stroke).

Deficits in Age-Related Macular Degeneration

Nearly 6 million Americans have been diagnosed with age-related macular degeneration (ARMD). It is the leading cause of visual dysfunction for individuals over the age of 60.[55,56]

In ARMD, the *macula* (the central area of the retina. It has as its center point the fovea which allows for the detailed vision needed in activities such as writing, setting an oven dial, and reading) gradually deteriorates with age. This causes central vision loss while leaving peripheral vision intact.[55,56] ARMD may be either *dry* (characterized by scar tissue or drusen on the retina. There is presently no known prevention or intervention for this type of macular degeneration) or *wet* (affects 10% of individuals with ARMD). In wet ARMD, the growth of abnormal blood vessels (known as *neovascularization*) may leak blood into the macular area. Laser intervention can be performed to cauterize the neovascularization and retard its development. However, the laser intervention cannot be performed if the neovascularization is around the fovea or if the hemorrhaging is extensive. Although laser intervention in the early stages is important, it cannot stop this disease's progression.[55,56]

Ophthalmologists use several tests to evaluate the progression and extent of damage caused by ARMD:

1. The Amsler Grid, a checkerboard pattern, tests the central 20% of visual field abnormalities—such as darkened spots, distortion, or areas where nothing is seen.

2. The fluorescein angiogram provides photos of the retina, macula, and fovea to detect neovascularization and the hemorrhage source. The photos can guide the laser interventions and document the disease's progression.

3. Macular perimetry is a scanning laser ophthalmoscope (SLO). With the use of this instrument, *scotomas* (non-seeing areas) can be precisely mapped out.[56,57] It can also determine retinal areas that are most viable for focusing on details. This spot is termed the *preferred retinal locus* (PRL).[56,57] *Phantom vision* (Charles Bonnet syndrome), at times, may become a side effect of vision loss.[56,57]

There are three basic levels of visual impairment:

1. *Moderate low vision.* With this level visual acuity is between 20/80 and 20/160. These individuals experience near-normal reading performance with magnifiers and other vision-enhancing devices.

2. *Severe low vision.* With this level visual acuity is between 20/200 and 20/400. These persons can read slower-than-normal with magnifiers and other vision-enhancing devices (e.g., such as talking aids, tactile cues, and machines such as the Video Eye Millennium [a machine whose power magnification system is helpful with reading and other everyday tasks] [Video Eye, Boise, ID]).

3. *Profound low vision.* At this level visual acuity is between 20/500 and 20/1000. These order adults are able to experience limited reading ability with high powered aids and other vision enhancing devices.[56]

Occupational therapists and occupational therapy assistants specializing in visual rehabilitation have an outstanding opportunity to provide services to this rapidly growing population of late life adults, diagnosed with ARMD. First, we clinicians possess an understanding of the disease process and the aging body. Second, we have had a long history of utilizing adaptations for daily living activities. Third, we possess an awareness of the unique needs of the geriatric population.[56]

Intervention in Age-Related Macular Degeneration

Visual impairment due to ARMD can have a profound effect on most activities of daily living. However, vision-enhancing devices and compensatory techniques are helpful in enabling the client to adapt and remain independent. The tasks most often compromised are those that deal with reading, functional mobility skills, and writing.[56]

Reading occurs within a range of lighting and distances (and with varying sizes and types of materials). Some examples include reading information from food labels and directions, price tags, clothing labels, clocks, wrist watches, appliance dials (e.g., dryer, microwave, washing machine, stove), telephone dials or buttons, financial statements, street and store signs, elevator buttons, weather bulletins on the television and pleasurable materials (such as sheet music, books, newspapers, and magazines).[56]

Eye-hand coordination activities such as those needed for coordinating one's hand and pen tip with the line on which a person is writing is another area of difficulty for those with ARMD. Likewise, functional mobility activities (e.g., moving around the house and yard; negotiating curbs and stairs; negotiating obstacles and people in the house, the doctor's office, the store, or any other area; meal preparation; housekeeping; self-care tasks; and shopping) are difficult due to varying levels of contrast and lighting.[56]

Training the client to utilize the PRL, often termed *eccentric viewing* or *eccentric fixation*, can improve the performance of many daily living tasks. By using the PRL (the area of clearest viewing on a retina with a damaged macula), an individual with ARMD is taught to look around the *scotoma* (the scarred or damaged macular area). Clinicians trained in eccentric viewing methodologies (such as eye exercises, card exercises, saccades [jumping between two objects], eye-hand coordination techniques, and scanning using the PRL) usually teach clients to use their PRL within a few sessions.[56] Clients need to practice these techniques so that they readily become accessible to them.

Low Vision Technology

Much of the intervention with clients who are diagnosed with ARMD involves training in low vision techniques and devices. This should take place in the environment where they will be utilized.

There are three variables that can be manipulated to increase the independence of an older adult with ARMD (and other vision disorders). These are size, contrast, and lighting.

Size involves using different types of magnification. First, there is relative-distance magnification. This involves moving the object closer to the client's eyes (e.g., moving closer to the television set instead of sitting across the room). A second method involves the use of angular magnification using a magnifier to make an object appear larger. Most clients require training with these instruments due to the variety of focal distances and types of optical devices. Low vision optical devices are specific to task. Clients may need multiple magnifying aids to meet their needs. For instance, they may need a hand-held magnifier to read price tags; magnifying eyeglasses to read magazines, newspapers, and books; television magnifiers; and a telescopic device to read bus signs from a distance. Clients may also need to be taught how to handle magnifying devices. For example, if a client is using magnifying eyeglasses, he or she may need to be taught to hold the reading material much closer than the individual was accustomed to and to learn to move the reading material rather than one's eyes. Also, repeated instruction may be needed in how to keep the print in focus. When using a telescopic device, a client may first need to be taught to practice locating a stationary object.[56-58] A third way includes relative size magnification. With this method the object itself is made large (large-print books and magazines, large print address books, oversize kitchen timers, large print playing cards, enlarged checks, and computer software that can increase the print size on most computers). A fourth method involves electronic magnification (use of a copy machine, increasing the letter size and words by increasing the print size of a computer, and closed circuit television that uses a device to enlarge the image onto a television screen).[56,58]

Contrast is another variable that can be easily manipulated to increase the visibility of objects. Many older adults with low vision experience difficulty with contrast sensitivity. This involves being able to detect differences between shades of grey and sensitivity to detect the background from the foreground. Examples of the effective use of contrast are: bold, lined paper and black felt-tipped pens can facilitate writing and reading; in the kitchen a dark-colored cutting board can be used with light-colored food substances such as chicken, onions, and potatoes; and a light-colored board can be used when slicing green peppers, tomatoes, red meat, or carrots. Tea and coffee can be poured into a light-colored mug. Colored liquid-level indicators can be used to prevent overpouring. White, black, or orange raised dots or lines can be added to appliances that have dials; colored toothpaste, when applied to white bristles, aids in helping the toothbrushing process; and to achieve the best possible contrast in photocopies, all copies must be made from the originals (copies of a copy are low contrast and difficult to read).[56,58]

Lighting is the third variable that can be used to improve the visual functioning of the older person with ARMD. Lighting is a critical factor for maximizing the retina's function. Clients with ARMD require two to three times more light than was needed when this same individual was younger. Brighter overhead lighting in the kitchen makes seeing food in a pot or plate or finding a can in the cabinet easier. Increased lighting on the stairs or in the bathroom is helpful in preventing falls. Task lighting (for reading, writing, and mending clothes) is also helpful in empowering the older adult with ARMD to complete everyday tasks. Penlights and/or flashlights are helpful in providing extra lighting for menus, price tags, appliance dials, thermostats, hot water heaters, and house heaters.[56,58] Manufacturers have recently begun to sell voice operated light switches to the public.

Glare (caused when light reflects from a shiny surface) reduction also needs to be addressed. Glare can be controlled in a number of ways. First, one can decrease glare by changing the surface from which the light is being reflected (e.g., place a desk blotter on a shiny table or desk or put a non-glare placemat or towel upon a shiny kitchen counter). Next, one can wear sunglasses with light colored lenses (amber is helpful) to ward off glare. Third, reduce glare by positioning the individual's body or the light in relation to the light in a different manner (e.g., ask the client to sit with his or her back to the window; have the light from a table lamp shine directly on the page from the side of the client's better eye; and ask the client to place the table lamp behind him or her when reading). Sheer shades, curtains, or blinds can be adjusted to decrease glare while at the same time maximizing the amount of sunlight coming back through the window. To reduce glare, the client can try several shades of sunglasses for use in a number of lighting situations (e.g., a sunny day versus a day when there is a lot of cloud cover) before a pair or two can be found that works adequately and/or wear a large brimmed hat or visor to counteract glare.[56,58]

There are other devices helpful to those elders with impaired vision that use sound. Some examples include talking calendars, clocks, and scales. Computer software is available that can convert text to speech.

"With an increasingly elderly population in need of low vision services, the opportunities for low vision specialists in developing comprehensive rehabilitation programs for this population will continue to expand."[52, p. 23] In working with clients who are diagnosed with ARMD, Anne Toth-Riddering reminds us that, "In many instances, simple manipulation of an environment and enhancement of the residual vision allows the client to complete tasks more independently."[56, p. 23]

The following are resources that are useful with low vision technology:

- ✧ Cole, R. D. & Rosenthal, B. P. (Eds.). (1996). *Remediation and management of low vision.* St. Louis: Mosby.

- ✧ Gentile, M. (1997). *Functional guide to evaluation and treatment options.* Bethesda, MD: The American Occupational Therapy Association, Inc.
  1-800-SAY-AOTA

- ✧ Low Vision Gateway
  www.lowvision.org

- ✧ *Occupational therapy practice guidelines for adults with low vision.* Bethesda, MD: The American Occupational Therapy Association, Inc.
  1-877-404-AOTA

- ✧ Warren, M. (Ed.). Self-paced clinical course. *Low vision: Occupational therapy intervention with the older adult.* Bethesda, MD: The American Occupational Therapy Association, Inc.
  1-877-404-AOTA

- ✧ *Resource guide: Treatment of adults with low vision.* Bethesda, MD: The American Occupational Therapy Association, Inc.
  1-800-SAY-AOTA

- ✧ Special Equipment
  ▲ Eschenbach Portable Low Vision Kit (Contains a variety of low vision magnifying aids in a broad range of powers, that are most commonly dispensed to ARMD clients.)

Eschenbach: Innovators in Low Vision
904 Ethan Allen Hwy
Ridgefield, CT 06877
1-877-422-7300
www.eschenbach.com

⌃ The Video Eye Millennium 11
Video from
Video Eye Corporation
Department MM
10211 West Emerald St.
Boise, ID 83704
1-800-909-7052
www.videoeyecorp.com
A power magnification system that aids clients to continue reading and doing everyday tasks

✧ Catalogs Selling Adaptive Aids
⌃ Independent Living Aids (ILA)
1-800-537-2118

⌃ Lighthouse Catalog
Information and Resource Service
1-800-334-5497
Products Catalog: 1-800-829-0500

⌃ Maxi Aids
1-800-522-6294

✧ Communication (Reading) Aids
⌃ American Printing House for the Blind (*Newsweek* and *Reader's Digest* on tape)
1-800-223-1839
www.apn.org

⌃ Doubleday Large-Print Library
1-800-688-4442
www.JoinDLP.com
(enter online Code PB2)

⌃ Large-Print Cookbooks

612-540-2311
⌃ Large-Print *Literary Reader*
1-800-216-5893

⌃ Large-Print *Reader's Digest*
1-800-877-5293

⌃ National Library Service for the Blind and Physically Handicapped (Free Talking Books)
1-800-424-8567
www.loc.gov/nls

⌃ *New York Times Weekly*
Large Print Edition
1-800-631-2581

⌃ *Time Magazine* Large-Print Edition
1-800-881-2137

⌃ Thorndike Press and G.K. Hall
1-800-223-6121
www.mir.com/Thorndike

⌃ Ulverscroft Large Print Books, Inc.
1-800-955-9659
www.ulverscroft.com

✧ Organizations
⌃ American Foundation for the Blind
11 Penn Plaza, Suite 300
New York, NY 10001
212-502-7600

⌃ American Optometric Association
Low Vision Section
243 N. Lindbergh Blvd.
St. Louis, MO 63141
314-991-4100

⌃ Macular Degeneration International
2968 West Ina Rd. #106
Tucson, AZ 85741
520-797-2525

PERCEPTION AND PERCEPTUAL MOTOR DYSFUNCTION

Perception involves the mechanism by which the brain interprets sensory information that is received from the environment.[59]

Optimally the test battery should include perceptual tests that require a motor response or have flexible response requirements from either of the modes. Observations of performance and the analysis of the perceptual-motor demands of functional everyday activities further serve to complement standardized evaluation procedures. This aids in relating test results to functional performance.[59] Before the perceptual evaluation is performed, the therapist must have completed evaluations of both motor and sensory functions as well as being aware of language deficits, general alertness, and responsiveness.[59]

Approaches to intervention can involve the remedial (this is characterized by seeking to cause some change in the central nervous system functions) and/or the adaptive/functional (this is characterized by the repetitive practice of specific tasks that can enable the client to become more independent in activities of daily living performance) methods.[59] Only the most common perceptual and perceptual-motor deficits that affect late life adults will be presented.

Stereognosis

Stereognosis involves the perceptual skill that allows the individual to identify common shapes and objects without the use of vision. It is dependent on intact parietal cortical function. Stereognosis is the skill that makes possible reaching into one's purse or pocket and finding keys or reaching into a dark room and finding the light switch. Proprioception and stereognosis enable the use of hand tools and the performance of hand activities without the need to visually concentrate on the implements being used (e.g., knitting while watching television, using a fork while conversing, and typing while looking at the computer monitor).

Deficits in stereognosis are termed *astereognosis*. Tests for stereognosis generally involve having the client's vision occluded (with the client's hand resting on its dorsal surface against the table). Objects are presented randomly. Manipulation of objects is encouraged. The client should be asked to name the object or describe its properties (if he or she is unable to name the object). Test objects can include common articles (such as a metal teaspoon or a plastic comb) that incorporate the client's ethnic and social background. To ensure that the individual being tested has not had previous experience, three-dimensional geometric shapes can be used to evaluate form and shape perception. In *Evaluation and Treatment of Perceptual and Perceptual Motor Deficits*, Pedretti, Zoltan, and Wheatly present specific stereognosis test procedures and the form for Recording the Test of Stereognosis.[59]

The intervention for astereognosis is initiated with the client being permitted to see and hear an object as it is being felt (to benefit intersensory facilitation). Vision is occluded during a period of tactile exploration. Next, a pad is placed on the table top. Visual and auditory cues are eliminated (which allows the client to rely on tactile-kinesthetic input solely). Re-education is initiated with the gross discrimination of very dissimilar objects. Then the client is asked to estimate quantities of the same items (e.g., the number of marbles in a box) through touch alone. Next, the client is directed to discriminate between small and large objects hidden in sand or rice. The client is asked to discriminate between two- and three-dimensional objects. Training is finalized when the client can pick a small object from several objects.[59,60]

Body Scheme

Body scheme involves a postural model that is related to the way an individual perceives the position of his or her body and the relationship of the various body parts. It involves one's knowledge of body construction, its spatial relationships, and its anatomic elements; a person's ability to differentiate between left and right; an individual's ability to visualize the body in movement as well as its parts in different positional relationships; and one's ability to recognize the difference between bodily health and disease.[59]

Asomatognosia is a loss of body scheme. It can be evaluated by asking the client to point to body parts on command as well as by imitation.[59] Body scheme disorders are usually associated with parietal lobe damage. Some therapists use body and face puzzles as well as the "draw-a-person" test. However with the two latter tests, the therapist must first rule out constructional apraxia as a cause of poor performance. Right and/or left discrimination deficits can occur in intrapersonal space and/or extrapersonal space. To evaluate right and/or left discrimination the therapist can ask the client to point to his or her own body part and specify the right or left side. *Unilateral inattention* (visual inattention has been discussed in the preceding section on visual dysfunction) refers to the inability to integrate perception from the left side of space or the left side of the body (left neglect is more prevalent than right side inattention). The most effective evaluation of unilateral inattention in terms of body scheme is for the therapist to directly observe the client dressing and performing other activities of daily living .[59,60]

The intervention for body scheme disorders can include a variety of approaches. Using the remedial approach for treating unilateral body neglect, the clinician can apply sensory input (e.g., rubbing a client's arm or leg) before the client dresses (it is always wise to observe precautions to prevent increased spasticity with this approach). The clinician can also engage the client in activities that focus attention on the affected side (e.g., conversing or treating a client from the affected side).

When using an adaptive or compensatory approach, the clinician can place work materials, food, and utensils on the unaffected side as well as provide instructions from that side. Repetitive cuing and practice can also be effective.[59] The transfer training approach is another type of useful intervention method. An example of this strategy might include the client practicing assembling human figure puzzles. The clinician would then quiz the client about the location of the body parts. At a later stage, the client may be able to appropriately touch and name his or her own body parts. The Bobath neurodevelopmental approach is yet another way to provide body scheme disorder intervention. With this method bilateral weight bearing activity can be applied to improve function. "Perceptual retraining is integral to the handling techniques and feedback about correct movement during the motor retraining program."[59, p. 232] It can help to stimulate total body awareness as well as enhance proprioception.[29,30,59]

PRAXIS AND APRAXIA

Ideomotor and Ideational Apraxia

"*Praxis* is the ability to plan and perform purposeful movement."[59, p. 235] *Apraxia* is an impairment in the ability to perform purposeful movement when there is no loss of coordination, motor power, sensation, or basic comprehension skills.[59] Apraxia is usually the result of a dominant hemisphere lesion. *Ideomotor apraxia* is characterized by the client being able to perform the act automatically but he or she is not able to perform willfully on command. It is important to observe the client in activity performance so that this deficit can be correctly identified. *Ideational apraxia* is characterized by the inability of the client to form the concept of movement and his or her inability to perform the act either automatically or on command.

The Praxial (Motor Planning) Procedure as described on page 237 of *Occupational Therapy Practice Skills for Physical Dysfunction* (Adapted from Zoltan and Associates: *Perceptual Motor Evaluation for Head Injured and Other Neurologically Impaired Adults* [Revised Edition]. San Jose, CA, 1987, Santa Clara Medical Center) is a screening evaluation that includes eight actions on command (e.g., blowing out a match, drinking a glass of water, brushing one's teeth, cutting paper with scissors, throwing a ball, saluting, washing one's hands, and acting like a boxer). These actions include asking the client to imitate the examiner (e.g., "I am blowing out the match—now you show me how you...").

The first five of these actions involve asking the client to use real objects (e.g., the examiner asks, after presenting a ball, "Show me how you throw a ball"). During this portion of the test the examiner should ensure that the client will be safe in handling any object. As the test proceeds the examiner should indicate the type of apraxia that is observed during the activity (e.g., blowing out a match involves buccal-facial movement abilities; cutting with scissors involves unilateral limb kinetic movement; drinking from a glass includes buccal-facial, unilateral limb, and kinetic movements). The examiner is asked to rate each item separately on a scale of 0 to 3. "0" indicates that the individual can perform the action in an intact manner. "1" indicates that the client is impaired but is able to approximate an accurate response for most of the task (the response is compromised or is greater than the allotted time [10 seconds for each time]). "2" indicates that the client is severely impaired (poor approximation of an accurate response, trial and error is used, and the response is greater than the allotted time). "3" indicates that the client is unable to attempt a response and unable to perform.[59]

Intervention of ideomotor and ideational apraxia involves providing concise, clear, short, and concrete instruction (aphasia may be present as well). The task needs to be broken down into clear and concise component steps. Providing the client with guidance through the correct movement (giving proprioceptive and tactile input with brief verbal instruction) is helpful. Once the client can perform each step of the task separately, the clinician can begin to combine steps—grading slowly until the task is completed.

For instance, with hair combing the clinician can break the task into steps:

1. Lift the comb.
2. Bring the comb up to the hair.
3. Move the comb across the top of the head.
4. Then bring the comb down the left side.
5. Next, bring the comb down the right side of the hair.
6. Then bring the comb down the back.
7. Replace the comb on the table.

To be effective, much repetition is necessary.[59]

Constructional Apraxia

In *constructional apraxia* the client is not able to construct a design, make a copy, or draw. The client is not able to assemble or organize parts into a whole (as in drawings that are two-dimensional or putting block designs together that are three-dimensional). This dysfunction is related to the parietal lobes (usually from a CVA or severe head injury).[59] Functional activities that are affected by constructional apraxia involve activities such as dressing, setting a table, and stacking a dishwasher. The following four tests for evaluating constructional praxis are recommended:

❖   The Test of Visual Motor Skills (TVMS)

Gardner, M. F. (1992). *The test of visual-motor skills* (TVMS). Burlingame, CA: Psychological and Education Publications.

❖   The Benton Visual Retention Test

Sivan, A. B. (1992). *The Benton visual retention test*. San Antonio, TX: The Psychological Corporation.

❖   The Rey Complex Figure

Lezak, M. D. (1983). *Neuropsychological assessment* (2nd Ed.). New York: Oxford University Press.

❖   The Three-Dimensional Block Construction Test

Benton, A. L. & Fogel, M. L. (1962). Three-dimensional constructional praxis: A clinical test. *Arch Neurol, 7*, 347.

In evaluating the client's performance for daily living tasks, the therapist should observe the client dressing. To perform this type of task in a successful manner, there needs to be integration of motor planning, visual perception, and motor execution.[29,30,59]

If one employs a transfer training or remedial approach to treating the client, then practice of constructional tasks, guidance, three-dimensional models, and demonstration will be necessary. Tasks can be graded in complexity (for instance, the number of places that are required to assemble a task).[59]

Dressing Apraxia

Dressing apraxia involves the inability to perform and plan the motor activities that are necessary for dressing. It is linked with problems of spatial orientation, body scheme, and constructional apraxia. In this disorder the client experiences difficulty in initiating dressing or may make errors in dressing orientation (e.g., putting on clothes upside down, inside out, and on the wrong side of the body).[29,30,59]

In intervention, the clinician should instruct by using set patterns for dressing that present cues to help the client distinguish the left, the right, the front, and the back. It is helpful to have the client position the garment the same way each time (e.g., slacks with the zipper facing up, a shirt with buttons facing up). Labels can also enhance the client's ability to differentiate between the front and the back of a garment. Another helpful method is to use color-coded small buttons or ribbons for the left, right, back, or front of a garment.[29] In general a functional or adaptive approach that is combined with the neurodevelopmental approach has been effective with those late life adults who experience dressing apraxia.[29,30,59]

The profession of occupational therapy has much to offer older adults who experience perceptual and perceptual-motor dysfunction. These deficits affect the client's overall functioning status. Through careful evaluation and purposeful intervention clinicians can provide this population segment with methods and technology to improve their self-care abilities—thus, increasing their feelings of self-worth as well.

CEREBROVASCULAR ACCIDENT AND OCCUPATIONAL THERAPY INTERVENTION APPROACHES

A CVA, commonly termed *stroke*, is the second most significant cardiovascular disease found in late life adults. This condition is the third most common cause of death in the United States and most other industrialized countries.[61]

Stroke, defined as a rapid onset of neurological deficits that last 24 hours or more, is generally the result of:

1. Intracerebral hemorrhage (a leak of blood from the vascular system)
2. Thrombosis and/or embolism (an obstruction of blood flow through the vascular system)
3. Vascular insufficiency

These conditions lead to the infarction of brain tissue.[61,62]

Common impairments include *hemiplegia* (paralysis that occurs on the contralateral side of the lesion); *hemiparesis* (weakness that occurs on one side of the body); visual/perceptual impairments, cognitive impairments, perceptual/motor dysfunction, *aphasia* (language difficulties which may interfere with expressive and receptive language, the understanding of nonverbal and pragmatic language as well as written expression); gross and fine motor impairment, and sensory disturbances.[62] Cognitive, visual/perceptual impairments, and perceptual/motor dysfunction (as seen in a CVA) have been discussed in the preceding components of this unit.

Many elderly clients with a CVA may be confused and/or suffer from some type of aphasia. Therefore, it is important to be clear when giving instructions or presenting an evaluation. Suggestions for facilitating communication and enhancing appropriate management and rehabilitation are as follows:

- ✧ Gain the client's attention before attempting to communicate.
- ✧ Face the person directly so that facial cues can be discerned.
- ✧ Use short, simple sentences.
- ✧ Keep to the topic; keep to one subject at a time.
- ✧ Speak distinctly and at a moderate rate.
- ✧ Do not move about while speaking because movement can cause voice level fluctuations as well as confusion.
- ✧ Avoid changing topics in a sudden manner. When subjects are changed, make certain that it is done gradually and that the client understands the change.
- ✧ Avoid asking the client to choose from a number of choices; often the client may have difficulty retaining the information.
- ✧ Gesture and demonstrate information that you are trying to convey.
- ✧ Try to use the same words each time you repeat the same or similar routine.
- ✧ If the client does not respond appropriately the first time, repeat the instruction or the question in a different way.
- ✧ Allow the client adequate time to respond.

❖ Do not shout at the client; speak with a normal vocal intensity.

❖ Use yes or no questions if this is the only manner in which the client can respond.

❖ Encourage and praise the client for each accomplishment.

❖ Anticipate and understand that the client might cry, laugh, swear without provocation, or lose control. When this happens, try to redirect the client's attention to other tasks.

❖ Avoid background sounds (e.g., turn off radios and television, discourage paper shuffling and chairs scraping).

❖ Encourage the client's communication adjustments by accepting his or her compensation modes and methods of communication.

❖ Avoid covering your face with your hands when conversing and doing any other distracting activity with your mouth (such as chewing gum, drinking, or eating while speaking).[10]

❖ Foster a positive attitude.

General Evaluation Recommendations

Evaluation of clients who have been diagnosed with a CVA should begin with performance areas (if this is possible). If the CVA is severe, the therapist may need to begin the evaluation focused upon performance components that may affect (at a later time) performance areas. Evaluation, at this stage, should include the following areas:

1. Sensory processing
2. Range of motion (active and passive as determined with a goniometer)
3. Muscular tone
4. Muscle strength
5. Presence of edema (may use circumferential measurements with tape or a volumeter)
6 Perceptual/visual skills
7. Cognitive skills
8. Psychosocial status

If the client is able to engage in some self-care activities, then the evaluation should begin with self-care and basic functional mobility involving everyday tasks (e.g., going to the toilet, getting out of bed). Many clients with CVA experience *dysphagia* (difficulties swallowing). Because dysphagia can lead to possible aspiration, a swallowing evaluation should be completed as soon as possible. This type of evaluation can be performed by either an occupational or speech therapist.[63]

Stroke rehabilitation may occur in an acute care hospital (where rehabilitation interventions are normally initiated during the acute phase), at an inpatient rehabilitation hospital or unit, in a skilled nursing facility, at an outpatient rehabilitation facility (may be free-standing or attached to an acute care or rehabilitation hospital), and in home-based rehabilitation where the client is treated within his or her own residence.[64] Most areas of intervention for stroke include remediation of the affected areas as much as is possible, instruction in self-care activities, education in mobility within the context of daily activities, and instruction in homemaking, home management, and driving.

Somatic Sensation Testing

Because of safety reasons, it is important to know as early as possible if there are any major sensory deficits (e.g., Would a client be able to tell if his or her hand were on a hot stove? Can an individual indicate that he or she needs warm gloves because the weather is severely cold? Is the client able to feel pressure in the sacral area when seated in a wheelchair?)?

When performing somatic sensation testing certain principles of methodology should be followed: explain the procedure to the client (allowing the client to ask for feedback or questions); always make certain the client's eyes are not occluded when giving instructions; always test non-affected areas as well as affected areas to establish what is normal for that person and to determine what the client understands; when occluding the client's vision for a test, ask the client to open his or her eyes in between tests to avoid disorientation or dizziness; all stimuli should be applied proximal to distal on ventral and dorsal surfaces and randomly interspersed with nonpresentation trials; if the client is not able to verbally respond, he or she can point to a picture, replicate a movement, or point to a duplicate stimulus; all scoring, recording methods, and definitions need to be constant; and all results should be entered on the appropriate form and dated.[65] All testing should be administered in a distraction-free, quiet setting with vision occluded.

Primary Somatic Testing

It should be noted that in all of the following types of somatic tests that are presented here, persons with receptive aphasia cannot validly be tested.

Light touch involves the ability to "feel" light touch. The stimulus involved is a light touch with an eraser tip or a cotton swab over small areas of the client's skin. With vision occluded, the client is to indicate when a stimulus is felt (usually by stating "yes" or "now" or pointing to the location).[65,66] The Semmes-Weinstein calibrated monofilament test (controls the amount of force applied to the client's hand via a calibrated hand-held instrument) is another method of testing light touch. It is especially helpful for those with peripheral nerve involvement.[65]

The ability to feel pain is another important aspect of primary somatic testing. As a stimulus the therapist can use a safety pin with one blunt end and one sharp end (the pin must be cleaned with an alcohol swab before testing and must be discarded after each test). The therapist should apply mixed sharp and dull in a random manner. The client responds by giving an indication when and which stimulus is felt—by answering "dull" or "sharp."[65,66]

Thermal sensation involves the ability to distinguish variations in temperature. The stimulus in this test is water capped test tubes; one is filled with ice water and the other with hot tap water. (Both are tolerable to normal touch.) The therapist then randomly alternates the use of each test tube. The stimulus should be kept on the body surface long enough to allow a temperature change to occur on the skin's surface (approximately one second).[65,66] Another method is the use of the Hot/Cold Discrimination Kit by Rolyan (available at the following address: Smith and Nephew Rolyan, Inc., One Quality Drive, P.O. Box 1005, Germantown, WI 53022).[66] In both procedures the client is asked to indicate if the stimulus that is felt is hot or cold.[65,66]

Discriminate Somatic System

Please note, again, that in somatic testing a person with receptive aphasia cannot be validly tested.

The ability to localize touch or "tactile localization" is tested by the therapist touching the client's skin with an eraser tip. Stimulus duration and intensity will influence the accuracy of the response. After each stimulus, the client will open his or her eyes and describe the area touched or place a finger on that area.[65,66]

Two-point discrimination is the ability to perceive two distinct stimuli when one is touched with two stimuli simultaneously. The therapist may use an aesthesiometer, a paper clip, or a Boley gauge as a stimulus. Two points are simultaneously applied along the longitudinal axis in the center of the area to be tested (with equal light pressure to the palmar surface of the forearm, hand, and fingers). During the testing the therapist adjusts the distance between the double stimuli in order to identify the amount of distance that is needed between the two stimuli before the client is able to perceive that two stimuli are present. One-point application trials are interspersed with two-point test trials. The client is then asked to identify the stimulus with the response of "two-point" or "one point."[65,66]

Stereognosis is the ability to tactually identify objects. This test has been described in a preceding component (Perceptual/Motor Dysfunction within this unit.

Proprioception is the ability to identify limb position in space. The therapist holds the body part that is being tested in a lateral position to avoid cutaneous input. Slowly, the therapist passively positions the joint being tested. Joints are tested in combination and in isolation. The client is then asked to reproduce the position with the opposite extremity. If the client is not able to copy the limb's position, he or she may respond with a gesture or point to directional arrows on a slate—"down," "up."[60,65]

Kinesthesia is the ability to be aware of movement in space. To provide the stimulus, the therapist holds the body part being tested in a lateral position so that the tactile input is reduced. Next, the joint is moved up and down. The level of kinesthetic detection is influenced by velocity. It is easier to detect kinesthesia when the movement is brisk. The client is then asked to indicate in which direction the body part was moved.[65,66]

There are several methods by which one can record sensation. First, sensation can be recorded as intact, impaired, or absent. Other recording options include graphs, diagrams, dermatome distribution, peripheral nerve distribution, the number of trials (such as in the stereognosis test), or the number of correct responses.[65]

Intervention for Sensory Dysfunction

Sensory loss inhibits movement. Thus, movement that is attempted may be uncoordinated or clumsy. The possibility of injury is a major concern. Therefore, the most major concern is the client's safety and ensuring that the client will not be injured by burning, bumping, or becoming snagged on equipment or furniture during performance of everyday activities. Compensation (teaching compensatory techniques) plays a big factor in promoting safety. The following are some examples of the use of compensatory techniques:

1. Utilization of the less affected hand to perform a variety of activities (eating, cooking, ironing)
2. Utilization of vision to observe motion and location of body parts

3. Utilization of the less affected hand to test bath water (or use of a bath thermometer)

4. Utilization of adaptive devices (e.g., one-handed cutting board to avoid cutting the affected hand, one-handed rocking knife, one-handed knitting needle setup)

The client who has been diagnosed with CVA needs to become aware of his or her sensory deficits. Safety issues during performance of activities of daily living must be continuously brought to the client's attention and reinforced. Depending on the client's specific condition, it may be possible to train the individual to check the position of the limbs by observing them. Clients need to be evaluated for safety awareness and trained to consider safety factors in a given activity (especially if a potential hazard exists such as can be found in cooking). The client who wishes to continue to be involved in home management activities needs to demonstrate safety awareness, to use good judgment, and to be able to utilize visual compensation techniques for sensory loss. The therapist frequently needs to repeat instruction and cueing to reinforce compensatory strategies. In cases where clients exhibit poor judgment, poor memory, the inability to understand cause-and-effect relationships, and preservation, it becomes difficult for these individuals to effectively attend to compensatory techniques. In these situations, supervision is needed.[66]

Remedial intervention is another approach in improving client performance. *Sensory bombardment* (which involves stimulating as many of the senses as is possible) has been found to be helpful in some clients. During regular therapeutic activities, the therapist can stroke or touch the affected parts and encourage the client to observe the touch stimulation and movement. Weight bearing on various body parts (arms, trunk, legs) increases proprioceptive feedback.[66]

Eggers provides a variety of interventional modalities for sensory retraining. As a prerequisite for intervention, the clinician must normalize the client's muscle tone and find the optimal position that is the most conducive for sensory re-education. Eggers is an advocate for integrating both motor and sensory retraining. This sensory retraining program focuses upon kinesthetic and tactile re-education. The therapist must find ways to provide stimulating sensation without increasing spasticity. Because many clients exhibit delayed processing of sensory information, sufficient time must be allowed for these individuals to make responses to sensory information. When retraining for tactile-kinesthetic functions, other deficits such as aphasia, visual/perceptual dysfunction and hemianopsia need to be considered. If these clients are to relearn sensation, variation and repetition of sensory stimuli are necessary.[60]

Eggers promotes a graded intervention program for sensory dysfunction. Initially, the client is permitted to hear and see an object as it is being felt (for the benefit of intersensory facilitation). Next, vision is occluded during tactile exploration. At the final stage of intervention a pad is placed on the table top so that both visual and auditory clues are eliminated. Thus, the client relies only on tactile-kinesthetic input. Tactile-kinesthetic re-education begins with the gross discrimination of objects that are dissimilar (e.g., round or square shapes, rough or smooth texture). A client may be asked to bilaterally roll large cylinders that are covered with different materials. The nonaffected hand is used to guide the affected hand during this process. Next the client is asked to estimate quantities (e.g., the number of marbles in a box) through touch. When this is accomplished, the client then begins training to learn to discriminate between large and small objects that are hidden in the sand—progressing to the point when the client is able to discriminate between two- and three-dimensional objects. As the final part of the training, the client is asked to pick a specific small object from among several objects.[60]

Dysphagia Management

Dysphagia is defined as being unable or having difficulty with swallowing. *Deglutition* is the normal consumption of liquids or solids. Eating, the most basic activity of daily living, also includes the ability to reach for food, place it in the mouth, and swallow it. The occupational therapist is trained to evaluate and treat all the components involved in eating: muscle tone and positioning of the trunk, head, and upper and lower extremities; motor control; oral and pharyngeal function; inhibition of primitive reflexes; and the intervention of perceptual, sensory, and cognitive dysfunction that may prevent the client from appropriately participating in the eating process. Older adult involvement in acquired dysphagia includes a variety of conditions. The most notable is CVA. Parkinson's disease, brain tumor, head injury, and anoxia are other conditions found in late life adults that contribute to dysphagia and failure to thrive.[67,68]

Deglutition is a complex sensorimotor process that involves the brain stem, the cortex, six cranial nerves (trigeminal-V, facial-VII, glossopharyngeal-IX, vagus-X, spinal accessory-XI, and hypoglossal-XII), 48 pairs of muscles, and three cervical nerve segments.[10,67]

Swallowing involves the following four stages.

THE ANTICIPATORY/ORAL PREPARATORY PHASE

This is initiated with the act of looking at and reaching for food. Olfactory and visual information stimulates secretions from the swallowing glands. It is at this point that the individual decides the type, quantity, and rate of oral intake that he or she will pursue. When the tactile contact is made with the food, the jaw comes forward to open. The lips then close around a utensil or glass to remove the food. The labial musculature acts to form a seal to prevent any food or liquid from leaking out of the oral cavity. Chewing begins as the mandible moves in a strong combined lateral and rotary direction. Saliva is produced when sensations of taste, smell, food texture, and chewing take place. The chewing action of the tongue and mandibles is repeated in a rhythmical fashion until a cohesive *bolus* (mass of chewed food) is formed. When liquids enter the oral cavity, the tongue forms a groove. The shape of this groove (which occurs along the dorsal surface of the tongue) funnels the liquid towards the pharynx.

In preparation for the next stage, the bolus (now a cohesive mass) is held between the anterior tongue and the plate. The tongue forms a cup around the bolus to seal it against the hard palate. The airway is opened, and the larynx and pharynx are at rest.[10,65,67]

THE ORAL PHASE

This is initiated when the tongue moves the bolus toward the back of the mouth. The tongue forms a central groove to funnel the food in a posterior position. The oral stage, which requires the individual to be alert, is voluntary. A normal voluntary swallow is needed to elicit a strong swallow response for use by the pharynx in the next phase.[10,65,67]

THE PHARYNGEAL PHASE

During this phase breathing is briefly interrupted. As the food enters the pharynx, the initiation of the involuntary components of the swallow begins. Once the swallow response has been triggered, it continues (without pause) in the movement of the bolus until the total act is completed. This swallow response is controlled by the medulla oblongata in the brain stem. As the swallow response is triggered, several physiologic functions occur that act to prevent regurgitation of the material into the nasal cavity. The entire pharyngeal tube elevates and peristalsis occurs, carrying the bolus to the top of the esophagus. This must be a rapid movement so that respiration is interrupted only on a brief basis. The larynx elevates, the vocal cords adduct, and there is a downward bending of the epiglottis. The closing of the epiglottis and vocal cords prevents food from entering the airway. Finally, there is a relaxation and opening of the upper esophageal sphincter. When this sphincter relaxes, food then passes from the pharynx into the esophagus. If the involuntary swallow response does not occur, there will not be a normal swallow.[10,65,67]

THE ESOPHAGEAL PHASE

This phase begins when the bolus enters the esophagus through the cricopharyngeal sphincter. Breathing is resumed, and the food is transported through the esophagus by peristaltic wave contractions to the stomach.[10,65,67]

Nelson recommends the following to be parts of the evaluation process:
1. Medical chart review.
2. Mental status review (e.g., is the client alert? oriented? able to follow commands?).
3. Physical status evaluation (involves head and trunk control which includes evaluating strength, tone, and quality of movement of the head, neck, and trunk. Head control is necessary to provide adequate jaw and tongue movement so that there is an optimal swallow response). Outer oral status (oral sensation, facial muscle evaluation, oral reflexes) and inner oral status (tongue musculature, motor control and movement, palatal function and swallowing, dentition [teeth, gums, inner cheek], and saliva formation) need to be functioning adequately in order to promote a safe swallow.[67]
4. The clinical evaluation of the swallow. During this process the client must be assured a safe swallow. The client's ability to protect the airway must be carefully assessed. The client needs an intact palatal reflect, intact elevation of the larynx, and the ability to emit a productive cough.[67] It should be noted that soft food (puréed) is more easily formed into a bolus than chopped food. Ground food allows the therapist to assess a client's ability to chew and form a cohesive bolus. Thick liquids (nectar blended with one-half banana for a 7-ounce drink) move more slowly from front to back. This allows the client with a delayed swallow more time to control the liquid until the swallow response is initiated. Thus liquids are the most difficult to control.[10,65,67]

In *Therapy Practice Skills for Physical Dysfunction* (4th Ed.), Nelson describes a complete Dysphagia Evaluation Procedure (which includes a Dysphagia Evaluation Form.)[67]

Other information regarding a dysphagia assessment can be obtained through videofluoroscopy (a radiographic procedure that uses a modified barium swallow recorded on videotape). This procedure helps the therapist determine the cause of any aspiration. It can also be used to determine intervention techniques and the safest diet level.[67]

Intervention in dysphagia includes positioning (e.g., the client should be positioned symmetrically with normal alignment between head, neck, trunk, and pelvis); appropriate diet selection (e.g., the food for a dysphagia diet should be of uniform texture and consistency, provide sufficient volume and density, be cohesive, provide a pleasant temperature and taste, and be able to be suctioned or readily removed when needed).[67] Foods to avoid are foods with multiple textures (e.g., salads and vegetable soup); stringy and fibrous vegetables, fruits, and meats; flaky and crumbly food; foods with skin and seeds; hard rolls; foods that liquefy (e.g., gelatin, ice cream); and garnishes such as parsley or lettuce.[67]

Diet selection also includes appropriate diet progression:[67]

❖ Stage 1 (puréed food). This is best for clients with little or no tongue or jaw control, decreased pharyngeal or jaw control, decreased pharyngeal transit, and a moderately delayed swallow).

❖ Stage 2 (mechanical soft food). This is best for clients with a beginning rotary chew, a minimally delayed swallow, and enough tongue control with assistance to propel food back toward the pharynx.

❖ Stage 3 (chopped ground food). This is recommended for clients who can chew appropriately, are able to produce a controlled bolus formation, and can maintain a fair swallow. After mastering Stage 2, the client may progress to a regular diet and a variety of strengthening prefeeding and feeding techniques.

Some prefeeding and feeding techniques include:[67]

❖ Prefeeding
  ▲ The facilitation and encouragement of trunk strength
  ▲ Promoting normalization of tone
  ▲ Providing a firm seating surface
  ▲ Facilitating strength through neck and head exercises (e.g., flexion, extension, and lateral flexion), if a client cannot move his or her head, reduce the tone of the shoulders and trunk—facilitate normal movement
  ▲ Providing lip exercises (blow bubbles into a glass of liquid with a straw, fanning lips so that the client can feel drool or wetness on lips or chin)
  ▲ Educating client in tongue exercises (improve tongue range of motion, normalize neck tone, normalize jaw tone)
  ▲ Asking the client for slow oral transit, asking the client to practice "ng-ga" sounds
  ▲ Teaching the client how to produce a voluntary cough

❖ Feeding techniques
  ▲ For slow oral transit, tuck chin toward client
  ▲ Teach the client to pat or wipe mouth and chin with every few bites
  ▲ Guide the client through a correct movement pattern—consider the use of adaptive equipment and utensils as needed
  ▲ Ask the client to drink liquids from a straw until control improves, assist the client to hold correct feeding position (e.g., consider lateral trunk supports)

⮝ Stroke the client's outside of cheek whenever pocketing of food occurs with index finger moving the finger back and up toward the client's ear

⮝ Teach the client to check cheeks for pocketing

⮝ Teach client to double swallow to ensure a safe swallow

⮝ Instruct the client to clear his or her throat immediately after each swallow so that residual food may be removed)

Overall, occupational therapy goals in the intervention of dysphagia include: facilitate appropriate positioning when the client is engaged in eating, improve motor control at each swallow stage through the facilitation of quality of movement and normalization of tone, maintain an appropriate and adequate intake of nutrition, prevent client aspiration, and finally, re-establish oral eating to the safest, most optimal level possible.[67]

THE NEW YORK PRESBYTERIAN HOSPITAL DYSPHAGIA PROGRAM

Wendy Avery-Smith describes an occupational therapist-coordinated dysphagia program that she helped to develop and enlarge at the New York Presbyterian Hospital on the New York-Cornell campus. This dysphagia rehabilitation program is currently directed by her.[68]

Because dysphagia care is an advanced clinical skill, postgraduate training is paramount before one can evaluate and treat dysphagia clients.[68]

Since its inception in the 1980s, the Dysphagia Program at New York Presbyterian Hospital has grown so that there are now several specialty areas within the intervention program. Originally occupational therapists assessed clients with dysphagia at bedside and designed individual intervention programs to remediate and manage swallowing deficits. A format for the swallowing team's (consisting of an occupational therapist [including a designated occupational therapy team leader], a speech-language pathologist, a gastroenterology attending physician, a dietitian, and a nurse clinical specialist whose focus was on hyperalimentation and alternative [not by mouth or NPO] forms of providing nutrition) rounds was developed so difficult cases were discussed.

The popularity of the program grew as physicians began to realize that the dysphagia program could aid in minimizing the risks of pneumonia and other morbidities in susceptible populations, as well as decrease client lengths of stay. Besides the inpatient programs, an outpatient program was developed (for those individuals with persistent dysphagia to be seen for further therapy after their hospital discharge). Clients are seen from every age and a variety of diagnoses. For our purposes, the geriatric population alone will be discussed. Some of the most noted diagnoses among older adult clients in this program include client's failure to thrive, CVA, pulmonary disorders, those with tracheotomies, and clients who require postoperative dysphagia intervention following pharyngeal and oral cancers.[68] The dysphagia program continues to expand. In 1991, approximately 250 referrals for swallowing evaluations were received. By 1997, approximately 600 referrals were issued.[68]

Avery-Smith describes the management of a typical stroke client in the program. First, the client is referred early (before any medication or oral food is attempted). Overall alertness is a prerequisite for the major part of the evaluation. The client must be awake enough to safely eat by mouth and participate in the evaluation. Since blood pressure may still be labile, it is checked before the client is positioned upright (in bed or preferably in a chair). At that time any necessary environmental changes are made to ensure that the client can best attend and is comfortable.[68]

All stroke clients are assessed using the Dysphagia Evaluation Protocol. This evaluation protocol is available as follows:

✧   Avery-Smith, W., Rosen. A. B., & Dellarose, D. *Dysphagia evaluation and protocol.*

Therapy Skill Builders

555 Academic Court

San Antonio, TX 78204

1-800-211-8378

It contains a 64-page soft-bound manual, a 40-page pocket spiral-bound manual, and a package of 15 record forms (four pages each).[68]

The assessment includes all performance components involved in swallowing (e.g., feeding history, nutritional status, respiratory status, cognitive perceptual observations, posture and self-feeding skills, sensorimotor skills of the oral-pharyngeal complex, and feeding time [with relevant liquids and food]). Modifications are made for clients with aphasia or those who are unable to understand or follow verbal instructions. If the client is at too great a risk for aspiration, the feeding trial is deferred. Instead, a program of overall rehabilitation and feeding exercises is initiated.[68]

At times a client may be sent for a videofluoroscopy (even if the feeding trial is delayed, this may be helpful for those clients whose stroke was recent).[68] Initially spontaneous neurologic recovery can occur. A reassessment within a short period of a few days may demonstrate a dramatic improvement. After the feeding trial is conducted, the occupational therapist can decide the most appropriate level of the aspiration prevention diet that the client can satisfactorily tolerate.[68]

Avery-Smith describes various intervention initiatives with specific cerebral lesions. First, clients with a left middle cerebral artery CVA need a longer oral and pharyngeal transit time than an unaffected person. They perform better in a natural eating situation than when given commands to eat and swallow. Therefore, intervention centers upon presenting a familiar natural eating setting with minimal verbal directions.[68] Those clients with a right middle cerebral artery CVA need a longer pharyngeal transit time and are at a higher risk for laryngeal penetration and aspiration than left CVA clients. Intervention procedures for this group focus upon increasing an awareness of deficits, simplifying the visual display at mealtime, limiting external distractions, and instruction in swallowing techniques such as a neck rotation or chin tuck to decrease the risk of laryngeal penetration. Both groups benefit from the aspiration prevention diet (provides boluses that require minimal oral manipulation and limits easily aspirated liquids). A repeated videofluoroscopy may be necessary to corroborate appropriate swallowing maneuvers and diet texture.[68]

In addition to the recommendations previously listed, Avery-Smith emphasizes a variety of intervention strategies. First, *proximal trunk control* is essential as it can aid in "priming" the distal oral-pharyngeal mechanism as well as distal upper extremity functioning so that self-feeding is enhanced. It is essential that the client can see and smell the food serving before introducing it into the mouth, as this serves to coordinate oral movement so that the bolus can be received and manipulated. Because upper-extremity and oral movements naturally occur together during self-feeding, facilitating these movements with each other aids in enhancing them both and encourages safe swallowing.[68]

Indirect therapy (exercises to improve pharyngeal, facial, and oral movement as well as sensibility) can be undertaken during evaluation, before a feeding trial, or before a meal. *Thermal tactile stimulation* to the faucial pillars to increase strength and frequency of the swallow can be done before a meal or a snack. If a client is designated NPO (high risk for aspiration), these procedures may be utilized in anticipation of feeding trials.[68]

Direct therapy (actual eating activities with the client) may occur only on a feeding trial basis with an occupational therapist, especially if it has been determined that the client is at high risk for aspiration. Manual techniques to improve neck and head control and swallowing during trial periods may be employed. Auditory and visual stimulation reduction are helpful for clients with perceptual or cognitive impairment to aid in improving their attention span while eating. Swallowing techniques such as the Mendelshon maneuver (elevating the larynx to prolong airway closure), neck rotation, and chin tuck may be used if they are effective in reducing aspiration risk. Other strategies such as presenting a simplified food tray and a plate of interesting food at the midline, or on the right side to a client with left neglect, may be initially helpful until the individual learns scanning techniques.[68]

At New York Presbyterian Hospital, a Four-Stage Aspiration Prevention Diet is used:
- ❖ Stage 1 includes soft formed boluses (requiring minimal oral manipulation) and no fluids. For nutrition's sake, intravenous fluids or nasogastric tube feedings may be needed.
- ❖ Stage 2 adds soft chewable food (e.g., well-cooked pasta and soft fruit—no liquids are still in effect).
- ❖ Stage 3 includes thick liquids (e.g., fruit nectars, and tomato juice) as well as ground meats, and similarly textured chewable food.
- ❖ Stage 4 involves a mechanical soft diet (with a wide range of cut-up chewable food) and a full range of fluids.[68]

Team interaction is a highly important aspect of this program. Family and nursing staff are instructed in diet, exercises, special positioning, swallowing, and eating techniques that the client is using. The occupational therapist works with the radiologist during videofluoroscopy. The occupational therapy clinician also works with the dietitian, the physical therapist, the psychiatrist, and the speech-language pathologist. At New York Presbyterian Hospital the speech-language pathologist works with those dysphagia clients who suffer from language and speech problems and with the occupational therapist in dysphagia interventions for those clients who have had neck and head cancers.[68]

Although teams may operate in a variety of ways, it is always important to develop a multidisciplinary approach that utilizes and respects the expertise of each member. "Because of their understanding of the many performance components involved in eating and swallowing, occupational therapists are appropriate professionals to act as team leaders and to coordinate a multidisciplinary dysphagia program."[68, p. 23]

Hemiplegia Management With Cerebrovascular Accident

Hemiplegia is defined as a paralysis that occurs on one side of the body. It is the result of a vascular insult that causes a lesion in the brain which results in neurological deficits.[63] A lesion on the right cerebral hemisphere (right CVA) produces a left hemiplegia, and vice versa.[69] The following represent possible problems that may occur after a CVA:[63,69]

✧   Motor paralysis may be accompanied by visual dysfunctions
✧   Perceptual disturbances
✧   Intellectual and personality changes such as depression, denial, repression, preservation, emotional liability, lack of motivation, rigid behavior (e.g., an inability to adapt to change)
✧   A reduction in evaluative and behavioral standards (e.g., inadequate products and poor performance may be acceptable to the client in contrast to standards previously held)
✧   An increase in frustration and stress (therefore, it is important that the therapist select meaningful activities that are difficult enough to present a challenge for the client to be able to improve his or her functional skills; at the same time the task must not be so difficult that stress or frustration is evoked by a task that is above the client's capacity for performance)
✧   Language and speech disorders

Goals of occupational therapy intervention in hemiplegia include:[69]
✧   Prevention of deformity caused by poor positioning and abnormal tone
✧   Achievement of maximal, voluntary, unilateral, and bilateral use of affected body side and extremities
✧   Achievement of maximal active range of motion, coordination and strength of the affected body side and extremities
✧   Inhibition of abnormal patterns of movement and posture
✧   Achievement of maximal functional independence in self-maintenance
✧   Facilitation and enhancement of the realistic adjustment to and acceptance of the disability
✧   Facilitation of a healthy balance between rest, work, and play
✧   Facilitation of the re-entry to meaningful roles in the community and family
✧   Improvement of functional social interaction and communication skills

ASSESSMENT AND EVALUATION IN HEMIPLEGIA

A simple self-care activities of daily living task can provide valuable screening information regarding sensorimotor functioning, cognition and perception, and range of motion. It can also identify problems that need attention immediately.[69]

A major purpose of the evaluation is to establish the client's assets and deficits. It also provides a baseline for progress. The evaluation process is continuous. It begins with a gross evaluation of motor, sensory, cognitive, and perceptual functioning, and its effect on self-care. Then, it progresses to more in-depth assessments of complex areas of performance.[69]

When dealing with motor function, it is important to establish the degree of hypertonicity in the client with CVA. Pedretti recommends the Brunnstrom test to determine the stage or level of motor recovery, the presence of synergistic movements, and any associated reactions.[69] The Hemiplegia Classification and Progress Record, as established by Brunnstrom is detailed (along with test administration instructions) on pages 406-408 of the fourth edition of *Occupational Therapy: Practice Skills for Physical Dysfunction*.[70]

Pedretti further recommends the Bobath method (neurodevelopmental) for determining abnormal movement patterns, abnormal motor patterns, the presence of primitive reflexes, righting reactions, abnormal coordination, protective reactions, equilibrium, and the postural mechanism.[69]

In the evaluation process (using the Bobath method) the emphasis is placed on the quality of movement. The occupational therapist observes changes of tone, coordination, and postural reactions rather than looking at specific joints and muscles.[71] In all evaluations the client must be observed from the back, the side, and the front. For symmetry, observations should be either *static* (client standing, sitting, or supine) or *dynamic* (client tries to move—trunk, both upper extremities, and his or her head and neck). Asymmetric observations include observing the client's posture, the pelvis, and the shoulder girdle while the client is in an upright position (sitting if possible). The client's shirt should be removed in order to detect asymmetries of the upper extremities, shoulder girdle, and trunk. Full privacy should be afforded to the client during this part of the evaluation. Davis recommends the use of reference lines in order to structure observation, as this will help establish deviations. The first reference line is the vertical midline. Questions to be answered upon observation include: Is the head centered at the midline position? Is the trunk shifted to the side? Are the medial borders of both scapulae equally distant from the spine?

Next, a horizontal line should be visualized at the top of the shoulders. Some of the questions to consider at this line include: Are both shoulders at the same height? Is one shoulder abnormally high or the other abnormally low?

The third reference is a horizontal line at the hips. Questions to be asked in this segment include: Is one hip lower or higher? Does the client bear weight equally over both hips? The therapist should also observe any folds or unilateral creases on the trunk (a possible indication of other problem areas).[71]

To determine underlying causes of asymmetries, the affected limb is taken through passive range of motion (within normal patterns of movement in normal alignment) and discomfort upon movement should be noted. The limb should never be moved past the point of pain. The client is then asked to describe the pain (e.g., dull, stabbing, pulling, aching) as this will demonstrate a specific location. This is helpful in determining the cause of the pain. If the therapist feels resistance, the client probably has a high tone (the limb must be slowly moved through range of motion to prevent a quick stretch that is usually followed by clonus). If no resistance is felt (and the arm feels heavy), the client probably has low tone.[71]

In performing a dynamic evaluation, the therapist observes any movement that is initiated by the client on the affected side. Sometimes the client will make *associated movements* (the non-affected side attempting the same movements on the affected side) or *associated reactions* (movement influenced by abnormal synergy patterns). Associated reactions should be inhibited or discouraged. Comparing the client's movement pattern with normal movement pattern is helpful in identifying problem areas that may be interfering with normal movement. A problem may have more than one cause.[71]

The Bobath Neurodevelopment Approach to Intervention

Intervention, using Bobath Neurodevelopmental (NDT) principles, is concerned with the "facilitation of movement on the hemiplegic side, trying to achieve symmetry of body and movement."[60, p. 8] In the "beginning the therapist guides the movements of the client through manipulation techniques, thereby preventing any recurrence of the abnormal pattern until the client is able to control himself."[60, p. 9]

It is the therapist's job to identify where the client displays abnormally low or high tone and to develop an intervention program that is designed to normalize tone. *Inhibition* involves decreasing abnormally high tone; *facilitation* deals with increasing abnormally low tone.[71]

Normalization of muscle tone involves one or more of the following techniques: weight bearing over the affected side, scapular protraction, trunk rotation, facilitation of slow controlled movements, anterior pelvic tilt/position pelvis forward, and appropriate proper positioning.[71]

Eggers' *Occupational Therapy in the Treatment of Adult Hemiplegia* provides a variety of intervention strategies useful to the client diagnosed with a CVA. Throughout the book she aptly details intervention that is helpful with motor problems.[60] She defines intervention approaches as follows: orientation toward the affected or hemiplegic side, use of symmetry in training for balance, selective hand and arm function, facilitation of normal movements, development of useful coordination of both hands, facilitation of automatic reactions, and facilitation of kinesthetic-tactile perception.[60]

Positioning is important in hemiplegic intervention. The hemiplegic arm should always be positioned in the client's field of vision so it can be visually controlled (not forgotten). For instance, when the client sits at the table, the hemiplegic arm should always be on the table (not under it). For best results, the client should be the one to position his or her hand.[60]

MANAGEMENT OF THE EDEMATOUS UPPER EXTREMITY

At this point it is important to describe various methods of dealing with the edematous hand. These methods are not specific as to a described theory, but are helpful solely in reducing edema of the upper extremity. Management of the hemiplegic hand that has become edematous involves a number of strategies to reduce serous fluid. Rich in fibrin, this fluid can cause the small finger joints to stiffen rapidly. The following are a number of approaches that can be used to reduce edema:[10,69]

✧ The use of retrograde massage. The therapist or assistant gently massages the affected hand to slowly push the fluid (starting distally with the fingertip and working proximally up to the forearm). This massage assists in blood and lymph flow.

✧ The use of an elasticized type of glove. This helps to compress and reduce the swelling.

✧ The use of pressure wraps that may be surgical gauze or Coban (3M, St. Paul, MN) elastic wrap. With this intervention the therapist or assistant wraps the affected hand starting with the distal tips of each finger and gradually applying the wrap until it is proximal to the edema. The therapist or assistant can work gently squeezing the fingertips (distal to proximal) until the forearm is reached. The wrap is in place for 5 minutes, and this may be repeated three times daily.

✧ The use of appropriate positioning. The hand is never left to dangle. When in bed, it is important to elevate the affected hand through the use of pillows or similar devices to avoid edema or increasing edema.

PRACTICAL STRATEGIES USING THE BOBATH METHOD

From the beginning of intervention the Bobath method (NDT) promotes the following three concepts. First, the therapist should enable the client to become more aware of the hemiplegic side. Second, integration of both sides of the body is essential. Third, it is important to increase sensory stimulation to the hemiplegic side.

In terms of bed positioning NDT strategy dictates that the hemiplegic side of the client should face the stimulation source (e.g., the door, the night stand, the television). In this way the client learns the value of increasing integration of both sides of the body. Bed positioning follows a specific theoretical basis. All clients should be properly positioned following these guidelines: weight bearing increases awareness of the hemiplegic side and increases sensory input, weight bearing normalizes tone and inhibits spasticity, lengthening of the hemiplegic side inhibits spasticity, and weight bearing of the affected side enables the client to be less fearful. Jan Zeret Davis specifies details and diagrams as to: lying on the hemiplegic side, lying on the non-hemiplegic side, and lying supine. These are well documented and can be found on pages 445 and 446 in *Occupational Therapy: Practice Skills for Physical Dysfunction*.[71]

When donning clothing, the three major principles (as stated earlier) still apply. Shirt donning will be considered first. One example stipulates that the shirt should be positioned across the client's knees. The armhole should be visible and the sleeve positioned between the knees. The client then bends forward at the hips (this inhibits the extension synergy of the lower extremity) and places the affected hand in the sleeve. As the arm drops into the sleeve, the shoulder protracts and gravity inhibits upper extremity flexion synergy. The collar is then brought to the neck. The client is asked to sit upright and dress the nonaffected side. Lastly, the shirt is buttoned from bottom to top.[71]

The hemiplegic shoulder can become a major problem for the client diagnosed with a CVA. The shoulder is composed of seven joints. In order to become pain free during range of motion, all seven joints need to work synchronously. If the arm is raised in shoulder abduction or flexion (without the scapula gliding along with the movement), joint trauma and pain can be the result. The scapula must first be mobilized, and spasticity must be reduced to promote range of motion and allow for selective movement. By protracting the scapula, hypertonicity of the upper extremities is reduced. This in turn, permits selective control and increases isolated movement. Reflex inhibiting patterns can be used to reduce and control spasticity.[71] If the muscles around the shoulder girdle are weak, the hemiplegic shoulder will often become subluxed. Slings are not effective with subluxation as they keep the arm in a poor position and often contribute to swelling and pain. Pain in the subluxed shoulder is caused by forcing the head of the humerus back into place. Performing standard range of motion procedures on hemiplegic arms when the scapula is not gliding can also be the cause of pain. Basic intervention includes proper positioning, mobilization of the scapula, proper sitting, and appropriate weight bearing.[71]

In addition to the NDT approach there are other methodologies that are frequently used in treating the hemiplegic client—these are the Brunnstrom approach, the proprioceptive neuromuscular facilitation approach, and the Rood approach to neuromuscular dysfunction.

THE BRUNNSTROM APPROACH

Signe Brunnstrom's approach to intervention of the hemiplegic client utilizes the concept that motor patterns are available to the client at any point in his or her recovery process. Brunnstrom viewed reflexes, synergies, and other abnormal movement patterns as a normal part of the recovery process that the client needs to go through before normal voluntary movement can take place.[70]

During the early stages of recovery the client should be helped to gain control of the limb synergies. Selected afferent stimuli (such as tonic neck reflexes, tonic labyrinthine reflexes, stretch and cutaneous stimuli, and positioning and associated synergy patterns) inhibit its antagonist by means of reciprocal innervation.[70]

Proper head positioning, the attainment of good sitting or trunk balance, and the achievement of pain-free range of motion at the glenohumeral joint are early goals of intervention.[70]

In the restoration of upper limb functioning a number of intervention procedures are performed. During the early stages of recovery (Stages 1 and 2) the arm is essentially flaccid. Some components of synergy patterns may begin to appear. At this point the major focus of therapy is to elicit muscle tone and synergy patterns by means of a reflex basis. In the next recovery stage (end of Stage 2 and Stage 3), synergies and/or their components are present. These may be performed voluntarily. Hypertonicity reaches its peak in Stage 3. Therapeutic goals during this period center around achieving voluntary control of synergy patterns by means of repetitious alternating performance of synergy patterns (first in the facilitation and later through the assistance of the clinician). Procedures during this stage may include: bilateral rowing movements (with the clinician holding one of the client's hands); weight-bearing on the affected arm may be utilized to reinforce elbow extension. During Stages 4 and 5 therapeutic intervention goals focus upon breaking away from synergies "by mixing components from antagonistic synergies to perform new and increasing complex patterns of movement."[70, p. 412] Skateboard or powder board motor activities that employ arcs of movement achieve elbow flexion which is combined with shoulder horizontal adduction and forearm pronation. This is then alternated by elbow extension with forearm supination and shoulder horizontal abduction.[70] Later in this stage of recovery the more complex figure-of-eight pattern can be performed with the use of the skateboard and/or powder board.[70]

Hand retraining is treated separately as hand recovery and remediation does not necessarily coincide with arm recovery. The first step of hand retraining is to achieve mass grasp. The second objective is to attain wrist flexion for grasp. The third goal is to attain active release of grasp. When finger reflex extension is obtained, then alternative fist opening and closing can commence. Voluntary movements of the thumb occur when semivoluntary mass extension is achievable.[70] For detailed information regarding hand retraining, please refer to pages 412-414 of Pedretti's chapter on "Movement Therapy: The Brunnstrom approach to the Treatment of Hemiplegia."[70] The following segment regarding splinting, although not specific to a developmental theoretical basis, is considered next as it deals exclusively with hand management (via splinting) in preventing deformities and promoting hygiene.

UPPER EXTREMITY SPLINTING FOR THE CLIENT DIAGNOSED WITH A CEREBROVASCULAR ACCIDENT

Antispasticity splints, resting hand splints, and soft splints (with a fiberfill foam or small cone interior) can be used to prevent or lessen contractor deformities. These aid in promoting a more appropriate hand position and hygiene (allowing cleanliness of the hand, preventing skin breakdown). Static type splints, such as described here, should not be worn continuously but should follow a schedule (e.g., a schedule could state 4 hours on and 2 hours off for morning, 4 hours on and 2 hours off for late afternoon, and 4 hours on at night). The schedule totally depends upon the individual's situation and condition. The clinician needs to educate the nursing staff or family members to constantly monitor the splint for comfort and cleanliness.

THE PROPRIOCEPTIVE NEUROMUSCULAR FACILITATION APPROACH

Proprioceptive neuromuscular facilitation (PNF) is based upon normal motor development and normal movement. This approach utilizes mass movement patterns that are spiral and diagonal in nature and that resemble the movement that is seen in functional activities. It is a multisensory approach that makes use of facilitation techniques which are superimposed on postures and movement patterns by means of the clinician's verbal commands, visual cues, and manual contacts (usually gently touching the client to guide movement). Besides stroke, PNF has been found to be effective with other disease states associated with the geriatric population such as Parkinson's disease and arthritis.[72]

In terms of evaluation, PNF follows a sequence from proximal to distal. Breathing, swallowing, voice production, oral and facial musculature, and ocular/visual control are considered first. Next, the head and neck region is observed (dominance of tone and alignment and stability are considered). Thereafter, the evaluation focus shifts to the upper trunk, upper extremities, lower trunk, and lower extremities. Each component is evaluated on an individual basis (considering specific movement patterns). Developmental activities involving the interaction of body segments are also observed. During the component of evaluating developmental activities, the therapist needs to consider the following issues:

✧   Is there a balance between the extensors and the flexors?

✧   Is one more dominant than the other?

✧   Does a need exist for more mobility or stability?

✧   Is the client able to move in all directions?

✧   Are there major limitations? Identify them.

✧   Is the client able to assume a posture and maintain it?

✧   If the client cannot do this, which postures or total patterns are inadequate?

✧   Are these inadequacies of a distal or proximal nature?

✧   Which techniques of facilitation does the client respond to in the most effective manner?

✧   Which sensory input (e.g., auditory, tactile, visual) does the client respond to best?

The last part of the evaluation involves observing activities of daily living to identify if performance of total and individual patterns is adequate within the context of functional activities.[72]

The diagonal patterns that are used in PNF utilize mass movement patterns that can be observed in most functional activities. Two diagonal motions occur in each major part of the body. Each diagonal pattern has an extension and flexion component along with movement away from or toward the midline and rotation.[72]

There are eight unilateral patterns and six (symmetric, asymmetric, reciprocal, ipsilateral, contralateral, and diagonal reciprocal) bilateral patterns. Total patterns of movement and posture (e.g., interaction between proximal [such as trunk, neck, or head] and distal [extremities]) are also an important aspect of PNF.

Procedures such as *manual contacts* (placement of the therapist's hands on the client to utilize pressure as a facilitating mechanism; stretch which is used to initiate voluntary movement, enhance and strengthen weak muscles, and increase the speed response in muscles) are helpful in improving functional movement; traction (facilitates joint receptions by means of creating a separation of the joints surfaces) promotes movement and is utilized for pulling motions; and approximation (facilitates the joint receptors through the creation of the compression of joint surfaces) promotes postural control and stability. It is utilized for pushing motions, and maximal resistance (applies the theory that stronger patterns and muscles reinforce weaker components) is useful for obtaining the client's maximal effort.[72]

There are a number of techniques that are utilized with the above mentioned procedures. The three that are mentioned here involve: agonist movement techniques are the reversal of antagonist and relaxation techniques; rhythmic initiation is used to improve the client's ability to initiate movement. This involves voluntary relaxation, passive movement, and repeated isotonic contraction within the agonistic patterns; and repeated contractions are based upon the repetition of activity that is needed for motor learning to take place. It is also believed to be helpful in developing and improving range of motion, endurance, and strength. This is brought about by facilitating the client's voluntary movement through stretch and resistance and the use of isotonic and isometric contractions.[72]

Reversal of antagonists techniques assumes that movement can reverse and change direction. It is believed that the stronger antagonist is able to facilitate the weaker agonist. This is done by causing the antagonist to contract (by means of the stimulation of isometric and isotonic contractions or a combination of both). *Slow reversal* (isotonic contraction against the resistance of the agonist) aids in increasing power in the agonist. *Rhythmic stabilization* is used to increase stability through eliciting simultaneous isometric contractions of the antagonist muscle group. This is contraindicated for clients with cardiac problems. No more than three or four repetitions should be performed at any given time. In this technique manual contacts are used on both antagonist and agonist muscles with resistance simultaneously. The client is not permitted to relax. This technique is helpful for clients with postural control problems due to proximal weakness or ataxia. If used intermittently when a client is performing an activity that requires postural stability (e.g., meal preparation), rhythmic stabilization can improve postural control.[72]

Relaxation techniques are helpful in improving and enhancing range of motion (especially when spasticity or pain is present) by means of passive stretch. *Contract-relax* employs an isotonic contraction of antagonistic muscle patterns against maximal resistance while only the rotational aspect of the diagonal movement is permitted to take place. This is then followed by relaxation and passive movement into the agonistic muscle patterns. This technique is repeated at each point in the range of motion where some form of limitation is felt to take place. This technique is utilized when there is no active range in the agonist muscle pattern. *Hold-relax* (performed in the same sequence as contract-relax) encompasses an isometric contraction of the antagonist that is followed by relaxation and the active movement into agonist muscle patterns. This technique is very helpful for the client who experiences pain or acute orthopedic conditions. *Slow-reversal-hold-relax* involves an isotonic contraction that is followed by an isometric contraction which is then followed by relaxation of the antagonistic muscle pattern. This is followed by active movement of the agonistic pattern. This technique is most helpful when the client has the ability to actively move the agonist. This particular technique is helpful in increasing elbow extension. *Rhythmic rotation* is especially effective in increasing range of motion and decreasing spasticity. The clinician passively moves the body part into the desired pattern. When restriction or tightness of movement can be felt, the clinician rotates the body part rhythmically and slowly in both directions. After relaxation is felt, the clinician continues to move the body part into the newly available range of motion. This technique can be very beneficial when preparing a splint that is to be fabricated for a spastic extremity.

THE ROOD APPROACH

Rood believed that appropriate sensory stimulation could elicit specific motor responses. It was Rood's contention that muscle movement could be facilitated, activated, and inhibited through the use of the sensory system.[73]

Rood also postulated that the demands placed on various muscle groups cause these muscle groups to be different from each other. She affirmed that "light work" muscles (known as mobilizers) were principally adductors and flexors. These muscle groups were involved in skilled movement patterns. On the other hand, "heavy work" muscles (known as stabilizers) were primarily the abductors and extensors. These muscles were needed for postural support.[73] Rood also postulated that voluntary motor acts are based on inherent reflexes and upon the modification of those reflexes at higher centers. Except for feeding and speech muscles, heavy work muscles are activated before light work muscles.[73]

In this approach the client is evaluated developmentally and treated sequentially. The cephalocaudal rule is followed as intervention begins with the head and proceeds from the proximal (segment by segment) until the sacral area is reached. Flexors are stimulated first, the extensors are next stimulated, the adductors are stimulated, and the abductors are stimulated last.[73] Movement is directed toward functional goals and repetition is needed for re-educating muscular responses.[73]

Rood affirmed that there are four sequential phases of motor control. The *reciprocal inhibition* (intervention) movement pattern subserves a protection function and is reflex governed by the supraspinal and spinal centers. *Co-contraction* (co-innervation) provides stability and is a tonic or static movement pattern. *Heavy work* is the next motor phase and is thought as mobility that is superimposed on stability. With this pattern the distal segment is fixed while the proximal muscles move and contract (e.g., creeping). *Skill* is the last and highest level of motor control. It combines stability and mobility. This pattern involves the stabilization of the proximal segment while the distal area moves in a free manner (e.g., the oil painting artist stands back from the canvas and with arms at full length is able to manipulate his or her brush freely).[73]

There are eight ontogenetic patterns that follow a specific sequence:[73]

1. *Supine withdrawal* (supine flexion) is a total flexion response toward the T10 vertebral level. This involves protective positioning because the neck is in flexion and the arms and legs are crossed. Thus, the anterior surface of the body is protected. This pattern is recommended for clients who are dominated by extensor tone and who do not have a reciprocal flexion pattern.

2. *Rollover* (toward side lying) involves the ability to roll over (the leg and the arm flex on the same body side). This movement activates the lateral trunk musculature and is a mobility pattern for the extremities. This pattern is useful for clients who are dominated by tonic reflex patterns when in the supine position.

3. *Pivot prone* (prone extension) is the full range of extension of the neck, shoulders, trunk, and lower extremities. It is both a stability and mobility pattern and plays an important role in preparing for the stability of the extensor muscles that are used in the upright position.

4. *Neck co-contraction* (co-innervation) involves the first real stability pattern and precedes co-contraction of the trunk and extremities. When the face is perpendicular to the floor, this pattern elicits the tonic labyrinthine righting reaction. This position and pattern promotes extraocular control and neck stability.

5. *On elbows* (prone on elbows) is weight-bearing on elbows, and it gives the client an opportunity to shift weight from side to side as well as provide better visibility of the environment. It stretches the upper trunk musculature, which influences stability of the glenohumeral and scapular regions.

6. *All fours* (quadruped position) involves stretching of the trunk and limb girdles which in turn develops co-contraction of the trunk extensors and flexors. Weight shifting (forward, backward, side to side, and diagonally) provides mobility that is superimposed on stability.

7. *Static standing*, a skill of the upper trunk, is the upright bipedal position, and it brings a higher level of integration (such as equilibrium and righting reactions) once weight shifting is initiated.

8. *Walking* is a sophisticated process that provides a gait pattern that unifies skill, stability, and mobility. It incorporates the ability to maintain balance, support body weight, and execute the stepping motion (a stance comes first which is followed by pushoff, swing, heel strike, and stride length).

With the Rood approach there are a number of facilitation techniques, including cutaneous facilitation and proprioceptive facilitory techniques. *Cutaneous facilitation* uses exteroceptive stimuli such as icing, light moving touch, and fast brushing (increases the fusimotor activities of selected muscles). Fast brushing should be applied over the dermatomes of the same area that supplies the muscle that is to be stimulated. Fast brushing is contraindicated for certain areas of the skin and should be used judiciously. For instance, facial brushing should be avoided with clients who have brain stem injuries, as autonomic dysreflexia may result (with the possibility of inducing a deep state of unconsciousness). Icing involves an extreme in thermal facilitation. It has been used for facilitation of the autonomic nervous system responses as well as muscle activity. Icing can be applied to: the lips to induce opening of the mouth; to the sternal notch to induce swallowing in dysphagia clients; and for the facilitation of autonomic nervous system responses and facilitation of muscle activity. Light moving touch or stroking can be applied with the fingertip, a cotton swab, or a camel hair brush to elicit neurological and muscular activity responses (may cause reciprocal innervation that can be seen as a phasic response or can be used to activate the superficial mobilizing muscles). Presently the frequency of this type of touch stimulus is to apply three to five strokes and allow a 30-second elapse period to prevent overstimulation.[73]

Proprioceptive facilitory techniques include:[73]

1. *Heavy joint compression,* which is used to facilitate co-contraction at the joint undergoing comprehension.

2. *Stretch* (quick), which is used to activate the proprioceptors in selected light work muscle groups.

3. *Intrinsic stretch,* which promotes stability of the scapulohumeral area.

4. *Secondary ending stretch,* which is often used to integrate the tonic neck labyrinthine reflex in the supine position.

5. *Stretch pressure* affects the Ia afferents and the exteroceptors of the muscle spindle.

6. *Resistance* is used in an isotonic manner within developmental patterns to influence stabilizer muscles. Heavy resistance is used to stimulate secondary and primary endings of the muscle spindle. Intermittent resistance which is graded to the desired motion can also be used for alleviating tight muscles.

7. *Tapping,* conducted by tapping over the belly of a muscle with the fingertips (three to five times over the muscle that is to be facilitated), acts on the afferents of the muscle spindle and results in increasing the tone of the underlying skeletal muscle.

8. *Vestibular stimulation* can be either facilitative or inhibitory depending on the stimulation rate. Slow rhythmic rocking relaxes while fast rocking stimulates.

9. *Inversion* involves therapy that uses the inverted position to alter muscle tone in selected muscles. This type of therapy should be used with extreme care and is contraindicated for most clients with cardiovascular disease.

10. *Therapeutic vibration* is a series of rapid touch stimuli that is used to desensitize hypersensitive skin and to produce tonal muscle changes. It is important to note that in older adults the skin is thin and the blood vessels, bones, and organs are more susceptible to vibratory stimuli.

11. *Osteopressure* involves pressure that is applied on the bony prominences and can be used to either inhibit or facilitate voluntary muscles.

There are eight inhibition techniques that Rood believes can be used in intervention. These include:

1. *Neutral warmth.* The client is supine and his or her body is wrapped in a cotton blanket for 10 to 15 minutes. This is useful for decreasing muscle tone and promoting relaxation.

2. *Gentle rocking or shaking.* This technique uses light joint compression, traction of the cervical vertebrae, and slow rhythmic circumduction of the head to promote relaxation.

3. *Slow stroking.* The client is prone while the therapist provides moving rhythmic deep pressure over the dorsal distribution of the primary posterior rami of the spine. This is useful for relaxation. However, it should not exceed 3 minutes.

4. *Slow rolling.* The client is in the side-lying position. The client should initially be with the uninvolved side down. Then, the clinician kneels behind the client and places one hand on the shoulder or rib cage and the other hand on the lateral aspect of the client's pelvis. The client is gently and slowly rolled from a side-lying position to a prone position and back again in a rhythmical manner. Some clients may require a pillow between the knees or under the head to prevent malalignment and friction. This technique is useful for promoting relaxation and decreased tone.

5. *Light joint compression/approximation.* This involves joint compression of body weight or less than body weight to inhibit spastic muscles near and around the joint. It has been helpful with clients in alleviating pain and temporarily offsetting muscle imbalance around the shoulder joint. This procedure compresses both the glenohumeral joint and the articulation between the humerus and the ulna.

6. *Tendinous pressure.* This is manual pressure that is applied across long tendons or to the tendinous insertion of a muscle to produce a dramatic inhibitory effect on spastic and/or light muscle groups where the tendons are accessible to pressure forces.

7. *Maintained stretch.* This involves positioning hypertonic extremities in the elongated position for various time periods to produce lengthening of the muscle spindles. Rood did not promote passive stretch for tight muscles. Instead, she recommended maintained stretch in the lengthened position for agonist muscles to increase the threshold of the muscle spindles. The antagonist muscle is next facilitated by cutaneous stimulation in an effort to offset any muscle imbalance).

8. *Rocking in developmental patterns.* An example of this can be seen with the client in the quadruped position. When the therapist applies pressure and stretch to the anconeus and triceps brachia, the client is assisted in the quadruped position as the clinician applies compression, greater than body weight, to facilitate co-contraction. The pressure that is exerted on the extended wrist and heel of the hand acts to inhibit the wrist flexors. At this point light moving touch over the dorsum of the hand is achieved to promote the extension of the fingers. Rocking in the quadruped position should initially be conducted with the neck in a straight and normal relationship to the body to prevent the proprioceptors of the neck from influencing the tonicity of the limbs. When the client moves in an anterior posterior plane, the pelvic and shoulder girdles are mobilized. Incorporation of flexion, rotation, and extension of the neck as a reflex inhibition measure may be utilized later in intervention.

Rood also recommended the use of gustatory and olfactory stimuli as a way of influencing the autonomic nervous system and facilitating cranial nerves. Banana oil and vanilla may produce a calming effect or evoke strong moods. Noxious substances such as vinegar and ammonia were utilized by Rood to stimulate the trigeminal nerve and activate the mastication muscles. Unpleasant odors (e.g., sulfur and fresh horseradish) can produce primitive protective responses such as choking and sneezing. Warm liquids can be calming to the oral musculature. Sour tastes and sweet food can stimulate the salivary glands.[73]

Occupational therapists and occupational therapy assistants use Rood techniques to prepare clients to perform purposeful activity. Ontogenetic motor patterns can be readily utilized with activities. For instance, in using supine withdrawal, an easel can be set up in such a way that the client can be supine and reach forward toward the midline to create an oil painting.[73] There is little doubt that "Rood's basic hypothesis, that sensory stimulation can elicit specific motor responses, continues to gain credence in the realm of physical medicine and rehabilitation."[73, p. 392]

These hemiplegic intervention methods have been presented in a summarized format. When implementing PNF, the Bobath, the Rood, and/or the Brunnstrom approaches, clinicians should first seek specific training (such as workshops, courses, and institutes) and then work under an expert clinician in any one of these areas before attempting these techniques on one's own.

A New Look at Hemiplegic Rehabilitation

According to the June 2, 2000 edition of *The New York Times*, a new kind of stroke rehabilitation therapy was realized. Scientists were able to demonstrate, for the first time, that the brain can be stimulated into reorganizing its circuitry so that individuals can regain nearly full use of their paralyzed limbs in 2 to 3 weeks, even if the stroke occurred years before.[74]

The rehabilitation involves immobilizing the nonaffected arm or leg "so that the client is forced to use the paralyzed arm or leg for familiar tasks. By intensively using the paralyzed limb, people can literally rewire parts of their brains."[74, p. A12] This technique has proved successful for clients who had their strokes decades ago and who have had limited use of their limbs since their CVA.[74]

These findings came from scientists at the Friedrich Schuller University of Jena in Germany and the University of Alabama in the United States. The study involved the arms of 13 clients and provided evidence that the adult brain has the capacity to reorganize itself after an injury. This intensive therapeutic method is termed "constraint-induced movement therapy." This study reported that maps were made of an area of the brain in 13 chronic clients before and after the intensive therapy. After the therapy, researchers found that the brain area that was responsible for arm movements had nearly doubled.[74]

Dr. Taub, a neurologist at the University of Alabama in Birmingham and an author of the study, said that after a stroke some cells die but many more are left in a state of shock. Many times the stunned cells, which might make up networks that control limb movements, remain stunned and in a state of permanent inhibition. Whenever the client tries to use his or her affected arm and fails, that failure is reinforced. The ability to perform mobility becomes suppressed (in a kind of learned helplessness). The ability to perform movements has not been extinguished, but the client has usually stopped trying. In the meantime clients begin to depend on their nonaffected arm to perform everyday tasks, and these movements then become reinforced.[74]

Constraint-induced movement therapy involves strapping down a client's nonaffected arm and forcing the affected arm to perform all the work. The therapy worked as the 13 women and men in Dr. Taub's study had a paralyzed arm from strokes suffered 6 months to 17 years previous to their involvement in the study. During the therapy the clients had their nonaffected arms secured in a sling or a splint 90% of their waking hours. They participated in the rehabilitation laboratory for 8 weekdays of intervention that lasted 6 hours each day. In therapy they practiced tiny movements that would enhance their ability to reach out, grasp, and move items. The clients regained three-quarters of their normal use of their paralyzed arms in just 2 weeks. It is the greatly increased use of the paralyzed arm that drives the brain to change and grow. Six months after the therapy concluded the clients' brains were remapped; the growth changes in the brain appeared to be permanent.[74] There are 250 clients who have been treated, nationwide, with this type of therapy in laboratories. Dr. Taub reported that these results have also been excellent.[74]

Other resources that are helpful when dealing with stroke rehabilitation are:

✧ Gillen, G., & Burkhardt, A. *Stroke rehabilitation: A functional approach imaginant*, 1-800-828-1376

✧ LaFeldt, L. The Occupational Therapist's Cognitive ADL Workbook (2nd Edition)
3990 Buttrick Ave. S.E.
Ada, MI 49301
616-682-5555, fax: 616-682-5556

✧ Reeves, R., Robinson, K. J., & Robinson, J. A. *Cooking again cook books.*

(Crockpot entries, one-dish meals, and cooking again—The beginning level—for brain injury, stroke and other neurologic disorders)
QHEST, Inc.
6929 Mayburn St.
Dearborn Heights, MI 48127
313-277-1516

✧   Rogeen, C. B. (Ed.). *Stroke—An AOTA self-paced clinical course*. Available from AOTA at 1-877-404-AOTA.

CHRONIC OBSTRUCTIVE PULMONARY DISEASE AND OCCUPATIONAL THERAPY INTERVENTION

Chronic obstructive pulmonary disease (COPD) affects nearly 16 million Americans. *Emphysema* (the destruction of the walls of the alveoli and bronchioles), *chronic bronchitis* (excessive mucous secretion in the bronchial tree leading to mucous plugging and obstruction of airflow), *bronchiectasis*, and asthma characterize this disorder. In COPD air can enter the alveoli during inhalation, but may not be able to be exhaled due to the collapse of air passages, which traps the stale air. The result is that there is a decrease of gas exchange, tiring respiratory muscles, increased CO_2 accumulation, and hypoventilation. COPD places a large burden on the heart, and the right side of the heart is forced to produce high pressures in order to push blood through the narrow blood vessels that lead to the lungs. The right chambers of the heart, then, thicken and enlarge. A condition known as *cor pulmonale*, in which the right ventricle of the heart is hypertrophied, is a direct result of COPD.[75,76]

COPD usually presents with the following symptoms: *dyspnea* (difficulty breathing), morning cough, expiratory wheezing, and breathlessness. In the later stages of this disease the breathlessness actually prevents the client diagnosed with COPD from lying down.[76]

The general intervention for this disease (depending on its severity) may consist of bronchodilators (which open air passages in the lungs), steroids, antibiotics, and exercise to strengthen trunk, shoulders, and hips (muscles most affected by the steroids).[75]

The Evaluation

The occupational therapy evaluation for COPD should be comprised of the following components:[75]

1. Review of the client's medical chart (e.g., Is the client on nasal cannula oxygen? What is the exact titration of the oxygen to keep the oxygen saturated at a desired level for activities of daily living? What is the client's use of medication and inhalers?).

2. Interview of the client (e.g., review of the client's daily routine at home, the types of activities that are difficult to perform, and if the difficulties are more difficult in the evening or in the morning; at this time of interaction the therapist can evaluate the client's cognition as well as observe the client's affect).

3. During the evaluation the client's resting heart rate, resting respiratory rate, and oxygen saturation rate should be noted as well as the current level of supplemental oxygen use (tracheal collar, ventilator nasal cannula).

4. Sensation, strength, and range of motion of the upper extremities should be observed and firmly evaluated. It is important to note any limitations, as these areas of weakness may cause the client to have difficulty with adaptive technology or to fatigue easily.

5. Whenever possible, evaluate the client while he or she is performing activities of daily living (e.g., donning or doffing a button-up shirt, lifting something very lightweight, walking 100 feet and performing a simple household task, and/or donning and doffing socks and shoes).

6. At the same time (while evaluating the client's functioning during activities of daily living) the therapist should note the amount of time required to complete activities; if there is inadvertent breath holding or interruption of regular breathing during and after activity; the client's respiratory rate during and after the completion of activities; the amount of accessory muscle use during and after everyday activities; the shallowness or depth of breathing during and after activities; and posture and physical limitations. The client should also complete a self-rating scale for activities that are performed (including how these activities affect the way that client breathes and any other self-observation in other bodily areas).

Generalized Occupational Therapy Intervention Program

The occupational therapist's role in pulmonary rehabilitation should include education in:[75-77]

1. Graded activities.
2. Activities of daily living, as described by the Health Care Financing Administration (HCFA)—now termed the Center for Medicare and Medicaid Services (CMS). *Activities of daily living* are defined as self-care and mobility; *instrumental activities of daily living* are defined by HCFA (now CMS) to be activities such as home management, check writing, and shopping.
3. Exercise training to increase activity tolerance. There should be at least a rest period for 60 minutes after eating a meal before beginning an activity or exercise program.
4. The principles of energy conservation and work simplification and body mechanics as it affects the performance of daily activities. This also includes prioritizing tasks so that the client's most important activities can be achieved.
5. Stress management, relaxation techniques, and pursed-lip breathing.
6. Education of other family members or significant others in the above-mentioned intervention areas.
7. Home visits prior to discharge and the development of a home program (including developing problem-solving strategies).[75-77]

Regarding home health and pulmonary rehabilitation, "The ability of the home health occupational therapy practitioner to be present in the client's home environment and to observe the client interacting within the environment adds another dimension to the practitioner's understanding of the client's story."[77, p. 1] Thus the practitioner is given the opportunity to structure intervention so that occupations and activities that are meaningful and purposeful to each client are part of the intervention program.[77]

Work Simplification, Energy Conservation, and Body Mechanics

Instruction in and performance of work simplification, energy conservation, and body mechanics are major issues for the client diagnosed with COPD. These include (but are not limited to) the following strategies:

- ✧ Balance rest and work.
- ✧ Pace oneself (allow time to complete a task before becoming fatigued or take frequent rest periods).
- ✧ Ensure adequate ventilation.
- ✧ Prioritize all tasks (eliminate steps that are unnecessary to complete a task, delegate where possible).
- ✧ Incorporate pursed-lip breathing techniques into one's daily routine (e.g., client breathes in slowly, as though smelling flowers, through the nose and then purses lips as if to kiss, whistle, or blow out candles. As a last step the client breathes out slowly).
- ✧ Avoid holding and lifting (e.g., slide pots from the sink to the range; when ironing, slide the iron rather than lifting it, and work in a sitting position; use helpful aids such as a multi-pocketed apron or use a cart on wheels to move items). Use lightweight pans.
- ✧ Work with arms close to the body.
- ✧ Do not plan meals when tired or hungry.
- ✧ Shop by phone or computer and use a delivery service when possible.
- ✧ When cooking, the exhaust fan should always be turned on to ensure adequate ventilation. Those clients who are bothered by heat can use a portable fan to cool themselves, and to help overcome shortness of breath that can be brought on by stress or exertion.
- ✧ Maintain adequate posture.
- ✧ Avoid reaching and overhead arm movements. Prearrange work stations which are at a comfortable level (e.g., the most used items should be placed within easy reach. Avoid extra reaching by using long-handled dustpans, sponges, and squeegees).[10,75,76]
- ✧ Avoid spray cleaners, as these are irritating and can cause breathing difficulties.

When performing activities of daily living, the following recommendations are helpful in reducing stress and fatigue:[75,78]

- ✧ Steam can be reduced in the shower by first running cold water before the hot water is turned on.
- ✧ In general, a tepid shower is best.
- ✧ Make one trip to the bathroom. Use a rolling cart.
- ✧ Use adaptive equipment such as long-handled sponge, a bath seat, and a hand-held shower head (as educated by the clinician) to conserve energy and provide safety when in the tub or shower.
- ✧ Use a shower caddy to keep all soap, shampoos, and washcloths in easy reach.
- ✧ Utilize a long terrycloth robe after bathing to eliminate the effort needed in drying (or wrap a towel around a long-handled sponge to help dry one's legs to avoid or limit bending).
- ✧ When dressing, the client should exhale when bending or flexing at the trunk.

Exhaling should also be used when bringing one's arms toward one's body or during any type of exertion or straining.

✧ Gather all clothing in one trip and place the items within easy reach. Assemble the clothes the night before to reduce overexertion in the morning when one is performing dressing.

✧ Clothing should be loose and simple. These items should not restrict the chest or abdominal expansion.

✧ Dress legs and feet first (as this requires the most energy). Bring feet up rather than down.

✧ Use long-handled dressing equipment (e.g., dressing stick, long-handled shoe horn, long-handled reacher) to reduce fatigue.

✧ When grooming, the client should prop his or her elbows on a table or countertop (e.g., during shaving, brushing one's teeth).

✧ Keep hairstyles as simple as possible.

In general, if the client is receiving oxygen, the use of pulse oximetry during therapy sessions provides information to both the client and the clinician regarding the correct or needed amount of oxygen that the client is receiving. Adequate oxygen saturation (including a decrease in dyspnea and decrease in fatigue) can be maintained during activities of daily living if good breathing techniques (such as pursed-lip breathing) and appropriate pacing of the activity is conducted.[75]

Stress management, breathing retraining, and relaxation techniques are other areas in which the occupational therapy clinician can provide service to the older adult with pulmonary disease. *Biofeedback*, which gives clients feedback on physiological events in the form of visual or auditory signals, is an excellent resource in facilitating relaxation and breathing training.

Biofeedback machines have transducers that can detect blood pressure, muscle tension, skin temperature, sweat gland activity, heart rate, and brain wave activity.

There are five operations in biofeedback. First, there is the detection and amplification of bioelectric signals (that otherwise would not be detectable). Second, bioelectric signals are converted to visual and auditory signals that the client can understand. Third, these signals can provide instantaneous feedback on the changes in and status of the older adult's biological state. Fourth, cortical awareness of the biological status is triggered. This enables the late life adult to learn volitional control of his or her biological state. Fifth, the skilled execution of the biological response can be reinforced. It is imperative for the biofeedback to be instantaneous, continuous, and directly proportional to the biological change that is taking place. The machine's feedback becomes the reinforcer—thus stimulating learning that is then shaped by the clinician to obtain the desired behavior. Although not an intervention in itself, biofeedback acts as an adjunct to other occupational therapy procedures and techniques. The intervention objectives in biofeedback are to decrease accessory muscle usage, to elicit relaxation, and to increase diaphragmatic breathing.[78] Clients can then use relaxation techniques (learned in biofeedback sessions) to enhance their daily routines.[78]

Other specific breathing techniques, besides biofeedback procedures, can also be employed to promote rhythmic, slow breathing. Pursed-lip breathing (which has been discussed earlier in this component) is used to slow the expiratory phase of breathing and maintain positive pressure in the airways so that they are kept open and able to improve ventilatory efficiency. When learning pursed-lip breathing, the clinician may hold a tissue loosely over the client's mouth to visually reinforce the slow and even exhaled air.[78]

A second technique is known as *diaphragmatic breathing*. This involves teaching the client how to coordinate the abdominal wall expansion with inspiration and to slow air expiration through pursed lips. The goal here is to increase tidal volume in the lungs and slow the respiratory rate. There are several ways to achieve this. One way is to ask the client to breathe out, contract the stomach muscles, and breathe in. This way the diaphragm will naturally expand and allow air movement. To achieve visual reinforcement, the clinician can ask the client to lay supine and then place a lightweight book on his or her abdomen. Then the client can be asked to watch the book rise and fall with each breath.[78]

Lower rib breathing is the final technique. This is accompanied by expanding the rib cage (this allows the lungs to fill up more). In this method the older adult places his or her hands on either side of the body on the lower section of the rib cage. With each expiration this provides some tactile resistance and allows the ribs to expand during inspiration.[78]

Finally, relaxation techniques including *progressive muscle relaxation* (which consists of a series of isometric tensions that are held for a period of 7 to 10 seconds. These are then followed by relaxation for 20 to 40 seconds); the use of tapes that include natural sounds such as rain forests and water flowing in a stream; meditation; imagery; and visualization allow the client to relax and focus.[78]

Occupational therapy has much to offer to the client with COPD in the way of improving his or her functioning capacity. "Occupational therapy is unique in that it brings holistic intervention to the pulmonary rehabilitation setting."[75, p. 28] Whether the therapist or the assistant are teaching a client how to feed him- or herself without becoming exhausted or if the practitioner is educating a homemaker in how to use adaptive equipment in order to resume a familiar and meaningful role, occupational therapy evaluation and intervention are a significant part of the pulmonary rehabilitation team.[75]

CARDIAC REHABILITATION IN LATE LIFE

Heart disease and related conditions have been discussed in Unit 2. This component will deal primarily with cardiac rehabilitation aspects.

The Evaluation

First and foremost is the evaluation process. This is initiated by reviewing the client's medical chart (e.g., the client's presenting primary diagnosis, the secondary diagnosis [if present], past medical history, any surgical procedures, medications and any supplements, and the results of laboratory and other diagnostic tests. Any information regarding the client's social support system and work history should also be noted. The chart review can usually provide the occupational therapy clinician with some information regarding what activity levels would be safest for that particular client).

Secondly, the client should be interviewed. Initially the therapist can begin the discussion with a review of the individual's functional performance level. Other information that the therapist will need includes preadmission roles, coping skills, the number of stairs in the client's home environment, and work (if that is applicable). During the interview process the occupational therapist should observe the client's posture, breathing patterns, level of discomfort, and information processing skills.

A functional evaluation (the client's current functioning level in activities of daily living—with close observation of the client's physiological response to functional tasks is an excellent way to glean information. These physiological responses provide a good indication of the late life adult's endurance or activity tolerance) is the next stage of the evaluation process. Evaluating the upper extremities' range of motion, strength, sensation, and gross and fine motor coordination may also be indicated. The therapist also needs to check with the medical staff concerning any special precautions or client needs before performing this type of evaluation.[76]

Vital Statistics, Cardiac Distress, and Physiological Symptoms

When working with the cardiopulmonary client, the clinician needs to be able to identify cardiopulmonary stress and any other changes on an immediate basis (e.g., rapid, labored, irregular, or shallow breathing that can be accompanied by coughing, wheezing, dyspnea, client cyanosis of the oral mucosa, fingers, and lips; chest pain; and anxiety). Physiological symptoms that directly relate to signs of cardiopulmonary distress also need to be recognized in a quick manner. These include fatigue, dizziness, chest pain, headache, nausea, palpitations, shortness of breath, anxiety, and profuse *diaphoresis* (sweating).[76]

A client's changing condition is indicated by a change in vital signs (e.g., blood pressure or BP; heart rate or HR—which is also known as the pulse, and respiratory rate or RR). *Tachycardia* (abnormally fast heart rate that exceeds 100 beats per minute [bpm]) and *bradycardia* (an abnormally slow heart rate that is less than 60 bpm) indicate that the client needs immediate medical attention. A pulse is evaluated for rhythm, strength, and rate. The respiratory rate refers to the amount of movement of the chest or abdomen (in and out) in one breath. *Tachypnea* is a respiratory rate that is above normal (normal being 12 to 22 breaths per minute), and *bradypnea* refers to a respiratory rate that is slower than normal.[76]

Blood pressure (the force exerted against the walls of the arteries as the blood moves through the arterial vessels) is another cardiac measure. The average systolic blood pressure is considered to be 120 mmHg, and the average diastolic blood pressure is considered at approximately 75 to 80 mmHg. *Hypertension* (high BP) is that which is consistently greater than 140/90. *Hypotension* (low BP) is consistently lower than 90/60. An *oximeter* (a non-invasive instrument that measures the percentage of hemoglobin that is saturated with oxygen) can indicate normal and abnormal O_2 saturation. The normal adult value for O_2 saturation is that which is greater than 95%.[76]

Oximetry is often used in the course of occupational therapy interventions to monitor the older adult's physiological response to a given activity. The oxygen saturation level should be maintained at 90% or greater during any functional activity. The heart rate should be limited to an increase of no more than 20 to 30 bpm above the heart's resting rate. Activity should be terminated with any client who has a heart rate less than 50 bpm. Blood pressure should be limited to a decrease or increase of no more than 15 or 20 mmHg.[76]

During cardiac rehabilitation it is important for clinicians to provide regulated activity and monitoring during the entire rehabilitative process (as this is a method of controlling or reducing the workload or stress that is placed on the heart).[76] *Graded activity* (activity that is modified according to the client's progress) enables the cardiac client to therapeutically proceed at the pace that is appropriate for him or her. It allows for very light activity at the beginning of intervention and then a gradually increasing activity load as safely needed.[76] The client's vital statistics must be measured before starting a therapeutic program or activity. Vital signs should then be measured 5 to 10 minutes into the intervention session and 5 minutes at the end of the session. If a client at any time exhibits an unsafe vital sign change or any symptoms of cardiac distress, the session should be ended immediately. A chart should be kept of all vital sign measurements as a way to monitor progress and increased endurance.[76]

Phases of Intervention

Cardiac rehabilitation consists of four phases. Phase 1 is the period of acute hospitalization. Activities during this phase are limited chair and bed transfers, very basic activities of daily living, and slow walking. Phase 2 consists of the time of discharge and extends to 12 weeks after the cardiac event. Intervention in Phase 2 centers around improving the client's activity tolerance and regaining endurance. It is at this time that risk modification and reconditioning programs are implemented. Mild endurance exercise training is initiated to increase aerobic capacity. Isometric exercise is contraindicated and therefore not permitted in this phase. Phase 3 involves the initiation of rigorous risk factor modification and strength training (to enhance and induce physiological adaptation to exercise, and the client is prepared to return to former activities as appropriate). At this stage, exercise training focuses upon lowering the heart rate and blood pressure so that the myocardial work load is decreased. Phase 4 is the maintenance phase. During this period risk factor modification continues to be ongoing and exercise habits are established.[76]

The Metabolic Equivalent System

Based on the client's physiologic responses to activities, activity levels are increased as the client proceeds through the various phases of cardiac rehabilitation. Every purposeful task places an energy demand on the cardiopulmonary system. Energy expenditure is best measured by the *metabolic equivalent system* (MET). The MET is the energy that is expended while an individual is in a resting state. 1 MET is equivalent to 3.5 mL of oxygen per kilogram of body weight per minute. The energy expenditure of activities is then rated based on the resting MET. For instance, if an activity is rated at 6 METs, that means that the activity requires six times the oxygen that is expended when at rest.[76]

The metabolic equivalent system divides energy expenditure (when involving activities) into several categories. Very light or minimal cardiac activity is considered to be 1 to 2 METs, light cardiac activity utilizes 3 to 4 METs, and heavy cardiac activity requires the use of 4 to 5 METs. Some examples of appropriate functional activities for specific inpatient cardiac activity levels are as follows:

✧ 1.5 METs—Early state of recovery (e.g., bed mobility, transfers to the commode, sedentary leisure tasks with the arm supported while reading or playing cards)

✧ 1.5 to 2 METs—Ongoing recovery (e.g., unsupported sitting [half-hour], standing tasks of 3 to 5 minutes, bedside bathing [clinician assists with feet and back], bathroom privileges)

✧ 2 METs—Progressive recovery (e.g., upper extremity sustained activity of 2 to 5 minutes, total body bathing at sink, standing tasks of 8 to 12 minutes)

- ✧ 2.5 to 3 METs—(e.g., standing tasks of 10 to 30 minutes with intermittant upper extremity activity, upper extremity sustained activity of 5 to 30 minutes, total body mobility, moderate leisure tasks)
- ✧ 3 to 3.5 METs—Continuing recovery (e.g., shower transfers, total showering [total body washing—including hair washing, total body drying], total body dressing, simple homemaking tasks, ability to perform energy-conservation techniques, and home preparation—daily activities using guidelines and recommendations for devices and equipment as appropriate)
- ✧ 3.5 to 4 METs—Most self-care activities fall (e.g., making beds, vacuuming, and mopping the floor) into the 4 METs category.[76,79]

Intervention

Work simplification and energy conservation (as described in the COPD section of this unit) is also an important aspect of cardiac rehabilitation. For example, adaptive equipment such as tub seats and long-handled sponges for bathing can enhance and increase bathing independence for the client who has limited activity tolerance.[76]

The use of relaxation and stress management (e.g., visualization, biomechanical techniques as discussed in the COPD section of this unit) are also highly recommended cardiac remediation.[76,79] It is also important for the client to learn to minimize situations and/or conditions that contribute to emotional stress.

Counseling as to lifestyle changes (e.g., appropriate exercise, pacing one's activities during the day; appropriate nutrition such as making use of a low sodium diet, reducing cholesterol intake, and cessation of smoking) is also part of cardiac rehabilitation.[10,76,79]

The ultimate goal of intervention and education is improving the client's self-management. The following guidelines (some previously referred to) are important aspects in helping the late life client with a cardiac condition achieve his or her fullest functional capacity. These include:[10,76,79,80]

1. The client should know how to utilize energy conservation and work simplification techniques when performing day-to-day activities.
2. The client needs to make use of proper body mechanics as applied to his or her cardiac condition.
3. The client should be made aware of how to distinguish between abnormal and normal cardiopulmonary responses to activities (e.g., shortness of breath, dizziness, chest pain, and chest palpitation).
4. The client needs to be made aware of stress and ways to reduce this factor through relaxation techniques.
5. The client should be educated in how heat and cold can adversely affect the cardiopulmonary system and ways to avoid this (e.g., in cold weather dress warmly, avoid going outside if the weather is severe, and keep the home at a comfortably warm heating level. In hot weather drink fluids, dress in cool comfortable clothing, avoid going outside at the hottest times of the day, and keep the home as cool as possible), enhance the client's knowledge as to how environmental adaptation can improve space efficiency (e.g., keep supplies in an organized and orderly fashion and place them in an accessible area), and reduce the energy that is required to successfully complete a task.

6. The client should be educated in how to reduce environmental irritants (e.g., reduce dust, avoid spray cans).

7. The client needs to recognize the importance of positioning for energy output and increased task accomplishment.

8. The client must learn to pace his or her daily schedule.

INTERVENTION FOR PARKINSON'S DISEASE

Parkinson's disease, a movement disorder caused by the loss of pigmented nerve cells of the substantia nigra, has been described in Unit 2. In the early stages of the disease, preventing musculoskeletal changes, managing the tremor, preventing the loss of mobility, preventing pulmonary complications, preventing abnormal posture, and promoting independent living skills can be achieved through medical management (anywhere from 4 to 8 years). However, in the late stage of this disease balance becomes impaired (e.g., stooped posture, slow shortened steps with a linear progression); and many clients experience falls. The rhythm of movement becomes slowed and/or replaced by diminished amplitude. Handwriting becomes micrographic. Reciprocal lift and grip in fine motor activities becomes slow and ineffective. Defective proprioception and movement is reflected in difficulties buttoning a shirt or cutting meat. Fatigue is a major complaint.[81]

Occupational therapy intervention involves: providing guidance to prevent musculoskeletal impairments, using graded activity to facilitate function (despite symptoms that fluctuate), educating the client to accommodate to the symptoms of the disease and adapting the environment to provide the greatest effectiveness and to maximize sensory input.[81]

The Evaluation Process

The occupational therapy evaluation procedure for the late life client with Parkinson's disease is initiated with a chart review. This also includes a review of the neurologist's report and the results of the magnetic resonance imaging (MRI). A baseline videotape (a recorded image of functional mobility that includes posture, balance, speed of movement), and the functional use of the hands (such as writing a sentence, retrieving an offered object, and reaching to tie shoes) is very helpful in the evaluation process. Specific functional mobility aspects should include rising from a chair, walking approximately 20 feet, returning to the chair, turning one's body around, backing up to the chair, and sitting down.[81]

For those elderly clients who have Parkinson's disease and who also suffer from dementia, the ADL-oriented assessment of mobility scale is recommended.[81,82] The physical dysfunction evaluation can include active and passive range of motion, posture, strength, and functional mobility. A videofluoroscopy examination may also be helpful to rule out silent aspiration. Other pertinent information relating to the evaluation should include an assessment concerning fatigue (the Fatigue Severity Scale is recommended),[83] activity configuration, depression, cognitive status, general awareness about the disease, medications being used, and if there is any participation in support groups (for the client and the caregiver).[81]

Intervention for the Late Life Client With Parkinson's Disease

Hooks contends that there are seven basic occupational therapy goals. These are:[81]

1. Educating and directing the performance of independent living skills by means of therapeutic techniques, sensory stimulation, and movement facilitation
2. Developing a routine for self-care activity within the limitations of functional mobility
3. Establishing an adaptive environment that maximizes sensory stimuli and accommodates immobility
4. Establishing a repertoire of behaviors and adaptive techniques to stimulate movement
5. Educating the client, the care partner, and other family members as well as significant others about Parkinson's disease and the therapeutic process
6. Providing guidelines for habits that facilitate and enhance good posture and movement (e.g., stretching, relaxation, cognitive and physical activity)
7. Helping to develop relationships with a support group[81]

Specific strategies in establishing a routine for activities of daily living includes:

✧   Developing consistent medication times (e.g., take medication upon rising in order to ensure the highest functional level that is currently possible).

✧   Toileting facilities should be accessible and adapted to meet the needs of compromised balance (e.g., a raised toilet seat [or levator] with arm rests, grab bars).

✧   Slippers (with a nonskid surface) and simple clothing should be readily available.

✧   The task of dressing should wait until the medication has had ample time to affect coordination and intricate use of the hands.

✧   The most demanding activities should be attempted during "on" times (when the client is most likely to be able to cope).

✧   Stretching key muscles several times a day can prevent muscle spasms.

✧   Increasing proprioceptive feedback and retaining active range of motion is necessary in order to meet every day challenges (e.g., dressing and bed mobility).[81]

Information booklets on activities of daily living written by occupational therapists are available without a fee to clients with Parkinson's disease by the American Parkinson's Disease Association:

✧   American Parkinson's Disease Association, Inc.

    60 Bay St., Suite 401

    Staten Island, NY 10301

    1-800-223-2732

Sensory stimuli that is carefully selected can aid in helping clients focus on a movement task. An example of one such technique to stop *festination* (shortened steps in a forward direction) is to change the motor program that is in progress. In this case, to restore balance, the clinician asks the client to stop and then places his or her forearm in the client's hand. The proprioceptive cues that are received from the client's hand and arm are enough to supply the brain with sufficient information to facilitate a balanced and upright posture. Other such techniques useful in improving posture are to apply pressure at the low back and fore-shoulder. This feedback facilitates thoracic extension. To elicit lateral weight shift, the clinician can apply gentle pressure via the opposite hip with one hand while using his or her hip to touch the client's adjacent hip. In combatting "freezing," the clinician may ask the client to straighten his or her leg and take a deep breath. Then the clinician will ask the client to step forward as long as the client's feet are taking long steps. A firmly spoken command of "toe up" or "lift" can often break the "freezing" while saying "long stride" may help the older adult move forward in a stride fashion.[81]

Practicing appropriate movement patterns (e.g., reciprocal arm swings or lifting the head and the eyes while walking) can be helpful. To facilitate thoracic extension and improve head position, the client can be taught to take deep breaths while feeling the spinal column straighten. Dynamic activities that demand visual tracking and upper body control should also be encouraged by the clinician (e.g., regulation horseshoes, volleyball, or kneading bread).[81]

Specific instructions in body mechanics to facilitate standing up (such as the clinician asking the client to move forward in the chair, position the hands and feet appropriately and then chanting "rock-two-three" with arm movements for each client as the client rises) are helpful in enhancing correct body mechanics. To promote upright standing, a high stool is preferable to an overstuffed chair.[81]

Rhythm is useful in helping the late life client to continue movement toward the end range (e.g., the rhythm of walking is paced between a march and a waltz). Listening to music while walking aids in heightening and lengthening the client's stride. Similarly, music is also helpful when the client is practicing handwriting using a series of movement patterns. Callirobics (Callirobics, Charlottesville, VA), a 10-week handwriting program, has been successfully used to improve handwriting ability of clients with Parkinson's disease in a Washington University Occupational Therapy Program.[81]

Proprioceptive neuromuscular facilitation movement patterns have been helpful in keeping kinesthetic memory intact for independent daily living skills as well as for stretching. For example, drying off after bathing can be accomplished by using reciprocal extension/flexion patterns of the upper and lower body. Caregivers can participate in the activity by guiding the client's hands to the limits of movement stating "push" for extension and "hold" for 6 seconds, and then signaling the next pattern. In time the tactile and verbal cues can be withdrawn, and sequencing and timing by music (using a waltz tempo or a verbal chant) can be developed.[81] Schenkman and associates suggest another therapeutic model that uses a progression of intervention. These are relaxation, breathing exercises, passive muscle stretching and positioning, postural alignment, active range of motion, weight shifting, balance responses, gait activities, and home exercise programs.[84]

Mat activities that help with the practice in lying down and getting up from the floor as well as rolling from side to side are effective in improving the bed mobility of the client with Parkinson's disease. Other mat activities that utilize reaching across, looking over the shoulder, and turning one's head to stimulate proprioceptive and vestibular information are also useful for improving bed mobility skills.[81]

Late life adults with Parkinson's disease also need to practice slow stretching movements to combat rigidity. Tai chi, volleyball, horseshoes, and other activities that are followed by a short stretching program can help to prevent muscle spasms. Balance practice that includes imagery of the directions of the compass (with visual cues from the clinician to lean north, south, east, and west) is also helpful in maintaining the client's functional abilities.[81]

Relaxation and deep breathing techniques are important components of the thera-peutic program as they raise the threshold at which the muscle can be stimulated to contract. Imagery and progressive muscle relaxation assist in preventing muscle tight-ness during the day. A stretching program can be done with a towel several times a day to prevent metabolic by-products build-up.

Stretching the large muscles of the hips, back, and shoulders frequently during the day and just before bed may aid in alleviating night muscle spasms.[81]

There is much that occupational therapy has to provide late life clients with Parkinson's disease in the variety and richness of intervention offerings.

CANCER AND OCCUPATIONAL THERAPY INTERVENTION

Cancer, a malignant neoplasm, can form a solid mass (known as a tumor) or as in leukemia spread as lymphocytes. These malignant tumors can metastasize (send abnor-mal cells to other body parts via the lymph or blood system). Cancer, as a disease state, has been described in Unit 2.

The Grading System

Clinicians come into contact with clients who are in various stages of tumor growth. Therefore, it is of utmost importance to understand the grading system that is used in this disease. Cancers termed as *low-grade tumors* (slower growing with cell structures that are more consistent and uniform) often respond well to surgery, radiation, chemotherapy, and hormone intervention. By contrast, high-grade tumors (rapidly growing with a tendency to metastasize) are usually more resistive to standard onco-logical intervention. Another way of categorizing cancer statistics is through the use of the *tumor metastasis node* system (TMN). The number of primary tumors is represent-ed by "T," "M" represents the number of metastases, and "N" represents the number of positive lymph nodes. As an example, T1, M1, and N0 indicates that there is one detectable tumor present, the number of metastases is one, and there are no positive lymph nodes present.[85]

The Evaluation Process

The evaluation process of late life cancer clients should include a chart review (e.g., medical management, radiation, chemotherapy, and surgical intervention; mobility [all of the subsets of movement such as range of motion, muscle strength, dexterity, speed of movement, coordination, and purposeful movement]; sensation [both discriminative and protective]; cognitive abilities; vision [visual perception and acuity]; self-care activities; homemaking/home management; and work [volunteer work to be included as well as leisure interests and abilities]).[85]

Intervention

Occupational therapy intervention that occurs immediately after surgery most often focuses upon improving general mobility, basic self-care skills, and swallowing abili-ties (if there is neurological damage, if surgical resection exists that involves the oral or oral pharyngeal cavity, or if there are fungal infections of the oral pharyngeal cavity).[85]

Depending upon the client's medical status, occupational therapy may receive refer-rals for: *lymphedema* (this is edema that is caused by an obstruction of the lymphatics), limitations in joint mobility (e.g., the early onset of adhesive capsulitis); instability that involves the limbs or the trunk, scar management, positioning, or splinting; impairment or loss of an upper extremity or hand function; the fabrication of cosmetic devices; if there is soft tissue compromise, depression, and/or adjustment disorder; somatosensory pain syndromes; and alteration in body image.[85]

If the disease progresses or if there are progressive conditions that are associated with medical interventions, the emphasis of intervention may center upon supportive care (e.g., positioning—to reduce poor functioning or to optimize functioning), rehabilitative approaches that substitute for loss of function, and counseling concerning changes in one's life roles. In this situation the development and support for self-esteem and the enhancement of hope can make a difference in whether the client will resume a "sick" or "well" role.[85]

If the cancer continues to advance, palliative and comfort care may become the main objective. In this case hospice care may be offered. This form of intervention has been discussed in Unit 2.

Preventative care in which wellness strategies are presented to at-risk cancer clients is highly important. Occupational therapists have been successfully involved with smoking cessation and stress reduction strategies in a variety of occupational therapy settings.[85]

Specific intervention techniques and strategies involved in the active occupational therapy management of older adults who are diagnosed with cancer vary as to the specific condition of the client. Foremost, the clinician needs to be aware of the client's level of pain and pain control regimen; the client's ability to tolerate maximal resistance (if there is metastasis to the bone); the side effects of drugs, chemotherapy, and radiation, and if there are isolation procedures that need to be followed.[27]

There are a variety of recommended intervention techniques. The clinician should incorporate functional activities into intervention whenever this is possible. All intervention approaches must be approved with doctor's orders. The maximization of functional independence in self-care activities is of prime importance. As the client's condition demonstrates improvement, training in daily routine tasks should be initiated. These include dressing, bathing, hygiene, grooming, self-feeding, and intervention techniques that involve energy conservation, work simplification, adaptive equipment, repetition, and compensation. It is important to access independence and recommend safety procedures in homemaking and home management activities (e.g., shopping, meal planning, preparation, cleanup, laundering, housekeeping, banking/checking, budgeting, and community mobility).[27]

Another important aspect of therapy is to provide the client (when appropriate) with vendor sources for adaptive equipment such as a bath bench; a toilet riser; grab bars; a rocker knife; a button aid; long-handled bathing, dressing, and cleaning devices; and elastic shoelaces. The maintenance of passive and active range of motion of both upper extremities is important in promoting joint integrity. Therefore the clinician should provide the client with graded activity and exercise programs of passive range of motion that are followed by gentle stretching of tight muscles, active assistance, and active range of motion. In terms of the early post mastectomy client, this individual can begin active range of motion exercise while supine with isometric exercises to the biceps, triceps, and more distal muscle groups. Once the sutures, clips, or staples have been removed, the client can progress to range of motion exercises of the scapula and shoulder. If edema is present, edema control techniques can be initiated (with physician approval) with the use of venous pressure gradient support, air splints (with elevation), Jobst pump, and the elevation of the involved extremity on pillows. The clinician should also become involved with correct posture and positioning (e.g., bed positioning; upright positioning in the wheelchair with the use of assistive positioning such as lapboards, lateral supports, and cushions).[27]

Other techniques useful with cancer management include:

❖ Increasing voluntary use of the involved upper extremity (e.g., muscle re-education, neuromuscular facilitory and inhibitory techniques)

❖ Increasing muscle strength and endurance of the upper extremities (e.g., progressive resistance exercise and graded activities)

❖ Increasing the client's awareness of sensory deficits (e.g., educating in compensatory techniques)

❖ Teaching safety factors (e.g., selecting appropriate water temperatures, avoiding exposure to extreme cold or hot environments, emphasizing consistent skin care, instructing in weight shifts every 15 minutes throughout the day to ensure skin integrity in compressed areas)[27]

More helpful techniques include:[27]

❖ Maximizing the client's tolerance for functional activity (e.g., provide graded activities to promote trunk control as well as increased tolerance for sitting; increase the amount, resistance, and the duration of the activities that the client performs each day—according to the client's tolerance level)

❖ Increasing the client's ability to compensate for visual decline (e.g., provide low vision aids such as large print books, magnifiers)

❖ Instructing clients in safety procedures (e.g., instruct the client in use of environmental methods to ensure safety such as using contrast colors at the stairs, on the stove, and at light switches)

❖ Maximizing cognitive functions (e.g., emphasize intervention strategies that can aid in reducing impairment such as orientation, sequencing, the ability to follow commands, memory, comprehension. These have been described in the section on cognitive intervention within this unit.)

❖ Instructing the family/caregiver/significant other in the client's rehabilitation regime, and assure accessibility in the home (e.g., assess home safety and accessibility in the home setting)

❖ If needed, recommend home modification(s) to the client and caregiver/family/significant other

Occupational therapy has much to offer in the rehabilitation of cancer clients. With our emphasis upon the holistic approach to intervention and our full array of methods and strategies to combat decline, we clinicians can effectively apply our skills and knowledge to aid this population segment.

DIABETES MELLITUS TYPE 2
AND OCCUPATIONAL THERAPY INTERVENTION

Diabetes mellitus type 2 affects 15 to 16 million Americans.[86] This is usually a late life onset condition (although younger persons are presently being diagnosed with this disease).

Evaluation

Suggested components for an occupational therapy evaluation include the following:[27]

1. The chart review
2. Client interview (avocational and vocational history, role history, interests, and present perception of the disease as it affects the client)
3. Self-care skills
4. Upper extremity active and passive range of motion
5. Upper extremity muscle strength
6. Upper extremity muscle tone
7. Upper extremity dexterity and coordination
8. Sensation assessment of the upper extremity (e.g., hot/cold, light touch, deep touch, sharp/dull)
9. Skin control (e.g., presence of skin lesions/ulcers, general skin appearance)
10. Cognitive function (e.g., judgment, orientation, memory, problem solving, following commands as related to daily activities and attention span)
11. Visual/perceptual functioning
12. Home safety and accessibility
13. Endurance
14. Architectural barriers within the client's community setting

There are some major precautions for clinicians, the client, and the family to be aware of when treating the diabetic 2 late life adult:[27]

❖ Be aware of the symptoms of *insulin shock* (known as *hypoglycemia*). This occurs when there is an insufficient amount of glucose for energy metabolism and an overabundance of insulin. Signs and symptoms of this condition involve headache, lassitude, drowsiness, shallow respirations, tremulousness, and nausea. In the event of a reaction (and if the client can swallow) utilize some form of sugar as found in orange juice, sugar water, cola, or a teaspoon of honey.

❖ The clinician, the client, and the family should also be well aware of the symptoms of *hyperglycemia* (a condition in which too little insulin is present in the blood, and the blood sugar level remains too high). Extreme thirst, fast and deep breathing, heartburn, excessive urination, nausea, headaches, blurred vision, constipation, and abdominal pain are symptoms of this condition. Medical and nursing services should be notified immediately of these signs and symptoms as they may lead to diabetic coma.

❖ Avoid injury. The client is subject to infections. Therefore, all cuts or abrasions should be reported and intervention rendered as needed.

✧   Be aware that the client's skin heals less readily and is susceptible to damage. Protect ulcers and lesions, particularly of the foot.

✧   Avoid excessive fatigue.

✧   Reinforce diet regulations.

✧   Prevent edema in the extremities that are poorly vascularized or after amputation by the use of elevation techniques and procedures.

✧   If the client is receiving injections, be aware of the site. If the muscle under the injection site is able to exercise, the insulin can metabolize more quickly. This can lead to a rapid decrease in blood sugar that is due to increased insulin circulation or a rise in blood sugar levels after exercise due to depleted storage of insulin.

Intervention

Occupational therapy intervention and management of diabetes 2 involves a number of strategies and modalities:[27,28]

✧   Increase functional independence in self-care (e.g., dressing, bathing, feeding, grooming).

✧   Educate the client in the use of energy conservation, work simplification, and time management.

✧   Instruction in adaptive equipment and in compensatory techniques for sensory and visual loss (e.g., low vision aids such as magnifiers).

✧   When needed, provide vendor sources for adaptive equipment.

✧   Promote independence and safety in home management activities—and in all activities whenever possible (e.g., use of long-handled dust brush and dustpan to prevent bending and possible falls).

✧   Foster appropriate meal planning (with the assistance of the dietitian or nutritionist).

✧   Educate the client in calorie counting, the weighing and measuring of food, and food exchanges.

✧   Ensure easy access and safety in the home by developing home modification recommendations as needed.

✧   Increase strength, endurance, range of motion, and activity tolerance (e.g., encourage the client to perform activity that is regulated in order to assist in insulin regulation).

✧   Provide aerobic exercise programming and graded upper extremity activities in a graduated fashion.

✧   Instruct the client in monitoring his or her blood sugar before and after exercise. There should be a "warm-up" and "cool down" phase as a part of every exercise program.

✧   Instruct the client to take his or her own pulse and identify his or her own target rate.

✧   Promote exercise that is appropriate in the community setting such as walking, cycling, and swimming. On average, the late life adult should be able to increase his or her exercise tolerance to approximately 20 to 30 minutes at least three times a week.

✧ If the client has had a recent below-the-knee amputation, ensure that he or she will receive a posterior knee conformer as soon as possible to minimize potential joint contractures.

✧ Increase the amount and duration of the activities that the client participates in each day.[27,87]

Other occupational therapy strategies that are useful for older clients with a diabetic 2 diagnosis include:[27]

✧ Increasing the individual's awareness of sensory problems (e.g., instruct the client in safety factors such as the appropriate use of the stove, selection of appropriate water temperature).

✧ Emphasizing the importance of consistently taking care of one's skin, use a mirror for inspection, dry skin thoroughly after bathing (especially the feet).

✧ Involving the client who has decreased sensation of the lower extremities to become aware of the fact that he or she may benefit from especially made shoes.

✧ The client should also be made aware of the possible benefits from the fabrication of shoe inserts so that pressure is evenly distributed over the sole of the foot during weight-bearing and ambulation.

✧ Ensuring and instructing the client and family in the knowledge of the rehabilitation process (e.g., provide instruction in the appropriate use of body mechanics in order to minimize or avoid injury).

✧ Ensuring the safe administration of insulin and medication management.

✧ For those clients experiencing diabetic retinopathy problems (which may vary from day to day and person to person), the clinician needs to address lighting, glare, and contrast issues.

✧ Encourage appropriate foot care as follows:
   1. Change socks daily.
   2. Do not wear socks that have darns or holes.
   3. Cut toe nails straight across.
   4. Do not cut calluses or corns.
   5. Break in new shoes slowly.
   6. Always wash feet in warm water (never hot) and pat dry with a soft towel.
   7. Do not walk barefooted.
   8. Wear only well-fitted shoes.

Stress management is another area of intervention that needs to be addressed. Instructing the client in relaxation techniques to decrease stress, fear, and tension (e.g., guided imagery, progressive relaxation, breathing techniques, and autogenic relaxation) is important. Assisting the client, the family, and significant others with the psychological adjustment to the disease (e.g., provide constructive outlets for frustration and anger through the use of therapeutic activities) is another important aspect of occupational therapy intervention. The clinician can also introduce support groups and help develop avocational interests and skills (including the assessment of and recommendations for adaptations that are needed so that the client can continue to participate in former and present avocational pursuits).[10,27]

One can readily see that occupational therapy can play a vital role in enabling older adults who are diabetic to improve their general health status, enhance their quality of life, and gain a sense of personal control over their lives.[10]

Osteoarthritis and Occupational Therapy Intervention

General Description

Osteoarthrtis is a degenerative joint process in which the cartilage on the end of the bone wears down (a pathological deterioration of the articular cartilage). The bone starts to grow around the margins of the joint (formation of the new bone at the bone's margins of the joint and in subchondral areas—resulting in the formation of osteophytes) which causes a "lumpy" enlarged appearance. This degenerative process can be caused by genetic heritage (known as "primary osteoporosis"). All other types of osteoarthritis degeneration are defined as "secondary osteoporosis." These include: impaired blood supply, wear and tear of daily living, continued minor trauma, excessive strain and wear and tear on specific joint areas (e.g., obese persons might develop osteoarthritis in the hips and knees; desk workers might develop the disease in the wrist, spine, and neck), and a single severe injury.[10,88]

The most affected areas are the weight-bearing joints (i.e., knees, hips, and lumbar spine). Total hip and knee replacement are major avenues of intervention for individuals affected with this condition. The role of occupational therapy with his type of remediation will be considered in the section entitled Orthopedic Rehabilitation later in this unit.

Hand Management

The focus for this discussion will be upon osteoarthritis as it affects the hand. Involvement of osteoarthritic joints of the upper extremities and digits can compromise the fine motions of the fingers. Common complaints and symptoms include joint pain on rising, stiffness after immobility (such as any type of static positioning such as sleeping, sitting, etc.) during damp weather and periods of fatigue, and limited range of motion in the affected joints.[10]

In the hands, the degenerative process of osteoarthritis can continue for years without any stiffness or pain. Then, at some point, an individual can develop inflammation in the joint. This causes pain, stiffness, and, at times, swelling and redness. It is the pain that ultimately limits one's activity level.[88]

Osteoarthritis can affect all of the joints in the thumb. The base of the thumb (known as the carpal-metacarpal [CMC] joint) is most commonly affected. However, osteoarthritis can occasionally spread to the adjacent joints of the trapezium bone within the CMC. This condition is termed pan-trapezial or STT (because it affects the scaphoid, trapezium, and trapezoid bones as well as the joints between them). In osteoarthritis the CMC is affected most often because the thumb is used very often and because its wide range of mobility makes it vulnerable to stress.

Symptoms of osteoarthritic problems with the CMC joint involve:[88]

1. Aching or pain around the base of the thumb, up the forearm, or down the thumb toward the tip. The pain may become worse when the thumb is used to pinch something.
2. The CMC joint may become stiff in the morning or after it has not been used in a while.
3. Tenderness over the CMC joint is common.

4. If the inflammation is severe, there may be redness, warmth, or swelling.

5. In time, the motion in the joint may become limited. For instance, it may be difficult to spread the web space between the thumb and index finger as wide as possible (making it difficult to grasp large objects), and it may become difficult to place the palm flat on the table.

6. The thick ending around the joint margins may give the joint a square or protruding appearance.

7. The adjacent joints of the CMC joint may develop STT arthritis.

In terms of occupational therapy remediation, an *orthosis* (customized splint) that immobilizes the wrist and the thumb can reduce motion and stress on the CMC joint. This provides the CMC joint with "local rest" to the joint that allows the tissues inside to become less inflamed. This way, the client can perform activities and still protect the thumb so that it can heal. Adaptive equipment or tools can be helpful in lessening stress on the CMC joint. Specifically, enlarging or padding a handle and making it non-slip, and enlarging the head of keys (especially the ignition key of the car, which makes a lever force and using lever faucets) are excellent ways of reducing pressure on the CMC joint. The client can also be instructed in reducing the amount of tightness that he or she may be using to hold a tool. If inflammation does occur, a cold compress may be applied.[88]

Osteoarthritis of the thumb's metacarpal-phalangeal (MCP) joint presents symptomatically as the inability to spread one's thumb away from the hand. This results in the difficulty of not being able to grasp large objects such as books, milk cartons, files, or thick catalogs, and the activity of using squeeze bottles (e.g., liquid detergent, contact lens solutions, shampoo bottles, or lotions) places stress and resulting pain on the MCP joint. Occupational therapy remediation, in most instances, calls for the fabrication of the CMC orthosis.[88]

Osteoarthritis of the thumb interphalangeal joint (IP) as well as the distal interphalangeal (DIP) joints of the fingers is very common and tends to be related more to genetics than to trauma, strain, or overuse. Symptoms in these joints are:

✧   The IP joint of the thumb or the DIP of the fingers may develop a painless bony enlargement which may cause a loss of motion.

✧   The joint may become inflamed, painful, and enlarged.

✧   The joint may become unstable (e.g., the pinching motion may cause the joint to collapse backward).

✧   The joint may become bent at an angle.

Occupational therapy remediation calls for wearing an orthosis that blocks motion that decreases inflammation and pain and stabilizes the joint to allow motion. The figure eight orthosis is recommended for these purposes.[88] If a joint does not respond to orthosis immobilization, steroid injections, or medication to decrease pain and increase function, surgical interventions may be utilized.[88]

Osteoarthritis of the fingers most often occurs in the DIP and the proximal interphalangeal joints (PIP). Symptoms associated with this condition often include stiffness and inflammation. There are two basic reasons for stiffness in the fingers. First, there is a gel phenomenon. This is associated with morning stiffness and develops because fluid in the tissues and in the joint sets up like gelatin when they do not experience movement. This occurs after one has not used his or her fingers in a long time (e.g., sleeping or watching television or a movie). However, once movement is initiated, the joint area begins to "loosen up."[88] The second response involving stiffness occurs when there is permanent loss of motion. This can make the fingers feel extremely stiff. Bending or straightening one's fingers fully becomes difficult or impossible to perform. This is due to bone growth (osteophyte formation) around the edge of the joints (not due to ligament or tendon problems or muscle weakness). When the bones hit the edge of the thickened bone, they are unable to move further. This is technically known as "bonyblock."[88]

Occupational therapy remediation of the fingers, in most instances, calls for the reduction of inflammation that is associated with stiffness and pain. First, there is the use of therapeutic stretch gloves at night which are effective in reducing morning pain and stiffness. There are two types of gloves that are available for consideration. Futura Thermoelastic Gloves™ are knit elastic gloves that are tight at the fingertips and less tight in the hand. These are designed specifically for the reduction of swelling. Esotoner™ gloves (made of nylon) are lighter and do not provide gradient tension. After usage of both, the client with the help of the clinician can determine which is most helpful. A second form of remediation is to ask the client to fill the bathroom sink with comfortable warm-hot water and squeeze a large Nerf ball or a large very soft sponge in the water. Using something soft will encourage a lot of finger motion.[88]

Next, the following exercises can also be conducted in the warm water:

✧ Ask the client to straighten and stretch his or her fingers as much as is possible.

✧ Then ask the client to make a complete fist as much as possible.

✧ Then ask client to spread his or her fingers as wide as possible.

If there is a problem specifically with the DIP joints, it may be due to bony cysts (often painful while they are forming and then painless after becoming bone). To combat inflammation and pain in the DIP joints, the clinician can:

1. Fabricate a slip-on (plastic cylinder splint) that is specifically designed to immobilize the DIP joint (thereby reducing inflammation and subsequent pain).

2. Recommend joint-protection techniques.

3. Wrap the joint with nonadhesive tape that is self-adhering (such as Coban Wrap). This will keep the joint warm and act as a reminder to the client to be gentle with the joint.

When there are problems (especially in the finger PIP joints), splinting with an orthosis for more than a few days is not recommended as these joints are used to manipulate tools and equipment. Also, the ligaments of these joints are prone to stiffness (if immobilized in any one position). For severe inflammation a steroid injection or surgical joint reconstruction with a Silastic implant (Wright Medical, Arlington, TN) is recommended. Occupational therapy intervention includes the use of joint protection techniques: wearing a glove (golf or driving is helpful) with the fingertips cut out to keep the joint warm; wrapping the joint with a Neoprine sleeve or Coban Wrap to keep the joint warm and remind the client to be gentle with the joint; and if there is severe inflammation, a cold compress can be helpful.[88]

In general, there are times when cold is best to be used and times when warmth is best. Melvin suggests the following guidelines.[88]

For application of cold:

✧ Cold works best when there is severe, acute inflammation (e.g., the presence of redness, warmth, and swelling).

✧ Cold should only be used if there is improvement (even if the joint is inflamed).

✧ If the joint feels worse after initiating cold intervention, discontinue the intervention.

✧ In the thumb, where there has been inflammation caused by excessive use of the CMC and the MCP joint, cold is helpful.

✧ If all DIP joints are warm and inflamed, dip them in ice water for approximately 1 minute.

✧ Place the DIP joints between two cold gel packs (apply only to the affected joints).

✧ Apply a thin plastic bag that is filled with crushed ice.

✧ Place a thin wet cloth such as a handkerchief or thin dish towel between the client's skin and the ice.

✧ Apply a cold gel pack that has two layers of thickness for 10 to 15 minutes. If the client's hands are thin, less time will be required.

For application of heat:[88]

✧ Warmth is best when the major problem is stiffness as heat loosens up the joints and increases circulation. This in turn reduces stiffness.

✧ Heat also tends to increase fluid or swelling in the joint, and as such is contraindicated for use if the joint is inflamed or swollen.

✧ Place the hands in warm water that is of a comfortable and helpful temperature.

✧ Use gel-filled mitts (that can be heated in the microwave—make certain that these are not too hot prior to intervention).

✧ Ask the client to wear plastic gloves while performing housework (alleviates discomfort by keeping the fingers warm).

✧ If there is a single painful joint, one can wrap a two-layer strip of plastic food wrap around the joint (wrap firmly but not tightly). This acts like a mini-sauna and increases circulation to the joint. This is helpful at night if one or more of the joints are painful, and wear a warm mitten or glove for a half-hour.

Reducing muscle tension is another helpful strategy. If muscular guarding exits (when a client becomes cautious concerning the use of his or her hands due to pain), this produces a natural reaction to protect the hands. These subconscious protective measures can result in muscle tightness of the shoulders, neck, back, arms, and hands. Most people are unaware of this situation until they stop to notice it. The clinician can educate the client to become aware of neck or shoulder discomfort when he or she is performing a specific activity. Once the client has recognized this, he or she can be taught to check positioning and the amount of tension experienced. At this point, the client can begin to "loosen up" and try to continue the activity with the arms more relaxed. With effort and awareness, this habit can be changed with the resulting loss of pain in both the neck and the hands.[88]

Joint Protection and Energy Conservation

Joint protection techniques are another important aspect of occupational therapy remediation with osteoarthritic hands. Performing an activity with less pain is a sign that the joint is not being aggravated.[88] The following joint protection and energy conservation measures (utilizing assistive devices and adaptive measures to reduce joint pain) are recommended to alleviate or decrease joint stress:[10,88, 89]

✧ Use adapted handles (adhesive foam, foam tubing, or custom-made handles [out of orthotic materials]). These may have adapted, narrowed, or built-up handles. They are also available on the commercial market. Adapted handles are very useful with items such as utensils or toothbrushes to enhance grip with less tension.

✧ Utilize non-slip pads such as Dycem™ mats to reduce the force that is needed to stabilize items (e.g., under a dinner plate or a bowl).

✧ Use commercial key holders that increase leverage.

✧ Utilize leverage type fixtures for faucets or taps to reduce strain.

✧ Use lamp switch extenders that increase lever force (making turning on the switch easier). Touch-sensitive lamps are also available.

✧ Utilize leverage handles on doors instead of doorknobs to aid in opening and closing doors.

✧ Use the strongest joints available for any activity.

✧ Silicone spray such as WD-40 (WD-40 Company, Northbrook, IL) can ease the operation of locks, hinges, and sliding doors.

✧ Soaped runners on kitchen drawers increase the ease of sliding.

✧ Lightweight dishes, kitchen utensils, and pots should be utilized.

✧ Under-counter or wall-hung jar openers that permit bilateral palmar holding of the container are exceedingly helpful for individuals with active hand inflammation.

✧ Wipe spills immediately to avoid baking onto stone surfaces.

✧ Use a full teakettle to stabilize a saucepan against when one is stirring food in saucepan.

✧ When making a bed, make only one trip around the bed to save energy.

✧ Avoid sideways pressure on the fingers.

✧ Spring-load clipping scissors require no pressure for performance.

✧ Avoid tight grasp.

✧ Round bowls with a rubber-stabilizing ring permit the bowl to be positioned in a variety of angles.

✧ When performing a task such as cleaning out the refrigerator, divide the task into small sections, such as cleaning out one shelf a day (and remember to sit while doing so).

✧ Use commercial shoulder pads for straps on handbags, shopping bags, or suitcases to reduce hand tension.

✧ Avoid taking any item that involves the use of heavy weight on the fingers.

✧ Respect pain so that the undue strain is not placed on the joints.

✧ Sit while working.

✧ Sit and support the elbows on a counter or table when combing one's hair or shaving.

✧ Pace work periods.

✧ Slide objects instead of lifting them.

✧ Dress the lower extremities first as this takes more energy. Sit as much as possible while dressing.

✧ Always face one's work.

✧ Avoid positions that have the potential to cause deformity.

✧ Keep bulk foods in small containers.

✧ Set up efficient work areas (e.g., cooking, dishwashing) and rearrange tools and equipment as well as readjust working heights to promote comfort and efficiency.

✧ Organize items so that the most used articles are within easy reach.

✧ Avoid sustained (static) positions (using muscles in one position for long time periods).

✧ Maintain good body mechanics and good body positioning. Avoid positions of flexion if possible. Avoid twisting at the waist.

✧ Use straight-back chairs with a firm seat.

✧ Avoid clutter. Throw away things that are not needed.

✧ Eliminate details and combine steps as appropriate.

✧ Breathe easy. Use slow deep breathing to promote adequate ventilation.

✧ Organize the day so that it will not be overtiring. Make use of regular rest periods.

Intervention in General

Utilizing relaxation techniques, getting restful sleep, and participating in exercises (that allow one's heart rate to go up but are not "hard" on the joints) such as walking, arm exercises while seated, swimming, and nonimpact aerobics are examples of safe exercise that should be encouraged. These kinds of exercises increase the oxygen within the system (including the tissues in and around the joints). Oxygen plays a central role in helping the cells to function better, including those of the immune system (so that they can aid in helping the body to better control inflammation). Using good nutrition (low in fat, moderate to high in complex carbohydrates, and moderate in protein) is another example of helping the body to maintain and improve healthy living. Together all these recommendations provide a healthful, good source of energy that uses a holistic approach so that one can function at his or her maximum potential.[88]

Reducing Pain in Joints Other Than in the Hands

There are a number of methods that can be used to alleviate arthritis pain (and stress) on the joints other than in the hands. These include:[89]

✧ For those with painful knees or for those who have difficulty balancing, a bath chair or stool can be helpful in ensuring safety. It also allows for independent bathing for those individuals who experience difficulty lowering themselves into a bathtub.

✧ Raising the height of a favorite chair (removing the casters and attaching furniture legs of the desired height) aids in allowing the client to rise and sit down in comfort (and without assistance).

✧ Storing pots at waist level helps to avoid strenuous lifting. Condiments should be kept within easy reach.

✧ Using a wheeled cart for transporting kitchen and laundry items decreases stress on the joints.

✧ Utilizing Velcro (Velcro USA, Manchester, NH) fasteners whenever possible will minimize joint strain.

✧ Using long-handled brooms, dustpans, and mops will save one from bending and stooping.

✧ A long-handled brush with a cloth wrapped around it can be useful when cleaning the back of an oven.

✧ Using a broom to close a bottom dresser drawer involves less energy than bending from waist level.

✧ Any lifting should be done with leg muscles rather than back muscles.

✧ When carrying an object one should hold it close to his or her body for ease and efficiency.

✧ Making use of carefully planned work routines as well as organizing daily work areas is helpful in promoting efficiency and endurance.

✧ Planning to do the most difficult tasks when one is at his or her peak energy level (e.g., a morning person) enhances one's ability to accomplish the task or tasks.

✧ Making lists of what one must do (a need) as opposed to what one would like to do (a want) can aid in prioritizing one's responsibilities. This list can be for each week and also for each day. Trying to take care of as many responsibilities from the "need" list and also allowing time for those things one enjoys is important in balancing one's day. It is important to be flexible and not to get upset if these activities cannot be completed.

Aqua Therapy and Osteoarthritis

Aquatic therapy involves the use of water in which rehabilitation interventions are rendered to improve function. Water's warmth and buoyancy can provide relaxation. This in turn can aid in decreasing stiffness and pain. Water engineering and physics principles of flotation equipment can be used to position both therapists and clients for a variety of interventions as well as reducing joint trauma and weight-bearing. Meditative stretching and relaxation through the clinician's use of in-water positioning and rocking can also be used to address psychosocial needs.[90]

For many clients aquatic therapy can offer an ideal occupational therapy setting as it allows them to engage in a variety of meaningful occupations that might otherwise be impossible or difficult to perform during land-base intervention. The water's physical properties can therapeutically increase and improve occupational performance for a variety of reasons. Some of these include:[90]

1. Buoyancy reduces the effects of gravity (allowing a greater amount of movement).

2. Water's neutral warmth also promotes relaxation for clients who experience pain, stress, or muscle tightness.

3. The water's resistance can also enhance endurance training, graded activities, and strength building.

4. Other benefits also include improved psychosocial factors (e.g., interests, self-esteem, trust, and social conduct).

Specific activities such as aquatic dancing can be used to facilitate contraction of upper extremity muscles and trunk to improve posture while participating with a family member, a friend, or a significant other.[90]

Pain control and relaxation are promoted through the buoyancy and warmth of the water as well as through stretching activities (e.g., tai chi). Endurance and low impact strengthening are promoted by means of the water's resistance during activities such as swimming, treading water, water games, and water dancing.[90] Aquatic therapy can serve as a unique yet familiar modality in enhancing and improving function with osteoarthritic late life adults.

The Arthritis Foundation provides a number of "no cost" educational brochures and information on local exercise programs as well as self-help courses:

✧ The Arthritis Foundation
  1314 Spring St. N.W.
  Atlanta, GA 30309
  1-800-283-7800

Falls, Fear of Falling, and Fall Prevention

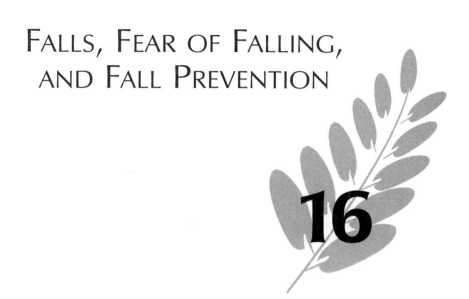

16

Description

Falling, an important health concern for late life adults, can lead to potentially serious injury, activity limitation, reduced functional ability, emotional distress, disability, fear, loss of independence, medical complications, depression, and an overall increase in health care costs.[91]

One in three people older than 65 falls each year. In 1998 approximately 9,600 older adults died from fall-related injuries. Those elderly who have fallen are two to three times more likely to fall again.[92] Falls cause 12% of all deaths for individuals 65 years or older. This makes falls the sixth leading cause of death among late life adults.[93] Falls occur in 32% of persons aged 65 to 74, in 35% of individuals 75 to 84 years of age or older, and in 51% of individuals 85 years of age or older.[94] Women are more at risk than men (42% of females who are 65 to 74 years old fall as opposed to 20% of males who are in the same age group).[94]

Falls can have a devastating effect on a late life adult's sense of safety and self-confidence. Because the fear of becoming dependent and of falling are so highly intertwined, many older adults will deny that they may have a problem falling. This makes it difficult to provide them with the help they need to continue living a healthy life style.[95]

Causes of Falls

There are two categories or conditions that cause falls. One is the *intrinsic* (or host) factor, and the other is the *extrinsic* factor. Intrinsic factors can encompass normal changes that occur in aging and in pathological states. These may include: cardiac problems; hemiplegia (a direct result of a cardiovascular accident); diabetes; osteo-porosis; osteoarthritis; orthostatic hypotension; reduced ability to notice an approach-ing car, siren, or bicycle; sensory losses or changes; syncope; progressive neurological disorders; postural instability; gait impairment; slowed reflexes; decreased muscle strength and range of motion; medication side effects; cognitive and/or perceptual impairment; incontinence, which can lead to the older adult taking risks to reach the toilet; addictive disorders such as alcoholism; any pathological state that can influence mobility; and psychiatric disorders such as depression, anxiety, and fear which may lead to a decreased ability to concentrate (and consequently a decreased awareness of the environment). Many elderly who are at high-risk for falls deny this, and as a result, they exhibit high-risk fall behavior.[91,96]

Extrinsic factors involve environmental conditions. These may involve clutter, the improper placement of furniture and supplies, existence of obstacles, pets under foot (as well as their food plates), inadequate lighting, throw rugs that are not secure, lack of safety devices in the bathroom (such as grab bars, or a bath seat in the shower, or a hand-held shower spray), slippery high-glossed floors, improper height of furniture, and lack of banisters on either side of the steps.[91,96]

OCCUPATIONAL THERAPY INTERVENTION REGARDING FALL PREVENTION IN THE COMMUNITY

Occupational therapy intervention includes several aspects. Some of these are ther-apeutic exercise programs to increase muscle strength and improve balance, instruc-tion in the use of assistive and adaptive devices to prevent falls, educating the client in appropriate nutritional and medication intake, and environmental adaptations and safety instruction in fall prevention. Occupational therapy can play a pivotal role in evaluating elderly clients to achieve as much independence as possible.

Increasing muscle strength, improving balance and gait, adequate monitoring of medications, the appropriate use of assistive devices, and the use of correct footwear were considered (by a recent study at Yale University under the guidance of Thomas Gill, MD) to be major factors in the prevention of falls.[97] In general, keeping fit and well conditioned not only enhanced good health but also aided in promoting the preven-tion of falls.[97]

Occupational therapists have been involved in a number of exercise programs with-in the community that promote wellness. Clinicians can readily incorporate standard style "fitness and well-being" programs within the umbrella of leisure time pursuits.

Late life adults need physical alerting exercises and activities to promote the use of daily tasks (e.g., dressing, bathing, carrying the groceries, and taking out the garbage).

Exercise has many benefits. Some of these consist of enhancing and improving car-diovascular function and endurance (such as decreasing blood pressure, developing auxiliary networks of small blood vessels which in turn decrease the load on the arter-ies; increasing the levels of high-density lipoprotein; and strengthening the respiratory muscles). Exercise consumes excess fatty tissue while at the same time it builds up lean body mass; increases glycogen in the muscles which helps to sustain activity, conditions muscles to work more before becoming fatigued; lessens the load on the nervous sys-tem by slowing electrical signals that are sent from the muscles; improves psychological well-being; improves general endurance; improves strength (the maximal power a person can generate); and *flexibility* (the ability to have full range of motion); improves body composition (e.g., the amount of fat versus lean body mass in the body); improves weight control; aids in digestion and reduces constipation; improves dynamic strength (also known as muscle endurance); and improves coordination and balance.

Weight-bearing exercise, for those who are diagnosed with osteoporosis, is thought to have a greater positive effect than nonweight-bearing activity. Walking, dancing, stair climbing, gentle jogging, and weight training are some examples of weight-bearing. All of these activities should begin slowly and increase gradually according to client tolerance. It is suggested that this type of activity take place three to four times weekly from 45 minutes to no more than an hour per session.[27] Practicing good posture, taking part in postural exercises, and the use of proper body mechanics are also recommended.[27]

In terms of aerobic exercises that encourage improved cardiac endurance, Herring recommends that intermediate exercise classes should consist of a warm-up of 10 minutes, a conditioning phase of 20 minutes, a pre-cool down phase of 5 minutes, a muscle strengthening phase of 10 minutes, and a cool down period of 10 minutes.[98]

Before promoting an exercise group, each clinician should receive a health clearance from the expected participant's physician. Awareness of the Safe Exercising Pulse Test is also recommended. This test is determined by the physician subtracting resting pulse rate from the maximum pulse rate (the greatest heart rate that the heart can safely beat) to ensure there is no overexertion. One should keep the heart rate within 10 to 13 beats of the safe exercising pulse.[99] With aerobic exercise the standard formula for a safe heart rate is 220 minus one's age multiplied by .70 to .85 of the individual's heart rate.

Whether the clinician is involved in a community group setting or providing individual consultation, exercise remains a powerful tool for improving function. An example of occupational therapy involvement in community-oriented exercise and wellness is Mary Borguard-Krenik's "Limited Class Exercise." This program was held at a multipurpose senior center in Greenville County, SC and is part of the Senior Action Program of Greenville County. The program meets three times weekly for a 45-minute session. A supportive atmosphere, flexible programming geared to the needs of the participants, and music were offered as part of the structure of the program. Specific exercises involved head rotations, wrist circles, finger dexterity motions, shoulder movements, and hip and waist movements. The three basic goals for this program were increasing circulation, flexibility, and endurance.[100]

Nutrition is an important aspect of any fitness or conditioning program. If one is a diabetic or has any other physical problems that affect food intake, it is imperative that the client follows the expected routine and be taught what types of food to eat, what types of food to avoid, how much to take, and when to eat (some disorders call for small meals that are served often). For most elderly a balanced diet includes proteins (e.g., legumes, fish, lean meat, chicken, or turkey), and calcium—especially if one is diagnosed with osteoporosis (e.g., nonfat milk, nonfat yogurt, tofu, collard greens, and turnips). Intake of vitamin D and potassium are also helpful for those with this condition; bread that has fiber, cereal and brown rice products, fruits and vegetables (e.g., citrus fruits such as oranges, tangerines, strawberries, cantaloupe; dark green vegetables such as broccoli, spinach, turnip greens; dark yellow vegetables such as carrots and yellow squash), and vegetables high in vitamin C (cabbage, baked potatoes) pro-vide a firm foundation for fueling the body with the resources it needs.[10] The clinician can supplement this information on nutritional food groups with easy-to-prepare recipes, instruction on how to read and understand nutritional content on food labels when shopping, and resources that describe how to cook with disabilities (e.g., arthri-tis, one-handed techniques for an individual with a dislocated shoulder).

Three resources that are helpful:

❖ Klinger, J. L., Frieden, F. H., & Sullivan, R. A. *Mealtime manual for the aged and the handicapped* (compiled by the Institute of Rehabilitation Medicine, New York Medical Center). Essandess Special Editions, New York.

❖ *Self-Help Manual for Patients with Arthritis.* Available from the Arthritis Foundation. 1-800-283-7800

❖ Lurio, D. (1983). *Special recipes for special people.* Philadelphia: Skylight Press.

Proper intake of medication and awareness of the side effects of each medication is important in promoting general well-being and preventing falls. This includes such aspects as being able to read medication labels; storing medication in the appropriate setting (e.g., in the refrigerator, out of sunlight); checking the date of the expiration of the medication and removing the prescription if the time has expired; being able to physically swallow the medication; awareness of any perceptual, sensory, or motor deficits that might affect the management of the medication; having the cognitive awareness to understand why the medications are needed and when to take them (e.g., morning, afternoon, evening); and how to take them (e.g., with food/without food/with water/without grapefruit juice). The clinician can be crucial in instructing in the use of adaptive type materials (such as pill containers that are easily opened and that are color coded for appropriate access), promoting finger dexterity exercises for strength-ening weakened muscles, educating in time management techniques (e.g., timers, written routines that are simple and enlarged visual aid in promoting the proper time for medication intake). These strategies are all part of occupational therapy's scope of remediation.

SAFETY ASSESSMENT TOOLS

Another important aspect of fall prevention is promoting safety and preventing fatigue when performing everyday activities. Assessments concerning safety and a "falls history" can provide valuable information which can be used to determine appropriate intervention.

An excellent instrument, useful in determining a client's "falls history" is:

❖ Falls Interview Schedule (FIS). This can be found on pages 662-663 (Appendix A) of the second edition (1996) of *The Role of Occupational Therapy With the Elderly.*[91]

Another excellent resource that is useful for determining safety in the home is:

❖ The Home Assessment Checklist for Fall Hazards. This can be found on pages 664-666 (Appendix B) of the second edition (1996) of *The Role of Occupational Therapy With the Elderly.*[91]

The original source for The Home Assessment Checklist for Fall Hazards is as follows:

✧ Berkman, C. & Miller, P. A. (1991). Fall Interview Schedule: Comprehensive falls questionnaire for community dwelling elders. In P. Miller (Ed.), *Programs in occupational therapy* (pp. 40-42). New York: Columbia University Press.

Tinetti recommends a performance-based mobility evaluation that looks at balance and gait. In this test the therapist observes the older adult walking and examines the sequences that are involved in his or her gait. The client is then asked to perform a number of functionality-oriented balance tasks while under the observation of the therapist. The client is asked to rise from a chair, stand balanced with his or her eyes closed, and then to complete a 360-degree turn while in a standing mode. The therapist rates the client's performance after observation and gives a numerical score for the normal, adaptive, or abnormal for each component that was assessed. A low score indicates that the individual may be at risk for falls.

This evaluation is available in the following article:

✧ Tinetti, M. E. (1996). Performance-oriented assessment of mobility problems in elderly patients. *J Am Geriatr Soc, 34*, 119-126.

It is important to know how to apply this information to occupational performance of daily tasks. For instance, an older adult who demonstrates difficulties with balance while standing with his or her eyes closed may be at risk for falls when trying to pull a shirt over his or her head while in a standing position.[91]

ENVIRONMENTAL SAFETY CONCERNS

In an institutional environment setting (such as a hospital or nursing home) late life adults were found to fall performing the following activities: getting in or out of bed, transferring into a wheelchair with the wheels unlocked, walking across the room with nothing to hold onto, leaning upon an object that moves such as a tray or bedside table, reaching for an object that is not within the client's reach (e.g., a light switch, toilet paper, a urinal, a telephone, or a call button), and walking with improper footwear.[96]

To remediate this situation a nursing home or hospital program needs to be established to prevent falls. Occupational therapists are usually members of these committees (e.g., fall prevention committee, restraint reduction committee). The following factors are recommended to alleviate or decrease at-risk fall conditions:

✧ Establish a fall risk classification for each client. This can be accomplished by reviewing the following conditions and factors of each client:

1. A history of falls
2. Mental status change
3. Agitation/anxieties
4. Sensory deficits
5. Mobility deficits
6. Communication difficulties
7. Urinary alterations
8. Medications that can affect alertness and mobility such as diuretics, laxatives, tranquilizers, hypnotics, narcotics, anesthetics, barbiturates
9. Debilitation

✧ Decreasing at-risk fall conditions can also be accomplished by:
  1. Providing a system to alert all staff as to who the high-risk clients are (color codes have been helpful)
  2. Educating staff as to fall prevention strategies
  3. Promoting frequent reassessment (since fall risk status may change)
  4. Educating all clients in fall prevention (e.g., instruct in appropriate transfer techniques; when a new client arrives, providing an orientation to the setting; instructing the appropriate way to get in and out of bed)
  5. Conducting environmental assessments
  6. Making appropriate recommendations (e.g., have light, telephone, call button, and TV remote control within easy reach)

Mobility devices such as a wheelchair, a cane, or a walker that the client uses should be readily accessible. All furniture should be nonmovable or locked. Have a commode adjacent at bedside if the client has poor endurance. High risk individuals should be at close proximity to the nursing station. They will need frequent supervision including being assisted in and out of bed and accompanied to the bathroom. An alarm system such as Ambularm™ or other devices can be used to signal staff that the client is beginning to rise and that assistance may be needed. Involving clients in exercise programs to build endurance and strength (especially walking type programs that stress ankle dorsiflexion strengthening) have been helpful in promoting balance and preventing falls.[96]

Safety and fall prevention in the home setting environment is a major concern for all those interested in maintaining independence within the community. The Falls Interview Schedule, the Home Assessment Checklist for Fall Hazards, and the Gait and Balance test recommended by Tinetti (described earlier in this component) are excellent ways to initiate fact finding and a baseline.

In terms of fatigue as a factor affecting safety, the following recommendations can be helpful. In the bathroom, the installation of grab bars allows the client to have support and increased ease in entering and exiting the tub area; a bath chair or bench will permit the client to sit while bathing (thus, reducing the energy needed to shower and at the same time promoting safety in balance). A properly fitting toilet seat will permit safety and ease of use. The seat may need to be raised (or a levator used at the base of the toilet), and armrests may also be needed to ensure safety. Other safety recommendations include: the installation of sturdy hand rails on both sides of the stairways to help break falls; hand rails can be textured at the end to signal a tactile warning that the last step has been reached; bright tape can be placed on the first and last step of each set of stairs; a light at the top and bottom of landings provides better visibility; there should be ample illumination throughout the home to ensure safety as well as easy-to-reach light switches; and porch steps can be covered with gritty, weatherproof-type paint to prevent tripping or slipping.[27]

Fall prevention in the home also involves a number of other concerns. Furniture should be of an appropriate height for the client. The following questions need to be asked:

✧ Does the chair the client is seated in have appropriate depth and height?
✧ Does the back of the chair allow the client to sit upright without the client having to lean back?
✧ Does the chair have arms that aid the client in rising?

✧ Is the carpet pile low and does the carpet have any loose threads that might cause one to trip?

✧ Are throw rugs tacked down?

✧ Is there any clutter (especially at walkways) on the floor or on top of furniture that might fall?

✧ Is a phone accessible?

✧ If the client has a walker, is it properly positioned to permit ready access?

✧ Does the client ever forget to use the walker?

✧ Is there a night light in the bedroom?[96]

✧ Does the client wear good sturdy footwear (discourage the wearing of only socks, loose-fitting slippers, or shoes that have slippery heels or soles)?

In order to lesson fatigue and where balance may be compromised, the client should be encouraged to dress while in a sitting position. To prevent tripping, discourage the client from wearing long robes or nightgowns or from wearing trousers that are too long. Be aware of appropriate temperature in the house (especially at nighttime in the winter when it is recommended that the thermostat be set no lower than 65°F, as prolonged exposure to cold temperatures may cause the body temperature to drop and cause drowsiness and lead to a risk for falls).[27]

Because nutrition and medication contribute to the welfare of the client and, subsequently, to falls, it is important for the occupational therapist to check where the client keeps his or her medications in the home and if they are being used appropriately. Also, an inspection of the refrigerator can reveal the cleanliness of food that is stored there as well as provide firsthand knowledge of what the client eats. Poor nutrition can lead to a number of problems, including confusion. This in turn can be a contributing factor for falls.[96]

For the late life adult who is at risk and who fears that he or she will fall, a telephone emergency alert system can promote a sense of security. In this type of situation a signaling device can be worn as a pendant around the neck or on a belt clip. When the older adult presses the recessed button, the telephone automatically dials a predetermined number (an operator, in many cases, will answer and speak to the client). In this way help is summoned immediately.[96]

Involving clients who are exceedingly fearful of falling when they participate in daily living tasks can be a challenge. The clinician needs to promote situations in which the client can begin to feel comfortable trying out new techniques. Fantasized consequences of feared behavior (such as transferring to the bathtub) can be examined and the intensity lessened. Goals that are realistic (ones that the client perceives as attainable) aid in instilling the hope that the client can learn new techniques. Grading activities to reduce fear of falling and teaching safer activities performance are other important occupational therapy interventions.[91, p. 659] Simulated activities can be utilized to establish confidence and self-trust. Once this has been established, the activity can be graded so that the older adult is gradually able to perform a desired but previously feared activity.[91]

There is much work ahead in the area of safety and the prevention of falls. With our knowledge base firmly planted in psychosocial awareness, physical disabilities, adaptation, and daily living skills, occupational therapy has a marvelous capability of helping late life adults remain safe and active in their community with a minimum of fear.

Occupational Therapy and Orthopedic Management

Hip Fractures and Total Replacement of the Hip

Description

Fractures occur in bone when the bone loses its ability to absorb compression, tension, or withstand shearing forces. Trauma is the major cause of most fractures. At the time of the fracture, blood vessels are torn across the fracture site. This causes bleeding and later clotting (known as *fracture hematoma*). The repair cells (osteogenic cells) form an external and internal callus. The callus initiates its growth from the time of injury. Its maturation rate is dependent upon the specific type of bone that is fractured. Generally, bone tissue occurs as two types: *cortical* (compact bone, found on the anterior bone surface that provides strength) and *cancellous* (spongy bone that surrounds spaces that are filled with bone marrow). As the fracture matures (termed *union*), the bone becomes more stable. Immobilization is a requirement throughout the maturation period. The time that is needed to heal a fracture varies as to the age of the client, the configuration and site of the fracture, the blood supply to the fragments, and the initial displacement of the bone. There are six types of fractures (actually six different categories or ways that a bone can be broken). These are termed: incomplete, complete, open, comminuted, displaced, and spiral.[102]

Medical Management

Medical management of fracture intervention consists of relieving pain, maintaining a good position of the fracture, permitting a bony union of the fracture to take place, and the restoration of the optimal functioning of the client.[102] *Reduction* is a term used to indicate the restoring of fracture fragments to normal alignment. This may be accomplished by a closed procedure (known as manipulation) or by an open procedure (surgery). With manipulation, force is applied to the displaced bone that is opposite to the force that produced the fracture. Reduction can be maintained in a cast, skin traction, skeletal traction, skeletal fixation, or a brace. *Open reduction* is conducted by exposing the fracture site to surgery so that the fragments can be aligned. These fragments may be held in place with internal fixation by nails, screws, pins, a rod, or a plate. An *open reduction with internal fixation* needs to be protected from excessive force or forces. Therefore, weight-bearing is restricted. In hip fracture, the articular fragment of the hip may need to be removed (needed when there are complications of a vascular necrosis, degenerative joint disease, or nonunion) and replaced by a prosthesis (known as endoprosthesis). With most instances, following a hip fracture soft tissue trauma, ecchymosis and edema can develop around the fracture site. This in turn can result in increased pain.[102]

Total joint replacement in the elderly is often indicated in: osteoarthritis, ankylosing spondylitis, chronic progressive polyarthritis, trauma, or diseases that damage articular cartilage. *Total joint replacement* (known as arthroplasty) is indicated when the goal is to alleviate pain and regain joint motion. The total hip replacement is composed of two parts--a high density polyethylene socket is fitted into the acetabulum, and a metallic prosthesis replaces the femoral neck and head. Acrylic cement is used to "fix" the bone's components. Hip precautions (with an anterolateral approach the client must avoid adduction, external rotation, and extension of the operated hip; with a postero-lateral approach the client must avoid specific ranges of flexion in the operated hip [usually 60 degrees to 90 degrees]; as well as adduction of the leg and internal rota-tion. Failure to maintain these precautions results in dislocation. With cement fixation, weight-bearing restriction need not be observed).[102] Recently biological fixation proce-dures involving the utilization of bony growth (instead of cement) to secure the pros-thesis have been conducted. With this procedure anterior or posterior hip restrictions can apply—with the additional restrictions on weight-bearing.

Occupational therapy intervention, in dealing with either a surgical repair of a frac-tured hip or a total hip replacement, can usually begin within 2 to 4 days after surgery has been completed (when the client is ready to start getting in and out of bed). It is the role of the clinician to instruct the client in the ways and means of safety and per-forming activities of daily living. At the same time the practitioner is to observe all movement precautions.

Occupational Therapy Evaluation and Management

A baseline evaluation should be performed to determine if there are any physical limitations not related to surgery that may impact on functional independence. Therefore, upper extremity range of motion, sensation, muscle strength, coordination, and mental status should be completed before conducting a functional evaluation. The client's pain and fear during movement and at rest should also be considered.[102]

A client with hip precautions will also need the following assistive devices when performing activities of daily living: a dressing stick, a long-handled reacher, a long-handled shoe horn, a long-handled bath sponge, elastic laces, and sock or stocking aid.[102]

Through the American Occupational Therapy Association, an innovative easy-to-read guide has been designed that instructs (with large drawings and print) the client in the appropriate ways to perform daily living tasks. First, in terms of sitting (if the ante-rior approach has been utilized), the client needs to keep his or her hip at 90-degree (right) angle or at an angle that is greater than 90 degrees. An abduction pillow may be used immediately following the operation and for several days after the completion of the operation. The operated leg may need to be elevated in order to control edema. Antiembolis hose may be worn (thigh-high hosiery that is worn 24 hours a day except for bathing) to prevent edema, to reduce the risk of deep vein thrombosis, and to assist in circulation. If a posterior approach has been conducted, the following applies. The hip must be kept at a right angle or at an angle that is greater than 90 degrees for 6 to 8 weeks. In both surgical approaches the client is not to bend forward more than 90 degrees while sitting. The knee is not to be lifted higher than hip height on the operat-ed side. It is also very important (in both anterior and posterior approaches) to not let the client cross his or her legs (at either the knee or ankle areas) until given permission to do so from the client's physician.[103]

When using a walker, the client must remember to keep his or her hip properly aligned and straight, and to be aware to not put more weight on the operated hip than was prescribed by the physician. There are several movements to be avoided at all costs. First, the client is not to rotate his or her hip in any way (the hip should not be turned outward or inward). The foot must be turned inward. Second, the walker must be flat on the floor before the client takes a step.

Chair positioning is very important when using the walker. Upon rising from a sitting position the client is advised to use a sturdy and firm chair that has armrests. This will promote using his or her arms to push up from the chair.[103] The hip must be maintained in an 90-degree position. This might mean that the client may need several cushions for positioning (one on the seat to sit higher and one at the small of the back to aid in utilizing the correct hip position). When positioning oneself for sitting, the client needs to back up to the chair until he or she feels the knees touching it. The operated leg is then moved out as the client reaches back for the armrest and lowers him- or herself down slowly, keeping the operated leg out straight. When preparing to arise, the client should scoot forward in the chair, keeping his or her hip positioned in a 90-degree stance. The client then pushes up, using the armrest (while keeping the operated leg out in front).[103]

Toilet transferring is another area of intervention focus. The client may use either a toilet commode with armrest, a raised toilet seat with armrests, or a levator (with armrests attached to the toilet). The methods for toilet transfer using a toilet commode with armrests are as follows:

- ✧ Before using the toilet commode with armrests, the walker legs should be adjusted so that the front legs are one notch lower than the back legs.
  - ▲ Ask the client to back up to the toilet until he or she feels the back of the knees touching it.
  - ▲ Ask the client to reach back slowly for the armrests and lower him- or herself onto the toilet (all the while keeping the operated leg out in front).
  - ▲ Ask the client to bend his or her knee and hip (on the nonoperated side) as the client lowers him- or herself onto the toilet seat.
  - ▲ Reverse this procedure when rising—utilizing the armrests to push up on.
- ✧ The client needs to be instructed to gain his or her balance before reaching for the walker.[103] The procedure (very similar to that of the toilet commode) for using a raised toilet seat with armrests or a levator with arm rests includes:
  - ▲ Asking the client to back up to the toilet until he or she feels the back of the knees touching the seat.
  - ▲ One hand should be kept on the walker while reaching back for the arm rests with the other hand.
  - ▲ Ask the client to bend the knee and hip on the nonoperated leg as he or she lowers him- or herself onto the seat. While doing this the operated leg must be kept straight out.
  - ▲ To reverse this procedure, the client should be instructed to place one hand on the walker and the other on the arm rest. On rising the client needs to achieve his or her balance before reaching for the walker.[103] The client should wipe between the legs in a sitting position or from behind when standing with caution to avoid internal hip rotation. In order to flush the toilet, the client should stand up and step to face the toilet. Safe walker usage is expected throughout this procedure.[102]

Other bathroom activities involve instruction for tub or shower stall transfer. While in the tub, a long-handled sponge (useful for washing the back and lower legs) and a hand-held shower spray are recommended. In both types of transfer a bath chair should be utilized.

For the tub transfer the following procedures are recommended:
1. The client is instructed to walk to the side of the tub (while using the walker) and to stop next to the chair and turn so that he or she is facing away from the tub.
2. The client is directed to reach back with one hand for the back of the tub/bath chair (at the same time one hand needs to be on the walker).
3. The client is instructed to sit down on the chair while keeping the operated leg straight out.
4. The client is directed to lift the legs (one at a time) over the side of the tub (using flexion precautions) and turn to be able to sit facing the faucet. Besides a long-handled sponge and hand-held shower spray, other items and methods such as soap-on-a-rope and a towel wrapped around a reacher (can be used for drying the lower legs) are useful in the tub/shower.

When transferring into a stall shower, the client should be instructed to ambulate (with the walker) to the lip of the shower and turn so that he or she is facing away from the shower stall. The client is then instructed to reach back with one hand for the back of the tub chair (which has been placed in the shower) and to leave the other hand on the walker. The client is then directed to begin to sit down slowly (all the while keeping the operated leg straight out). Finally, the client is instructed (making certain to observe flexion precautions) to lift the legs (one at a time) over the lip of the shower stall and turn to sit facing the showerhead. To prevent falling, non-skid strips should have previously been placed in the shower as well as the installation of a grab bar on the shower wall strategically placed where the client has easy access. Installation of a hand-held hose spray can also be attached to the regular showerhead. To rise and leave the shower, the procedures just mentioned should be reversed.[103]

Bed positioning is another major aspect of post hip surgery. To prevent improper positioning, there are a number of ways in which a client can effectively position him- or herself so that he or she can sleep without causing injury to the hip. While lying on one's side (the operated side is recommended to lie on), the pillow should be kept between the legs to help keep the hip from rotating inward. If the client prefers to lie on his or her back, a pillow should be placed between his or her legs. Be certain that the client is instructed to never point his or her toes inward.[103]

For a car transfer, the client is directed to back up (using the walker) to the passenger seat (bench type seat rather than bucket seats are recommended) and hold onto a stable section of the car. During this time the operated leg is to be extended as the client gradually sits in the car.[102] It is best to enter the side of the car that allows the operated leg to be supported (i.e., if the right leg received the surgery, then one should enter the car on the right side).[103] The client should then lean back onto the seat in a semireclining position. The client should then slide the buttocks toward the left side (using the upper and lower extremities to move as one unit to face in a forward direction). In preparation it is helpful to have the seat slide back and in a reclining position in order to maintain hip flexion precautions. Prolonged sitting in the car is contraindicated.[103]

Dressing is an extremely important component in occupational therapy hip rehabilitation. Before beginning to dress, the client should be instructed to sit on the side of the bed or in an armchair. Adaptive devices such as a dressing stick, a long-handled reacher, a stocking/sock aid, a long-handled shoe horn, and elastic type shoelaces are helpful. The underwear and slacks should be put on first. The client should be direct-ed to catch the waist of the underwear or slacks with dressing hook or a reacher. The stick should then be lowered to the floor, and the slacks or underwear should be slipped over the operated leg first. This process should be repeated for the nonoperat-ed leg. Next, the client should pull the underwear or slacks up and over his or her knees; when this is accomplished, the client is instructed to stand with the walker in front and pull the slacks up to the waist (using one hand on the walker and one hand to pull up).[103]

When doffing, the slacks and underwear should be taken off of the nonoperated leg first.

For donning and doffing socks or stockings, the following is recommended:[103]

- ✧ To don the sock or stocking:
  - ⊿ The item is slid onto the stocking/sock aid. The heel is to be at the back of the plastic, and the toe should be tight against the end of the aid. The top of the sock or stocking should not come over the top of the plastic piece. The sock/stocking can be secured with garters or notches in the plastic piece. This part of donning is accomplished with the client's two hands at the lap level.
  - ⊿ Next, the client holds onto the cords and drops the stocking aid in front of the operated foot.
  - ⊿ The foot is then slipped into the sock/stocking aid and then pulled on.
  - ⊿ The garters are released or the sock is removed from the notches with the assis tance of the dressing stick or reacher. Putting the sock on the nonoperated foot is performed in the usual manner.
- ✧ To doff the sock or stocking, the hook of the dressing stick or the reacher can be attached to the back of the heel of the sock/stocking, and the sock/stocking can be pushed off the foot.[103]

For donning and doffing of shoes, slip-on shoes or elastic type shoelaces can be used (so that the client does not have to bend over when putting on shoes or when tying the laces). A long-handled shoe horn or dressing stick can be used for the actual don and doff of shoes.[103]

Homemaking rehabilitation procedures are yet another important aspect of occu-pational therapy intervention of the post surgical hip client. First, heavy housework (bedmaking, lifting, and vacuuming) is contraindicated. In the kitchen commonly used items should be kept at the countertop level. Carrying items can be accomplished in the following manner:

1. Utilize large-pocketed aprons.
2. Slide items along the countertop (rather than lifting).
3. Attach a small bucket or bag to the front of the walker.
4. Use a wheeled utility cart (the cart should be pushed ahead of the walker).

Long-handled reachers should be used to prevent the client from bending down to pick up items. Scatter rugs need to be removed. The client should be instructed to sit on a high stool when doing countertop activities/tasks.[102,103]

Besides instructing and educating the client, the family, a designated caretaker, or a significant other needs to be made aware of and informed about the client's rehabili-tation program and any restrictions or hip precautions that may apply.

Upper Body Orthopedic Intervention

Description

Clinicians working with clients who have suffered a trauma to their hands or other upper body injury need to respect and understand that tissue has been injured. Following an injury, all tissues go through a similar repair process. There are three major purposes of tissue healing:

1. Eliminating pathological insult
2. Replacing the damaged tissues
3. Promoting regeneration to replace the injured or damaged tissue

Thus, the chances of functional restoration can be improved.[104]

Three sequential phases of repair constitute the process of normal tissue healing. Phase 1 (termed the *inflammatory phase*) may last from the onset to 5 days. During this phase the body tries to achieve homeostasis by limiting bleeding and removing debris (which would affect the wound). It is at this time that the body prepares the wound for healing. Symptoms at this time include heat, pain, swelling, tenderness, and loss of function. Intervention priorities in Phase 1 involve immobilization, wound management, and edema management.[104]

Phase 2 (termed the *proliferative phase*) may last from 5 to 21 days or longer. During this phase a deposit of collagen replaces lost tissue, as the resurfacing of the wound begins. The body strengthens the wound and rebuilds damaged structures. At this point *tensile strength* (also known as breaking strength), the force that is required to break a wound or tissue apart, is almost 15% to 20% of normal strength. Any load applied to the injured body part by splints or other devices must stay below the breaking strength of the tissue. Symptoms and observations during this phase include: the beginning of wound contracture, the presence of red granulation tissue, some pain, moderate swelling, and the beginning of the return to function. There are two options of intervention during this phase. One is referred to as *controlled mobility*. This intervention makes use of early motor programs for post-tendon repair (where tissue is allowed to move using less force than what would cause damage to the repaired tendon). *Immobilization*, the other intervention option, permits no motion until the wound or tendon is strong enough to withstand tension.[104]

Phase 3, termed the *maturation phase*, may last from 21 days to 2 years. This is the final phase. During this time the body modifies the scar tissue. The wound becomes less vascular as the capillary network retracts. Tissue strength is 50% to 70% of normal strength. Because scar tissue is not as strong or as well organized as normal tissue, the tensile strength of healed tissue usually does not go beyond 70% to 80% of normal tensile strength.[104] Intervention during this phase involves remodeling of the scar and improving its tissue structure by applying modalities such as exercise, gentle prolonged stretching, and splinting. All thermal modalities need to be closely monitored as scar tissue is less able to dissipate heat than normal tissue (due to its vascular nature). Strength training, task performance, and movement are administrated during this phase in a graduated manner that is consistent with the increasing tensile strength of any injured tissue.[104] Individualized intervention plans are highly important in establishing a program that has meaning to the client and that includes the client's disabilities as well as abilities and rehabilitation potential. This plan encompasses client-specific performance skills, areas of occupation, and contexts as it corporates the quality and the time of healing.[104]

Distal Radius Fractures

Distal radius fractures often occur when an individual falls on an outstretched hand with the wrist in extension. The fracture to the distal radius may be partial articular, extra articular, or complete articular. The radius carries approximately 80% of the axial load of the forearm. The ulna carries about 20% of the axial load. Articular distal radius fractures result in the disruption of both the distal radioulnar and radiocarpal joints. Changes in the forearm unit length ratio, as seen with the settled distal radius fracture, increase the radial load beyond its physiological limits.[104]

There are numerous types of distal fractures. The most common fracture pattern is the *Colles' fracture*. With this type of fracture there is a dorsal comminution of the distal radius with dorsal displacement of the distal fragment along an accompanying radial shortening. This angular disformation usually leads to a prognosis that the client will have limited dorsiflexion of the wrist (due to the fact that the carpal bones will run into the displaced radius when the client tries to dorsiflex his or her wrist). Other distal radius fractures include: Barton's fracture, Smith's fracture, chauffeur's or backfire fracture, the lunate load/die punch/medial cuneiform fracture. At present there is no general consensus on classification, and new classification formats are being promoted and developed all the time.

Fractures that occur at the lower end of the radius impact greatly as these fractures are more common than any other upper extremity fracture.[104] Early during the healing phase functional limitation may be due to swelling, pain, open wound or pin site, and often there is a decrease of digital range of motion. There can be, at a later time, additional limitations that are due to the decreased range of motion of the forearm and wrist, dexterity problems, and scar restruction. Other components that can affect overall function include: dominance of the involved hand, proximal joint mobility, and functioning capacity of the noninvolved hand. These characteristics represent the performance skills (known by the World Health Organization (WHO) classification system as impairment).[104]

Areas of occupation (known by the WHO classification system as *activity limitations*) are a major occupational therapy intervention area of concern. Throughout all of the healing phases of the fracture (e.g., the immobilization of the client's wrist to the introduction of modalities and home intervention planning), the clinician must determine how the injury will affect and is affecting the client's daily self-care activities, productive activities, leisure pursuits, volunteer activities, and work (as appropriate). The clinician should know and understand the client's goals for rehabilitation as well as what the client's normal functioning needs for that extremity are.[104]

Context and client factors (known by the WHO as *participation restrictions*) is the next area of concern. Questions are asked such as: Are there any life factors that might or will affect the rehabilitation process? Is the client living with someone who can assist him or her? Will the client's lifestyle be affected? Does the third party payer place any limitation on rehabilitation care?

When determining the intervention plan, client-centered goals should be formulated so that: pathology; the healing stage of the tissues that have been injured; the areas of occupation that are affected; the client's context, needs, and priorities; and the performance skills that are currently limiting functioning are considered and integrated into a holistic approach.[104]

The WHO classification system has been discussed in relation to occupational therapy terminology as a way for nonoccupational therapists to understand how our professional intervention is used in a worldwide context. Thus, occupational therapists can help others to better understand what we do and why we do it.

During the acute phase of intervention for a Colles' fracture, the client may require a volar wrist splint. After 2 weeks in a plaster cast (or internal or external fixation), the intervention for the Colles' fracture client is often initiated with range of motion exercises and activities of the wrist and forearm (once bony union has taken place). If needed, muscle strengthening in specific digits may be conducted with initial gentle gross grasp and pinch activities. Scar massage to healed incisions for the purpose of softening up the scar (gradually working up to deep circular motions as the client is able to tolerate) is a definite part of the rehabilitation process. Activities that promote increased prehension skills, hand dexterity, and other fine motor skills (e.g., graded activities that include buttoning buttons; using paper clips and tweezers; handling of pegs, small blocks, or coins) should be initiated. Desensitization techniques can be taught to decrease pain. Great effort should be focused upon increasing independence in everyday living skills (e.g., self-care, leisure pursuits). Adaptive equipment and techniques should be provided to facilitate self-care (as needed). Crafts and other activities may be introduced to promote improved function (e.g., using clay to facilitate gentle loading exercises, utilizing a light bag with a handle for carrying as part of a stress loading program).[27,104]

Intervention, depending upon the performance skills, the areas of occupation, and the client factors and context of each client, becomes an individual issue in which sound decisions, based upon these factors, are determined through the means of a client-centered approach. This is true for all areas of the curative process (and in any disease or fracture status).

Fractures of the Forearm, Elbow, and Humerus

Other upper body fractures that affect the elderly include forearm, elbow, and humerus fractures. During the acute phase (at onset and up to at least 2 weeks) of injury of the forearm a plaster cast or internal or external fixation is considered to be standard procedure. Any edema should be decreased (by elevation of the hand, retrograde massage to the hand, or an elastic support glove to reduce swelling in the fingers and thumb) as much as possible. At 2 weeks post-injury a forearm fracture brace or functional bracing are usually indicated. Once bony union has occurred, range of motion activities and exercises of the wrist and forearm should commence. Scar massage to healed incisions, desensitization techniques, progressive strengthening activities to promote dexterity and prehension activities, increasing independence in everyday living through instruction in the use of adaptive techniques and equipment, and splint provision (if required) with instructions in its use and care by the clinician are specific avenues in treating this type of fracture.[27]

Elbow fractures in the acute phase most often involve placing the elbow in an elbow conformer or a plaster cast with 90 to 100 degrees of flexion at the elbow. When the client is ambulating, the upper extremity can be placed in a sling for support. Any edema should be addressed by using edema control techniques (e.g., instruct client or significant other in positioning such as elevating the hand; instruct in hand exercise to reduce edema as well as provide and instruct in the use of external elastic support gloves). Gentle nonresistive range of motion can begin approximately 5 days after surgery. Active range of motion should be performed in a gravity-eliminated plane. Passive range of motion in the early stages of recovery should be avoided. Although a client may not achieve full elbow expansion, a useful arc of motion for everyday activities should be realized. The general course of intervention consists of scar massage, desensitization techniques, range of motion activities and exercises, progressive strengthening activities and exercises, dexterity and prehension activities, splint provision (if required—with instructions in its use and care), increasing independence in everyday activities by encouraging the use of the involved hand in nonresistive activities of daily living tasks, and providing adaptive equipment and instruction in the use of the equipment.[27]

Fractures of the humerus often require that the client's upper arm be initially placed in a shoulder immobilizer or, in some cases, in a plaster cast. After a brief period of immobilization (5 to 7 days, approximately), the upper arm may be placed in a fracture brace.[27] Some orthopedists may choose to keep the client in a shoulder immobilizer. Problems with edema should be addressed immediately by instructing the client in edema control techniques (as previously described). Active range of motion should begin as soon as the acute pain diminishes. This will avoid stiffness. Passive range of motion is contraindicated. Isometric exercises (both during and after immobilization) should be encouraged, as these act as a stimulant to fracture healing. Codman's exercises provide gentle active exercises of the shoulder. These pendulum movements are performed by asking the client to bend at the waist with the arm positioned away from the body (without the sling). The client is then instructed (while leaving the noninvolved hand on a table for support) to move the fractured arm into extension and forward flexion. Functional activities that allow forward flexion and extension movement (e.g., puzzles, tile projects, and board games are placed on a low table that requires anterior and posterior movement) are highly recommended. As a word of caution, if the client has an edematous upper extremity, Codman's exercises are to be avoided. Increasing independence in everyday living skills by utilizing adaptive techniques or equipment is recommended.[27]

The American Occupational Therapy Association offers two excellent "general" exercise booklets for the upper extremity. Each one of these exercises should be conducted with the knowledge, consultation, and approval of the client's physician. These exercises are written in clear, accessible language and can readily be used by clients. These resources are entitled "Home Rehabilitation Exercises for the Hand" and "Home Rehabilitation Exercises for the Shoulder, Elbow, Forearm, and Wrist." They are available at the following address and telephone number:

❖   The American Occupational Therapy Association, Inc.

   4720 Montgomery Lane
   P.O. Box 31220
   Bethesda, MD 20824-1220
   1-800-SAY-AOTA

Splinting the Frail Elderly

Lynn M. Swedberg has written an excellent article, entitled "Splinting the Difficult Hand," that describes a variety of splints and techniques that are useful with frail elderly clients. Most of these clients were residents of nursing homes. Often nontraditional materials and techniques were used to effectively meet the difficult splinting needs of these individuals.[105]

The custom fabricated splint should not only fit well, but it should also be comfortable and attractive to the client as much as possible. A major key to good splinting is to evaluate and identify the position that is tolerated by the client. If a joint is extended beyond this point, the result most often is increased pain and tone. On the other hand, if the joints are not extended to a position that can readily be achieved, the client may develop increased contractures that conform to the shape of the splint. Factors to consider when fabricating a splint include the risk of contractures versus the risk of negative side effects.[105]

Understanding the needs of the care setting is equally important when planning to construct a splint. In nursing homes fire codes are very strict. Materials must be fire retardant or self-extinguishing. For the purposes of infection control, splints must be easy to clean. All splints should be made from nontoxic substances (in anticipation of the client who might chew on splints).[105]

Only the joints or digits that are involved should be splinted. Active parts of the hand should be allowed to function freely. All splints need to be padded (as staff may place bulky liners or washcloths into the splint to "protect" the client). Splints need to be modified only by the clinician (not by the client or other staff because easily adjusted splints can be inadvertently bent out of shape). To accomplish this, all straps are riveted to the splint and firmly attached. A durable custom fabricated splint allows for modification by the clinician to accommodate the inevitable changes occurring in the degree of extension that can be achieved and tolerated.[105]

The following is recommended for hand-based splints that are used for the client who does not have wrist involvement:[105]

- ✧ Closed-cell cylindrical foam, carved to fit the client's hand, may be used.
- ✧ If finger abductors are needed, a palm protector with carved closed-cell foam or molded low-temperature thermoplastic and cut slits for fabric finger tabs can be utilized.
- ✧ A silicone elastomer can also be used as an insert (if the hand is more complex).
- ✧ As long as there is a firm base, soft materials against the skin will not cause increased spasticity.
- ✧ If a client cannot tolerate the thickness of laminated closed-cell foam, a nylon tricot open-cell foam laminated material or neoprene can be sewn into a shape that gently separates and extends the fingers.
- ✧ All styles can be trimmed so that the index finger and thumb (in cases when only the ulnar digits are contracted) are permitted free movement.
- ✧ Hand-based splints can be used as resting night splints.

Wrist-hand-finger splints are utilized when the wrist is involved. The following is recommended for ease, comfort, and effective intervention:[105]

- ✧ Often, a low-temperature thermoplastic is used to form a base (either of volar or dorsal design). The edges are folded over to eliminate any sharp edges and to reinforce the shape.
- ✧ For most clients a volar pattern with the thumb in abduction is effective.
- ✧ For clients with high tone (usually due to a CVA or head injury), a dorsal splint is used for added leverage.
- ✧ Custom carved thin, closed-cell foam triangular pieces are used to fit between and abduct the fingers.
- ✧ Self-adhesive fabric-foam padding and padded straps are added to promote comfort and a good fit.

✧   If a client is unable to tolerate the hard splint (even with padding), laminated synthetic sheepskin and foam or neoprene can be attached to a thermoplastic stay under the soft splinting material for reinforcement.

✧   Curved straps and double ulnar drift finger tabs can be incorporated into the straps, and sheepskin pads can be placed under the straps for comfort and effectiveness.

Elbow and shoulder components can be used to prevent injury or treat contractures. Custom carved forearm elevation, elbow extension, or a shoulder abduction splint from open-cell foam (leaving space for the hand splint to fit) provide an excellent way to promote a healthier alignment. In order to protect the skin and promote skin integrity, fabric covers can be sewn for the foam pieces.[105]

Specific recommendations and criteria for good splint design that promote appropriate positioning for the difficult frail elderly hand include the following:[105]

✧   For high muscle tone, the splint should provide for the abduction and extension of the thumb to tolerance, the extension of the wrist to tolerance (no more than 10 degrees to 20 degrees), flexion of the MCP joints to tolerance, and extension of the IP joints to nearly neutral.

✧   For contractures, the splint should promote the extension and abduction of the joints to a pain-free position (but no further than the position of rest).

✧   For arthritic deformities, the splint should provide the extension and support of the wrist and MCP joints as tolerated in the approximation of the functional position. If needed, gently correct ulnar drift, promote the extension and support of the IP joints (if passive range of motion is greater than the active range of motion). Permit the thumb to be able to move freely.

✧   For fragile skin, the split fabrication should follow these guidelines: place the straps carefully and use extra padding. Separate the thumb and the fingers with soft material.

✧   For edema, the position of the hand (in splint care) should incorporate the following: elevation of the extremity, extension of the wrist to 40 degrees, no restrictive strapping should be utilized, and there should be allowance for flexion of the MCP joints to at least 60 degrees (or allowance to permit the client the freedom to flex actively).

Goals for each of these described conditions (for which the splints would be fabricated) include:[105]

✧   *High muscle tone*—To reduce tone without causing a rebound into a flexor synergy pattern, thus preventing contractures and improving function.

✧   *Contractures*—To provide prolonged steady stretch in order to maintain or increase range of motion (without causing discomfort).

✧   *Arthritic deformities*—To accommodate and support the involved joints so that there is a reduction of pain and an increase of the functional use of the hands.

✧   *Fragile skin*—To promote skin integrity and hygiene as well as to protect the skin.

✧   *Edema*—To decrease edema and improve circulation so that there is a decrease in pain and contracture formation as well as an increase in function.

An excellent audit tool is also described in Swedberg's article. This document is useful in helping to facilitate sound decision making and for promoting quality assurance in the area of splint design and fabrication.[105]

SEATING, POSITIONING, AND WHEELED MOBILITY INTERVENTION

17

Addressing positioning and seating needs is essential in promoting optimal functioning in late life adults. One major focus of positioning and seating intervention is the promotion of appropriate biomechanical alignments in the older client.

In nursing homes the most commonly observed postures among late life adults consist of lower cervical flexion, capital extension, forward rounded shoulders, thoracic kyphosis, loss of the lumbar curve, and posterior pelvic tilt. Because the pelvis is the base of support for human beings in the seated position, it is essential to promote as close to normal positioning as possible.[106] The optimal sitting posture begins with the pelvis. There should be no pelvic obliquity, no pelvic rotation, and there should be a slight anterior pelvic tilt. In the trunk area there should be a slight lumbar lordosis, a slight thoracic kyphosis, and a slight cervical extension. Lower extremities should be in a neutral internal/external rotation, with flexion at the hip, knees, and ankles to 90 degrees, and a slight abduction at the hips. Upper extremities consist of allowing the elbows to be slightly forward of the shoulders, with the forearms supported and the hands placed toward the midline. The head should be in midline with the eyes facing forward.[107]

PROBLEMS INVOLVING SEATING SYSTEMS

Any deviation from the normal position of slight anterior tilt to neutral can cause total body alignment problems as well as general systems problems.[106] In many cases poor seating may be responsible for developing deformities. The result of improper seating on the body systems can be understood from the following discussion. The presence of posterior tilt may precipitate bladder and bowel complications; it may also prevent sit-to-stand transfers and maneuvers as well as functional ambulation activities; and it may preclude adequate heel strike during lower extremity propulsion. Conditions that cause malalignment and pain of the lumbar spine may be responsible for postural deviations at the cervical spine, thoracic, or pelvic regions. The presence of a scoliosis has been known to decrease internal body organ function. A thoracic kyphosis can inhibit gastrointestinal, swallowing, and cardiopulmonary function. Increased cervical flexion can affect language, speech, swallowing, and visual-vestibular functions.[106] If an individual is not supported in his or her own optimal position, the biomechanical alignment can be seriously compromised. If a person has a flexible deformity that is not corrected, it can become fixed over time. Changes in soft tissue, bone tendons, and muscle can shorten; the joint capsules can become tighter; and bone can actually bend. Fixed deformities can become worse without appropriate support.[107]

The development of skin problems (due to improper positioning) is another area that the clinician needs to address. Abrasion, pressure, and shearing are examples of the major skin problems that the older adult faces when poorly positioned. *Abrasion* takes place as a consequence of the skin rubbing against a surface with resultant skin damage. An abrasion caused by a scraping of the skin that bleeds or bruising may result in a raw area of the skin. Rubbing against any sharp edge (e.g., a client repeatedly rubs over the edge of a seat or wheel while performing a lateral transfer) can cause an abrasion. Therefore, it is important that these areas be smoothed and that any other potentials for abrasion be padded. Individuals with fragile skin are easily bruised and are at higher risk for abrasion with their seating, positioning, and wheeled mobility base than those with less fragile skin. Padding areas and smoothing edges are of major significance to this population segment.[107]

Pressure is the result of two objects pressing against each other. The force with which these two objects press will determine the amount of pressure. Within a positioning system the goal is to have low peak pressures and to evenly distribute the pressure (spread the pressure over a large surface at the same time, keep the greatest pressure as low as is possible). There are two reasons for developing pressure sores: (1) there is low pressure over a surface for a long period of time, or (2) there is extremely high pressure over a surface for a short time period. Pressure sores develop as a result of the pressure closing off the blood circulation through the capillaries. Once the blood stops, circulation to a certain area, nutrients, and oxygen are not delivered to the cells.[107]

Cells that are not provided with nutrients will die (known as *necrosis*). If the pressure continues, the necrosis will spread to surrounding areas. The longer this is allowed to occur, the greater the area of the pressure sore. The amount of pressure it takes for blood circulation to cease is generally agreed to be between 30 and 100 mmHg. Pressure sores develop from inside. The highest pressure is found in the flesh that is closest to the bone, and this is the first area to develop a necrosis. When the pressure sore finally creates a small opening in the skin, the sore beneath the skin can be very extensive. There are various ways of treating pressure sores. For the most severe cases, surgery may be required to remove the necrotic tissue and repair the damage. For less severe situations, changing positions may suffice.[107]

The prevention of pressure sore development is the prime reason for position changes. Positioning aids and cushions are also used to evenly distribute the overall pressure over a large surface and to lower peak pressure.[107]

Shearing occurs when two surfaces rub over each other. It differs from abrasion because the damage occurs under the skin (rather than on its surface). When shearing occurs, the flesh underneath the skin becomes stretched (blocking the blood flow of the capillaries). It can even tear the capillaries (preventing blood flow to the area). Intervention calls for decreasing the intensity and frequency of the shearing. Individuals who are wheelchair and positioning aid users may experience shearing when the client moves or slides out of position and is moved back. Shearing may also occur when the reclining back of a wheelchair is lowered or raised or in hospital beds when the head of the bed is lowered or raised. In terms of wheelchairs, some manufacturers now offer low-shear or no-shear backs for reclining wheelchairs (although some shearing may still occur).[107]

When determining what type of seating and positioning is needed for a client, a comprehensive positioning and seating evaluation is essential. Composed of many parts, it should include background information (e.g., medical diagnosis, age, activities of daily living status, history of skin problems, living situation, transportation resources, environmental accessibility, and third party payers). The most important consideration when determining positioning is comfort, as this will ensure usage as well as proper alignment.[107] The goals for wheeled mobility intervention and seating must be mutually agreed upon by all the participants (with the client's input and wishes taking precedence in order to ensure good follow through).[107]

EVALUATIONS, ASSESSMENTS, AND MEASUREMENT IN SEATING

When selecting an appropriate seating and wheeled mobility system, measurements need to be considered. Head height, hip width, chest width, shoulder width, elbow height, shoulder height, thigh length, calf length, inferior angle of the scapula, hip flexion angle, knee flexion angle, and ankle dorsiflexion angle are the specific areas that need to be measured for appropriate full bodied seating. Depending on an individual's needs, some of these measurements may not be needed. For details of how to specifically measure these areas, please refer to Anita Perr's article "Elements of Seating and Wheeled Mobility Intervention."[107]

Stinnett includes an evaluation that involves sitting at the side of the mat as well as asking the client to be supine on the mat. Observations of the client's functional ability in supported and unsupported seating are also conducted at this time. The client's reactions to supported sitting during simulated propulsion and weight-shifting as well as his or her ability to perform transitional movements through space are also observed. When the mat-side observation is being conducted, the therapist needs to determine scapular-humeral control during reach and the level of functional mobility (especially emphasizing the client's status for participating in daily living activities). Furthermore, if the client already has a wheelchair, Stinnett recommends asking the individual to stand at or sit in the wheelchair seating system that he or she is currently using.[106] At the same time the occupational therapist should also note the client's neurological status (e.g., any tonal influences or abnormal reflexes).[106] During the entire seating and positioning evaluation the client's posture needs to be observed while the client is in all the above-mentioned positions. The supine mat evaluations that Stinnett recommends involves observing and determining any type of orthopedic posture that might affect seating (e.g., fixed deformity vs. flexibility, past and current musculoskeletal abnormalities, body contours and the integumentary system). Stinnett also includes measuring the trunk width, limb lengths, range of motion, and joint angles while in the supine position.[106]

There is a useful assessment entitled "A Wheelchair Positioning Assessment Form" that can be found on pages 13 and 14 of Mayall and Desharnais' book, *Positioning in a Wheelchair*.[108]

MOBILITY BASES

There are basically two types of wheelchair mobility bases: manual and powered (scooters and powered wheelchairs). Any powered wheelchair consideration must focus upon the cognitive capabilities of the user (e.g., does the potential user have a basic understanding of cause and effect relationships as well as an ability to grasp safety considerations?). If the client's cognitive abilities present a safety problem and he or she is also unable to comprehend cause and effect actions, then powered wheelchairs should not be considered.

In determining if a client would benefit from a scooter (or another type of three-wheeled powered device), it is important for the therapist to evaluate the client's upper extremity function and endurance, as this type of mobility base involves adequate strength, good range of motion, and good dexterity so that he or she is able to manage a tiller and a lever that is squeezed for forward movement and pressed away for reverse. While squeezing the tiller, the user must be able to turn the tiller to steer the scooter.[107] Scooters also present issues such as: (1) transfers to and from scooters are often more difficult for some individuals than transfers to conventional powered wheelchairs; and (2) positioning may be more complex than a conventional wheelchair (although some manufacturers now provide some back supports and cushions for scooter use).[107]

Manual Mobility Bases

Manual mobility bases can be propelled by the arms and hand, with the legs and feet, or with the aid of another individual. They usually consist of large wheels in the back and smaller wheels (termed casters) at the front. When determining the use of a positioning aid, the occupational therapist should always be aware of the effect of its placement over the wheels. If there is excessive weight over the casters, the wheelchair will become more difficult to turn. The position of the user relative to the overall wheel base also affects the performance and the stability of the system. The further back over the wheels the user rides, the more likely tipping the wheelchair will become; the higher an individual sits, the higher the center of gravity becomes. This can cause the system to become less stable. If an individual is too far forward or too high from the wheel and push rim, he or she will be unable to reach the wheels effectively for propulsion. If the client sits too low in relation to the wheels, he or she may need to raise the shoulders in an awkward position in order to reach them). In general, the wheelchair user should reach back only slightly and push forward one-fifth of the way around the push rim.[107]

WHEELCHAIR ORIENTATION

There are three types of wheelchair orientation—standard, reclining (semi-reclining and fully reclining), and tilt-in-space.[107,108] Orientation refers to the seating system's position relative to gravity. In most instances the standard wheelchair positions the user in an upright position with the force of gravity pressing straight down through the head and the trunk. In order to tolerate this upright position, the client must be strong enough to overcome the gravitational force.[107] Hemi-wheelchairs, amputee wheelchairs (an amputee adapter can be adjusted to a standard adult wheelchair), and anti-tippers, using a standard wheelchair base, are also available from suppliers.[107,108]

If an individual is tilted in space or reclined, gravity will press more directly on the trunk and may aid in maintaining a beneficial posture. With a reclined seating system, the seat-to-back angle is widened. This allows the individual's hip angle to be open. A reclining backrest is most useful when the intended user is unable to flex sufficiently at the hips to be able to tolerate a 90-degree seat-to-back angle and when an open seat-to-back angle is needed for catheterization. Situations where the reclining wheelchair should be avoided include: when the reclining movement triggers extensor spasticity and when the client (who has a number of positioning aids such as lateral supports or headrest) is moved in and out of the reclined position. The positioning will change in relationship to the individual's trunk.[107]

The tilt-in-space chair offers a seat-to-back angle that remains constant. This means that the user's hip angle does not change. The seat and the back tip forward or backward as a unit. Tilt-in-space chairs have excellent pressure-relieving qualities. Also, with the tilt-in-space system, the postural supports remain in the appropriate position in relation to the client's trunk. This adds another benefit in that it is able to reduce the likelihood of shearing.[107] Tilt-in-space chairs are also helpful in offsetting decreasing muscle tone, as they reduce the force of gravity on specific areas.[106]

SEATING SYSTEMS

Seating systems are composed of various components such as a seat, a back (contoured or planar), and any attached components (e.g., lateral chest or trunk supports, headrest, lateral hip guides, and cushions). The back support should permit the user to move while supporting the trunk and at the same time maintaining the curves of the spine. These systems can be made from a variety of materials such as foam, air, or gel.[109]

A wheelchair can be ordered: with a sling seat and back, without a seating system (allowing for the placement of custom seating), or with a seat pan that supports a variety of commercially available seat cushions.[109] Drop seat bases, low seat bases, and long seat bases are available commercially and can also be custom made to fit onto a standard adult wheelchair (depending on the client's needs).[108]

Linear Seating

A *linear* (planar) system is made of flat surfaces. These systems are lower in cost than contour systems and provide easy movement for more active clients as well as having the ability to adapt to adjustments. The main disadvantage of flat surfaces is that most individuals do not have flat bodies.[109]

The following basic measurements can be taken by the therapist and then provided to a variety of companies who manufacture linear systems:[109]

1. Seat depth and width
2. Asymmetrical seat (for leg length discrepancy)
3. Back height and width
4. Seat-to-back angle
5. Biangular back (used to allow for natural spine contours and is composed of two linear surfaces)
6. Component placement

Cushions

Wheelchair cushions are placed under the thighs and buttocks to promote postural support for the thigh position and the pelvis as well as to increase the surface area for weight distribution (which aids in preventing pressure sores). Some cushion manufacturers use soft materials such as water, air, or viscous gel-like substances. However, it should be noted that the force of the cover or the shell against the user may also cause blood circulation disturbances. Specialty cushions such as above-the-knee amputee cushions and lumbar back cushions are also available from suppliers. Many cushion manufacturers combine soft materials with a contoured shape for postural support and pressure relief. In dealing with contoured seating it should be remembered that the contoured system, in general, provides better pressure distribution and better postural support than linear systems by increasing the surface area in contact with the body.[109]

Contoured Seating

Contour seating systems are designed to contour to or replicate the body shape of the client after he or she is seated. These contoured cushions offer the containment of the tissue around the bony prominences to prevent the obstruction of blood flow. Cushions made of foam become contoured when the user sits down. Foam, however, offers resistance when the client pushes against it. This might present a problem, depending on the properties of the foam used in the cushion and the amount of pressure pushing against the user. These two factors, if not in an adequate ratio, can cause blood circulation disturbances.[107]

Generic contours are available from manufacturers in backs, seats, and components. Some seating systems can be made of foam with a preischial bar or wedge board with a foam cushion. The Jay Cushion (Sunrise Medical, Carlsbad, CA) and the Stimulate Contoured Cushion (Supracor Systems, Inc., San Jose, CA) are manufacturers who readily supply contoured cushions. Sunrise Medical also supplies a Jay Back.

If a client's body shape does not match generic contours (and a linear seat is not adequate), a molded seating or aggressive contoured system may be indicated. Common aggressively contoured seats include the following: carved foam, the Matrix (Peach Medical: 1-800-253-6217, www.concentric.Me/~Matrix) and the Symmetrix Back (Crown Therapeutics: 1-800-851-3449, www.crownthera.com). The Symmetrix is made of a number of pods, placed at various angles and locations to support the trunk. This system has the ability to be reshaped any number of times.[109]

Molded Seating

Molded seating systems are actually molded to the client's body by means of a variety of methods. These systems are used mostly with clients who manifest significant orthopedic deformities as well as to provide better control to individuals with severe athetosis. The most common molded seating systems include Pin Dot Contour U (Invacare, Elyria, OH), foam-in-place, and sitting support orthosis.

The Contour U and other similar foam molded systems are made with a specialized simulator. The client is placed on bags of small beads, and a vacuum is used to remove the air from the beads as well as tighten the beads around the client's contours. The seat, made out of foam from this mold, is skinned to make it watertight. If for any reason the foam needs to be recarved at a later date, the seat must be reskinned.[109]

Foam-in-place molded seating systems are made by pouring liquid foam into a plastic bag that is behind the client, under the client, or both. The foam expands quickly to fill in any gaps that might exist and then hardens. There are various levels of firmness available. The foam-in-place does not work well for clients who are unable to hold still.[109]

The sitting support orthosis, made by a few suppliers in the United States, consists of a bag of beads which is placed over the client. During this process the client is placed on a form in a prone kneeling position. A cast is then made of the molded bag, and the final seat is then made from plastic. This can be padded, as needed, and the plastic can be heated and changed somewhat if deemed appropriate for the changing needs of the client.[109]

Armrests

The armrest should be used when the arms are not being used. While in the wheelchair, the client should be able to maintain a position with the hands free to perform other activities (such as self-feeding, reading). Armrests should not be used for upper body support for any long-term situation, as cumulative trauma disorder and deformities can develop in the shoulder complex. In general, armrests are grouped as full length or desk. The full-length armrest runs from the backrest of the wheelchair to the front edge of the seat surface. This full-length type of armrest is useful when using a lap board, for support when the client is moving from sitting to standing (and back), and when any other seating supports result in the forearm and the elbow resting forward. The desk-length armrest is useful when the client needs direct access to tables or a desk. These types of armrests are usually sufficient for the client who does not use his or her armrests on a full-time basis.

The armrest pad (usually provided by the wheelchair manufacturer) can be replaced with a pad of a different shape or custom designed for a client who has special needs. A number of manufacturers offer adjustable-height or fixed armrests. The thickness of the cushion and the client's position need to be considered when determining the optimal height for the armrest. This measure should be determined while the client is seated in the system that he or she intends to use.[107] In terms of specifics, different clients have different needs. To meet these needs there are a variety of styles available that can be attached to most wheelchairs. Some of these include a padded armrest, a flat padded armrest, elevating molded armrests, and elevating armrests designed to combat edema. Otto Bock makes a wide variety of armrests (e.g., a modular channel armrest that allows for three sizes of the forearm to be combined with four different types of hand pads). These are available from:

✧   Otto Bock Orthopedic Industry
     4130 Highway 55
     Minneapolis, MN 55422

Footrests

The front rigging is the entire complex that supports the lower leg. The main function is to support and protect the client's feet. The front rigging consists of the footplate and legrest or footrest. A footrest is a nonelevating foot support that consists of a footplate and footplate hanger. The footrest is essential for leg support. For example, if the footrest is too low, the foot will hang (causing excessive pressure or buildup under the distal thigh) and pressure sores can develop. Contrarily, if the footplate is too high, the knee will be raised and the weight then shifted back to the pelvis. This will cause excessive pressure on the proximal thighs and buttocks. If the knee is higher than the pelvis, sacral sitting (caused by the pelvis dropping back into a posterior pelvic tilt) with a kyphotic posture may develop. This posture adversely affects postural alignment, sitting tolerance, and function. Legrests (often termed elevating legrests) have a calf pad for lower leg support. These are used when the client is not able to flex the knees to tolerate the footrest position. This may occur in cases of arthritis, after knee replacement surgery, with other orthopedic conditions, and in addressing dependent edema. However, due to the fact that only limited elevation is attainable, treating dependent edema in this fashion may not be adequate.[107]

There are a number of specialty or custom made items (available from manufacturers) that have a specific focus on the lower leg and that are helpful for optimal sitting. Some of these include elevating blocks on footplates, knee protectors for elevating legrests, heel straps, legrest panels, the figure 8 foot strap, ankle positioning aids, and knee abductors.[108]

Seat Belts

Seat belts are sometimes referred to as pelvic positioning straps or lap belts. In pelvic positioning, the objective is to prevent the pelvis from sliding forward in the wheelchair while permitting the client to maintain the pelvis in a slight anterior pelvic tilt or in neutral. It is suggested that the seat belt be placed in such a way so that it pulls down perpendicular to the femur to prevent the pelvis from sliding forward while permitting the client to bend forward over it.[107] If the client's cognitive ability and hand dexterity are intact so that he or she can open the seat belt, a self-releasing seat belt will not be considered a restraint.

Lapboards

A lapboard (sometimes referred to as a tray table) is often added to the wheelchair seating system to promote additional upper extremity support. Clear lapboards, which allow the client and the caregiver to see through and view the condition and position of the lower extremities, can be helpful. However, if the client has visuoperceptual deficits, this may appear confusing. In that case a plastic opaque board may be the optimal choice.[107]

Trunk and Lateral Supports

A trunk support is used when the client is not able to independently maintain a posture that is upright. A reclining wheelchair or a tilt-in-space system can enhance support by changing the method by which gravity affects an individual.[107]

Lateral supports are usually placed on either side of the trunk to promote additional support. Depending on the situation and type of wheelchair, side cushions may be helpful in providing improved sitting posture.[108] In most instances the shape, location, and size of the lateral support can have a positive effect upon sitting. Three points of control are the most effective. One point of control is the side of the convexity. The force (support) should be applied to the rib that leads to the apex of the spine's curve. Most often it is necessary to provide a counterforce that has two points of control above and below that specific level. Without this counterforce single lateral support may result in pushing the client over to one side. It is important to note that lateral supports press on the ribs, which in turn can affect the spine.[107] A number of lateral supports are commercially available. Some of these supports can be identified as follows: spherical side thoracic support (with rigid rod assembly), lateral support with padded armrest, padded lateral support, and a firm contour back with lateral supports.

Headrests

Headrests are used when the individual has insufficient endurance, strength, or coordination to hold his or her head or neck in a neutral position. Headrests are almost always needed when the client is using a tilt-in-space or reclining seating position. Some of the types of headrests that are commercially available and that can be affixed to standard adult wheelchairs include foam headrests, back extension on a standard adult wheelchair, crown head support, headrest with combination head and neckrest, headrest support, and neck support.[108] For aesthetic reasons the headrest should be as unobtrusive and as small as possible.[107]

Problem Solving Involving Sacral Sitting/The Slider

Because the pelvis is the main foundation on which the trunk is balanced, pelvic stability is the centerpiece to performing all functional activities with the head, upper extremities, and lower extremities.

Sacral sitting, which promotes sliding, can be observed as the client slipping forward in the wheelchair, the buttocks on the front of the seat, and the weight placed out on the floor in front of the footrests. Another way to describe this is the client presents with a posterior pelvic tilt, poor trunk control, and the forward flexion of the lumbar spine.[108] Clients in these positions manifest several problems:

1. They are safety hazards and in a prime position for falling or sliding out of the chair completely.
2. Self-feeding and other self-care activities (such as washing one's face, brushing one's teeth, and combing one's hair) become compromised.
3. Deformities, pressure sores, shearing, and abrasion may develop.[108] A good seating system designed to promote appropriate posture can aid in providing this individual with improved functional abilities and a decrease in discomfort and hazardous sitting.

Possible solutions to sacral sitting include the usage of a wedge foam cushion, a wedge board with foam cushion, a foam cushion with a preischial bar, a 45-degree lap belt (secured appropriately to the wheelchair), and a drop seat with a wedge cushion.[108] Most often occupational therapy intervention involves fitting a solid seat insert and wedge seat cushion as well as using a 45-degree self-releasing lap/seat belt.

Stinnett recommends that clinicians provide sitting schedules (just like occupational therapists provide splint-wearing schedules to promote comfort and prevent skin breakdown). For elderly clients who use wheelchairs, "therapists must indicate the length of time in minutes or hours that the user should sit in a wheelchair as well as the amount of time that should be spent out of the chair."[106, p. 41]

Lynn M. Swedberg has written an excellent article entitled "Low-Tech Adaptations for Seating and Posturing" that details and describes how to provide low cost and low-tech seating adaptations used in her long-term care and home health practice. This is a marvelous resource for any clinician working with this population segment. To ensure a good fit, Swedberg relies on taking measurements of the client and the wheelchair and then comparing the results with an ergonomic seating system's standards—these include:

1. Chair width—1.5 to 2 inches wider than hips at their widest point
2. Seat depth—2 to 3 inches less than the distance from the back of the buttocks to the popliteal crease at the back of the knee (ensures that the hips are flexed and the trunk is upright when measuring)
3. Seat height—Same as lower leg length (from the popliteal crease to the heel of the shoe) for foot mobility in a wheelchair; 2 to 3 inches higher for other chairs for the ease of transfers (include the cushion's thickness in computations)
4. Armrest height—Add 1 inch to the distance from the seating surface to the underside of a bent elbow when the arm is held at the side (include the cushion's thickness)
5. Back height—Same as the measurement from the seating surface to mid-scapula (include the cushion's thickness in computations)

Adaptations can make a big difference in the lives of our clients. However, Swedberg cautions therapists to review their insurance policy and always consider the malpractice risks before making more wheelchair system modifications and/or adaptations. Throughout the article Swedberg discusses typical wheelchair seating problems and possible solutions using inexpensive materials. Possible improvements in seating outcomes (goals) can include:[110]

✧   Promoting safe swallowing
✧   Skin protection and/or healing
✧   Improved mobility and transfers resulting in reduced fall risk, increased respiratory capacity, increased ability to perform self-care activities, and normalized tone to enhance and improve function
✧   The ability to be out of bed without pain for activities and meals
✧   Increased socialization (being able to sit up and look at friends during conversation)
✧   Increased access and ability to go out into the community

Effective seating, positioning, restraint reduction (if the optimal seating system is used for the individual client, then restraints may not be needed to position the client safely in a wheelchair), and wound reduction (including the inservicing on the cause and prevention of abrasions, shearing, and pressure sores for frail elders in wheelchairs or in bed) can prove to be cost effective for many facilities. Occupational therapy, with its expertise in these areas, can prove to be a valuable link to promoting the maintenance of maximal mobility, safe swallowing, improved function in everyday activities, and an enhanced quality of life through the achievement of upright postural seated control.[106]

WHEELCHAIR TRANSFER
TECHNIQUES AND VEHICLE SAFETY TRANSIT

Appropriate wheelchair transfer techniques are essential in promoting safety within a facility or within the home setting. The basic guidelines for transfer training are provided as follows:[111]

✧ Utilize a secure gait belt around the client (usually at the waist).

✧ Move as close to the transfer surface as is possible and lock the wheelchair.

✧ Swing the footrests away and place the client's feet on the floor (or ask the client to place his or her feet on the floor).

✧ Remove the wheelchair's armrest that is closest to the transfer surface.

✧ The clinician/caregiver should then position him- or herself in front of the client.

✧ Scoot or ask the client to scoot his or her hips to the edge of the wheelchair.

✧ Ask the client to flex his or her knees so that the feet are slightly posterior to or below the knees.

✧ Ask the client to flex his or her hips so that the head is at or just anterior to the knees.

✧ Ask the client to place his or her arms on the armrest, on the knees, or reaching forward but not on the individual assisting with the transfer.

✧ Ensure that the clinician/caregiver guards the client's balance at all times.

✧ Ask the clinician/caregiver to place his or her hands securely on the gait belt at key points on the trunk or at the waist and hips to assist with the pivot (but not in a manner that would limit the client's ability to bend forward and not on the client's arms).

✧ Ask the clinician/caregiver to signal the client to pivot and to reach for the transfer surface.

✧ Ensure that the client is lowered to the transfer surface.

✧ Ensure that the client is assisted back into a stable seating position.

When instructing transfer techniques, the occupational therapy practitioner can verbally instruct the client concerning each step of the procedure. For those clients who manifest perceptual or cognitive deficits, tactile cues are the most effective. Transfer training requires demonstration and much practice.[111]

WHEELCHAIR/VEHICLE SAFETY TRANSPORT

In a *human vehicular collision* injury can occur when an individual hits something, something hits the individual, or the individual is ejected from the vehicle. At an impact speed of 30 miles per hour, the front of a vehicle is able to come to a complete stop within one-tenth of a second. However, unrestrained objects (e.g., purses, books, walkers, canes, crutches) and occupants (e.g., dogs, passengers who do not wear seat belts) will continue to move like projectiles toward the point of the impact of the crash at 30 miles per hour. To calculate the forward force generalized in a sudden stop/crash situation multiply the weight of the object (weight of the individual plus the weight of the chair) times the speed in miles per hour (force = mass x acceleration or deceleration; this is Newton's law of motion). For instance, a 130-pound client in a 60-pound wheelchair x 30 miles an hour is equivalent to 5,700 pounds of forward force.[112]

The principles of crash protection are threefold: (1) the crash forces need to be dissipated; (2) the occupant's impact within the interior of the vehicle can be prevented with a crash protection system; and (3) the individual can be prevented from vehicle ejection with an appropriate crash protection system in place.[112]

Although Mary-Ann Snell may have had a young child in mind when she wrote her article "Guidelines for Safety Transportation Wheelchair Users," her recommendations for safe wheelchair transport are useful with the older client as well.[112]

Her major recommendations for safe wheelchair transport are as follows:

✧   The wheelchair needs to be equipped with automobile type seat belts that fit snugly and securely over the bony structures of the pelvis—not over the abdomen.

✧   The seat belt must be firmly attached to the wheelchair frame (not to the insert or to any other removable part such as an armrest).

✧   The use of slides and triangular anchor end fittings serve to eliminate belt ends (in order to mount the belt to the frame).[112]

✧   The client's head and neck should be protected from whiplash injury. A headrest, therefore, is recommended for all wheelchair and other mobility devices (as well as for standard upholstered wheelchair backs). If a client does not need a headrest positioning device, the headrest should only be used during transport. Vehicle headrest's adjustments require that the item not be less than 1 inch from the back of the head. The middle of the headrest is to be in line with the middle of the ears.[112]

✧   The head should not be restrained during transport, as this leaves the neck totally unprotected.[112]

✧   Wheelchair lap trays should not be used during transport.[112]

✧   Reclined or tilted wheelchair position should not be used during transport. Ensure that the wheelchair is upright.[112]

✧   The seating insert must be well secured to the wheelchair's frame (at the back and at the base by using anti-gravity clips). Metal clips are usually recommended (webbing, buckle systems, and hook-and-loop fasteners are not recommended). When the seating unit does not have to be removed from the mobility base, it is best to permanently secure the seating system to its frame.[112]

✧   Rigid positioning devices, useful components for posture control, should not be used during transport as these devices do not dissipate crash forces. A belt system, soft neck collars, and foam trays can be used to promote upper trunk stability during transport.[112]

✧   "A tie-down system with an occupant restraint as well as wheelchair anchorage provides the best protection. Most companies now produce shoulder and lap belt systems for the occupant in addition to the four-point wheelchair restraint system."[112, p. 37]

✧   Any items that need to be carried in a vehicle must be tied down firmly. Do not use elasticized materials or cords as they could snap in a crash. This will prevent any loose objects from becoming deadly flying missiles if a crash occurs.[112]

✧   Because most crashes are frontal, rear-facing is considered to be the safest direction during transport. However, for the comfort of the client, front-facing transport can be utilized (if the appropriate restraint system is in place), as it is almost as safe as rear-facing. Never transport an individual in a side-facing position.[112]

✧   By providing these guidelines to the client, the family, and/or significant others, informed decisions as to how to safely transport a client in a wheelchair can be achieved.[112]

Arts and Crafts as a Modality and Leisure Skill Development

18

Characteristics

Arts and crafts have been traditionally associated with occupational therapy. A therapeutic crafts/arts program should promote the prevention of deterioration and the utilization of the client's remaining abilities.[10] The activities used need to be selected to meet each individual's physical and psychosocial needs as well as to provide value, meaning, pride, and satisfaction in the investment by the client. Decisions concerning the selection of an appropriate project need to be collaboratively discussed with both the client and the therapist.

Task-Focused Activity Analysis

Task-focused activity analysis should be utilized in every activity that a client engages in (whether it be in a physical, psychosocial, work, or leisure context). Task-focused activity involves clinical reasoning that enhances the clinician's ability to quickly identify the demands of activities and to use this information when working with clients. Task-focused activity analysis addresses three broad-based performance components such as sensorimotor development, psychosocial skills and psychological development, and cognitive integrative skills as well as cognitive development. Task-focused activity analysis is initiated with a description of the task (taking into account all aspects of performing the activity—from the initial planning to the cleaning up process). The following represent components of task-focused activity analysis:[113]
1. Description of the activity
2. Age range

3. The physical, social, and cultural context in which the activity will be used (such as "Where the activity will occur" and "Will it occur with others?")

4. The supplies and equipment needed to carry out the activity (also included is understanding the intrinsic nature of the materials—resistance, pliabilty, controllability, and the preparation time that is needed)

5. The awareness of any potential safety hazards (e.g., impaired sensation, suicidal precautions) and providing any necessary adaptations or preventative strategies that are needed to diminish potential hazards

6 The understanding of the sequential steps of the activity and how to present these appropriately to the client (e.g., clear instructions and directions)

7. The development of a summary of the performance components

8. The grading and/or adapting of an activity to meet the client's needs

During this entire process it is essential to consider the client (needs, goals, interests) and any occupational therapy theoretical concepts that would influence and promote a positive outcome.[113] To be successful, activities need to be client-focused. Arts and crafts remediation are particularly in need of in-depth task-focused activity analysis to promote appropriate and meaningful intervention.

Since therapeutic crafts and art approaches may often be misunderstood by the client and other professionals, it is of the most utmost importance that the practitioner seize every opportunity to explain intervention rationale (e.g., why a specific media is being utilized and how it will improve and enhance a client's ability to improve functional ability).[10]

INTERVENTION OBJECTIVES

Arts and crafts are modalities that can provide a variety of intervention objectives and initiatives. Some of these are:

✧ *Cognitive and intellectual objectives.* Improving one's ability to make decisions, increasing attention span, following directions, improving orientation status, improving concentration skills, and improving problem-solving abilities.

✧ *Psychiatric/psychological objectives.* Developing a sense of self-identity, self-concept, and self-esteem; coping with success or failure; dealing and coping with fantasy and symbolism; understanding cause-and-effect relationships; expressing creativity, originality, and need gratification; developing appropriate outlets for anxiety, frustration, tension, anger, aggression, and hostility; participating in reality testing; developing tolerance in a task and/or group situation; and improving and enhancing the ability to effectively relate in social and personal relationships and interaction.[10]

✧ *Physical rehabilitation and restoration objectives.* Increasing range of motion, increasing physical endurance, improving eye-hand coordination, improving the ability to perform motor movements smoothly, improving coordination abilities; learning to compensate for physical loss (e.g., one-handed skill training), learning to use adaptive devices/techniques to promote increased functional independence, improving muscle tone, strengthening specific groups of muscles, and increasing perceptual awareness.[10]

✧ *Sensory objectives.* Improving and enhancing the ability to be aware of body parts and the auditory, visual, tactile, olfactory, perceptual, and kinesthetic senses.[10]

✧ *Vocational objectives*. The development of crafts and arts skills for the purpose of seeking remuneration for products.[10]

✧ *Avocational objectives*. Increasing the client's potential for developing interests and hobby skills.[10]

Arts and crafts media can also be used as a vehicle to evaluate and assess client function through observation of a client's ability to understand instruction in this area and being able to perform the task or project at hand.[10]

PROJECTS

There are many basic projects that older adults can fabricate using crafts and arts skills:

✧ *Collages*. These may be fabricated out of wood, cloth, found materials, or any number of items a client might find interesting. These articles are glued together (on a panel) in an interesting design and can make handsome gifts.[10]

✧ *Paperweights*. Rocks of varying sizes can be painted and used as paperweights. Smaller rocks can be glued together to form an object (e.g., ladybug or butterfly).[10]

✧ *Stencil art*. A simple pattern repeated several times on a piece of paper can make attractive wrapping paper. This can be repeated on cork to make handsome coaster sets or on throw pillows and wall hangings.

✧ *Wooden toys*. Lumberyard cut off of 2-by-4's that are sanded and painted can make attractive cars and trains. Spool ends can be used to form the wheels.[10]

✧ *Stuffed toys*. Animal shapes made from colored fabrics that are later stuffed with washable material can make cuddly toys for grandchildren.[10]

✧ *Hand-fabricated blankets*. Knitted squares that are attached to one another can be assembled to form baby blankets (make nice gifts for grandchildren and are also useful as service projects such as blankets for AIDS babies).

✧ *Scrapbooks*. Scrapbooks that emphasize a particular theme such as flowers, a sport, a holiday, and family photos can be artistically arranged so that valued information can later be shared with family and friends.[10]

✧ *Photographic endeavors*. Photographs of nature, mounted on wooden panels, can provide pleasant and artistic gifts.

✧ *Yarn pompons*. A small pompon that is attached to a large pompon can serve as a base for a snowman, a mouse, a snow lady, a bear, or a toy mouse. Attaching buttons for eyes and felt pieces for ears (or eyes) adds to the creativity. These make excellent gifts for grandchildren, school children, grandnieces, and grandnephews.

✧ *Pictures printed from nature*. Objects such as a leaf, a feather, or bamboo dipped or brushed with paint and then pressed onto a fabric, printing paper, or rice paper can make effective and artistic wall hangings.

✧ *Rubbings*. Coins and metals are excellent sources for rubbings. The simplest method is with a pencil or a crayon. The object is taped down onto a paper. The paper is then turned over, and a pencil or crayon is rubbed over the area of the object. A heel ball (a more professional material) can also be used for this purpose. Rubbings of coins and metals can be used as decorative collages or mounted on wood panels in sets.

There are a number of arts and crafts media (e.g., enameling, copper tooling, water color, clay work, string art, paper art, Turkish knotting and braiding, weaving, batik and tie dying, charcoal drawing, colored pencil art, oil and acrylic painting, mosaics, needle work, leather work, wood working, quilting, tempera painting, felt tip marker art, and pen and ink art work) that can be used for therapeutic purposes. The utilization of these items depends upon the budget and work area that is available; the suitability of the project for each client; and a knowledgeable clinician so that instruction is clear, organized, and purposeful. Although projects may need to be simplified because of emotional, physical, or cognitive disabilities, they should never be childish.[10]

Information on crafts and arts is available at local libraries. However, there are several books that are especially helpful:

- ❖ Hamil, C. M. & Oliver, C. R. (1980). *Therapeutic activities for the handicapped elderly*. Rockville, MD: Aspen Systems.
- ❖ Smith, S. (1981). *How to draw and paint*. Secaucus, NJ: Chartwell Books.
- ❖ Spandorfer, M., Curtiss, D., & Snyder, J. (1996). *Making art safely: Alternative methods and materials in drawing, painting, printmaking, graphic design and photography*. New York: Van Nostrand Reinhold.
- ❖ *The best of colored pencil*. (1993). Rockport, MD: Rockport.

   (This book contains exquisite examples of colored pencil work and is suggested here because colored pencils are something that most people are familiar with. However, many people do not realize that there now is a colored pencil society, and that although this medium may have been used in early school years, it is now recognized as a mature, professional modality.)
- ❖ Wilkinson, V. C. & Heater, S. L. (1996). *Therapeutic media and techniques of application: A guide for activities therapists*. New York: Van Nostrand Reinhold.

LEISURE SKILL DEVELOPMENT

Leisure occurs outside of work obligations. *Leisure activities* usually provide opportunities for recreation, relaxation, personal growth and development, enjoyment, entertainment, a time for interaction with others, goal achievement, free choice of desired activities (which should be prioritized by the client), and challenge.[114]

Participation in leisure activities usually holds intrinsic value for the client, engenders increased self-esteem, and may have increased importance in the social life of the client, friends, family, and significant others.[115]

When assessing the leisure needs of a client, it is important to include previous activities (if the client is still interested in involving him- or herself in these), and new activities the client is willing to learn, and the older adult's abilities and potential for participating in these activities.[115]

INTEREST CHECKLISTS AND OTHER TYPES OF ASSESSMENTS

To determine an individual's interests, the therapist can use a variety of tools. First, there are interest checklists. Matsutsuyu's Interest Checklist examines the intensity of a person's interests in 80 different activities.

These are divided into five activity categories:[116]

1. Manual skills
2. Physical sports
3. Social recreation
4. Activities of daily living
5. Educational and cultural activities

In 1978, this checklist was revised to include factor analysis.[117]

Nystrom developed a questionnaire that measures active participation and includes questions concerning the definition of leisure (based on a study of activity patterns, leisure concepts, and the meaning of leisure time activity).[118] Gregory later adopted Nystrom's Activity Checklist so that questions that dealt with the meaning of the activities as well as questions related to life satisfaction were included.[119] Structured interviews can also be a helpful way to explore the role of leisure with the older adult.[120] An activities configuration and an occupational role history are also helpful tools in gathering client information regarding leisure interests. The activities configuration tool can be used to gather data concerning the client's education, work history, values, and other plans and interests.[121] The occupational role history is useful in determining a balance in activities.[122]

THE ROLE OF OCCUPATIONAL THERAPY

The occupational therapy practitioner often has many roles concerning leisure pursuits. Some of these are:

✧ As a resource person (referring the older adult to resources within the community).

✧ As a leisure task instructor. This can include:

  ⌃ Adapting tasks and modifying the environment to facilitate appropriate leisure performance

  ⌃ Ensuring safety

  ⌃ Using task simplification when needed

✧ As a consultant in a facility or community setting (assisted living, day care setting, or nursing home facility). When dealing with a client who experiences limited cognitive abilities and when educating staff, the therapist needs to ensure that the activity is pleasurable, safe, modified as needed, adaptable, familiar, routine, and dignified.

✧ As a consultant in the home setting. The clinician provides caregiver instruction. This is important as the client may be dependent on the caregiver to purchase materials that can facilitate participation in leisure pursuits, and the caregiver may need to learn new approaches and methods to enable the late life adult to get involved in leisure activities.[115]

✧ As a consultant in a facility or at home. The clinician introduces, educates, and helps procure adaptive equipment (e.g., provides catalogs) that can be useful with leisure activities. Some recommendations relating to adaptive equipment include:

  ⌃ Cardholders

⮝ Pneumatic video game controls

⮝ Slip-on keyboard aid (for limited grasp with computer work)

⮝ Adapted bowling equipment

⮝ Fishing equipment that can attach to a wheelchair or that can be used with one hand

⮝ Embroidery holders

⮝ Book holders

⮝ Rolling folding carts

⮝ Writing instruments that can be used with pencil, pens, and brushes.[115,123]

Activities that older adults participate in are varied as to each individual. Some of these are as follows:

✧ Music

✧ Entertainment (movies, plays, concerts, television)

✧ Painting

✧ Arts and crafts

✧ Traveling

✧ Educational experiences (courses, workshops, elder hostel, lectures)

✧ Service activities (religious service clubs, schools, hospitals, grandparenting)

✧ Puzzles

✧ Cards

✧ Board games

✧ Planned visits to a park, restaurant, or tavern

✧ Walking

✧ Driving

✧ Sports (golf, swimming)

✧ Dancing

✧ Pet care

Late life can be an enjoyable time. Leisure activities play a major role in determining an individual's quality of life and health. Occupational therapy practitioners "can modify or adapt elderly persons' lifelong interests to allow for their continued participation, and practitioners can explore and assist in the initiation of new interests in which the person can experience success, enjoyment, and satisfaction."[123, p. 734]

HOME HEALTH

DESCRIPTION

Home health care's major emphasis is upon promoting improved functioning so that a client can remain living at home either on an independent basis or with a family member, significant other, or employed caretaker. Most occupational therapy services are provided to a home client through a home health agency. However, occupational therapists may be in private practice or may also work for organizations that are not home health agencies (such as physical therapists, occupational therapists, or speech therapists who have developed their own business associations).

The really exciting aspect of home care is that it usually involves family members as well as the client to carry out the home care program. The home is the therapeutic setting. Therefore, the practitioner needs to improvise therapeutic programs from this setting. An example of this could be the use of soup cans to serve as weights (for therapeutic exercise programming) in promoting increased strength and range of motion of the upper extremity. It is important to realize that in home care the practitioner is a guest in the house, and as such he or she must be culturally aware and respectful of any customs and beliefs celebrated or displayed in the home.

Intervention can be varied:
- ✧ Instruction in activities of daily living or instrumental activities of daily living (using energy conservation techniques and/or body mechanics education as needed)
- ✧ Muscle re-education
- ✧ Perceptual motor training
- ✧ Fine motor training

◆   Neurodevelopmental training
◆   Sensory training
◆   Fabrication and training in the use of orthotics/splints
◆   Training in the use of adaptive equipment and/or techniques
◆   Home exercise programming to promote improved strength, range of motion, and coordination

In the area of physical dysfunction the client may have just come home from a hospital, rehabilitation center, or nursing home. In this case home care can serve as a bridge from the facility to the home. Besides physical dysfunction, home care programs are also available to mental health clients and developmentally delayed clients (as previously discussed in this unit). The opportunities for serving clients with many different needs, varied diagnoses, and diverse cultural backgrounds are other aspects of home care that make it a challenging and rewarding practice area.

Referrals are often transmitted by a fax machine, a phone answering mechanism, or a beeper. Most home health agencies have case managers and supervisors who are involved in ensuring that each client receives the care that he or she needs. A team usually consists of a physician, a primary care nurse, a nurse's aide (whom the occupational therapist may supervise when there are concerns of activities of daily living care), a speech therapist, an occupational therapist, a physical therapist, and a social worker. A psychologist or psychiatrist may be "called in" to provide services if needed. Interaction among the disciplines is stressed, and notes are required to describe any professional interface that has happened (be it a direct conversation or conference or telephone communication).

In most instances occupational therapists and other team members (except for nurses who are usually employees of the home health agency) are hired on a contract basis (home health aides may be employees of the home health agency or a separate contracting agency). Zahoransky speaks of the need for collaboration among team members and the use of the three "R's":[124]

1. *Recognition.* Occupational therapists need to educate the team as to our services as well recognize the merits of other team members. This recognition of each team member's unique role helps to avoid any duplication of service.

2. *Respect.* Respecting the rights of the client and respecting all team members' roles and interventions.

3. *Referral.* If each team member recognizes and respects the occupational therapy profession, then referrals will complement this respect.

The specifics for Medicare in home health care will be considered in a special appendix section entitled "Reimbursement Issues." However, some basics for therapeutic care are applicable to most programs in a variety of countries. First the client needs to be homebound and under a physician's care. There needs to be an occupational therapy referral, an evaluation, and a written care plan. Occupational therapy services (in the United States) must be certified by a physician. Services need to be reasonable and necessary. The client needs to demonstrate a potential for reasonable progress (make significant gains in functional tasks such as activities of daily living and other daily tasks) within a reasonable time frame. All home visits require a progress note documenting progress as well as such items as the client's desire to continue intervention and a discussion of discharge plans from the very initiation of intervention and at each succeeding session. At the conclusion of services there needs to be a discharge note—usually a summary of the client's status and future recommendations—in agreement with the physician who is in charge. All care must be provided by qualified personnel.[125,126]

Paulson suggests the following items that can serve as part of an "evaluation kit" (equipment and supplies that can be helpful in assisting evaluation and intervention). These include:[125]

- ✧ A goniometer
- ✧ A dynamometer
- ✧ A blood pressure cuff and a stethoscope
- ✧ A measuring tape (useful for measuring edema and sections of the home)
- ✧ Clothes pins (for pinch)
- ✧ Theraband and theraputty of various grades
- ✧ A rolling pin
- ✧ Nuts and bolts of various sizes
- ✧ Activities of daily living aids:
  - ▲ Elastic shoelaces
  - ▲ A long-handled shoe horn
  - ▲ A reacher
  - ▲ A dressing stick
  - ▲ A rocker spoon/knife
  - ▲ Foam tubing for building up handles on utensils
  - ▲ A plate guard
- ✧ Velcro
- ✧ Scissors
- ✧ Masking tape
- ✧ Foam rubber
- ✧ Duct tape
- ✧ A toolbox (for wheelchair repairs and assembling adaptive equipment such as a tub transfer bench)

The initial evaluation should include areas such as:[125]
- ✧ Functional mobility (to perform everyday activities)
- ✧ Balance (in performing daily care activities)
- ✧ Ambulation involving instrumental activities of daily living as well as daily care activities
- ✧ Upper extremity range of motion
- ✧ Coordination
- ✧ Grasp deformity
- ✧ Synergy
- ✧ Edema
- ✧ Pain

- ✧ Self-care activities
- ✧ Sensory and perceptual abilities
- ✧ Home management
- ✧ Interests and past work history
- ✧ Endurance and activity levels
- ✧ Medication management
- ✧ Structuring and time use
- ✧ Architectural barriers (including safety factors)
- ✧ The need for any adaptive equipment and/or devices useful in promoting independence
- ✧ Homebound status
- ✧ Precautions and contraindications
- ✧ Rehabilitation potential
- ✧ Intervention recommendations
- ✧ The plan of care with the collaboration of the client, the caregiver, the therapist, and the physician

Long- and short-term goals (with time frame) as well as frequency and duration are essential parts of the evaluation. During the evaluation, it is imperative that the client actually perform the task rather than accept a verbal report from the caregiver or the client.[125]

At evaluation, the therapist should be educating the client as to what home health therapy is (e.g., entitlements, requirements, expectations). Throughout the intervention process progress is constantly assessed. Progress notes are written after each visit, and the therapist continuously apprises and discusses progress with the client and the caretaker. In this way, the client and the caretaker can better understand the intervention program, and also better understand when goals have been achieved and when discharge is imminent. At discharge most forms include:

- ✧ The total number of intervention visits
- ✧ The modalities and methods used in intervention
- ✧ The discharge status of the client (e.g., discharged to home independence or discharged to home with a caretaker, discharged to outpatient therapy, client no longer homebound, client discharged to a facility)
- ✧ A statement as to when and how the physician was notified of discharge (and his or her agreement with this)
- ✧ The date that this occurred

EVALUATIONS

Paulson includes an example of a Home Care Evaluation (Visiting Nurse Association of the Sacramento Valley Division, Sacramento, CA).[125]

In *Occupational Therapy: Practice Skills for Physical Dysfunction*, Foti, Pedretti, and Lillie provide an example of an Activities of Daily Living Evaluation and an Occupational Therapy Department Activities Home Management Form, adapted from:

- ✧ Activities of Daily Living Evaluation Form 461-1

The Hartford Easter Seal Rehabilitation Center

Hartford, CT

✧ Activities of Home Management Form
  Occupational Therapy Department
  University Hospital, Ohio State University at Columbus[115]
A Home Evaluation Checklist is also presented, adapted from:
✧ Physical Therapy Home Evaluation Form
  Ralph K. Davies Medical Center,
  San Francisco, CA
  and Occupational Therapy Home Evaluation Form
  Alta Bates Hospital
  Albany, CA[115]

Another excellent resource is Trombly's Home Assessment Activities Checklist. This is a client-oriented functional assessment of activities in the home. Areas such as managing the site (e.g., getting in and out of the car, using a bus, driving, loading and unloading items in and out of the car, ability to move around the outside of the home, interests, hobbies, special needs outside of the home; managing the front and back door; climbing the steps or using the ramp; managing hallways and inside doors; managing inside stairs; and managing activities in the bathroom, kitchen, family room, bedroom, and laundry) are included.

This resource can be found in:

✧ Trombly, C. A. (1997). *Occupational therapy for physical dysfunction* (pp. 62-67). New York: Lippincott, Williams and Williams.

The General Occupational Therapy Evaluation for Geriatric Clients/Patients discussed earlier in this unit is another available evaluation tool that can be used in the home health setting.

Two other evaluation resources, available from the American Occupational Therapy Association, that are very useful in the home health practice as well as other practice settings are:

✧ *Canadian Occupational Performance Measure* (COPM) (3rd Ed.). This is a client-centered performance measure that is based on the model of occupational performance. The focus is upon performance in productivity, self-care, and leisure. It considers the client's environment, developmental stage, motivation, and life roles.

  1-877-404-AOTA

  www.aota.org

✧ *The Kohlman Evaluation of Living Skills* (KELS) (3rd Ed.). This evaluation determines a client's ability to function in basic living skills. It tests 17 basic living skills under five areas: self-care, health and safety, money management, work, and leisure.

  1-877-404-AOTA

  www.aota.org

While these evaluation recommendations are helpful, it should be remembered that many home health agencies develop their own therapy evaluation forms.

INTERVENTION CONCERNS

Joint Protection and Energy Conservation

Instruction in joint protection and energy conservation techniques is frequently utilized by home health occupational therapists when working with clients who need remediation with any type of self-care activities (e.g., self-feeding, dressing, bathing, grooming, toileting, functional transfers as associated with activities of daily living) and instrumental activities of daily living (e.g., home management such as meal planning, meal preparation, telephoning, laundry, cleaning, shopping, safety management, health management). This subject has been previously detailed in this unit.

Dressing

Dressing is a major part of the home health occupational therapist's technical expertise.

In general, dressing may be made easier by utilizing the following low technology aids and adaptive equipment:

- ✧ Front-opening garments that fit loosely can make donning and doffing garments easier.
- ✧ These items can be further enhanced by the use of large buttons, zippers with loops on the tab, and Velcro closures.
- ✧ A button hook with an enlarged weighted handle may also make dressing easier.
- ✧ Tying shoes can be eliminated through the use of elastic shoelaces, Velcro closures, and slip-on shoes.
- ✧ Slacks with Velcro closures for men and elastic tops for women help to make dressing less laborious.
- ✧ Brassieres with front openings and Velcro replacements for the usual hook-and-eye aid in facilitating donning and doffing of this garment.
- ✧ A pullover bra-slip is also helpful in enhancing the management of brassiere fastening.
- ✧ Clip-on ties can be used by men to eliminate knot tying.

All dressing should be performed sitting on a sturdy armchair, bed, or locked wheelchair. Adaptive equipment such as stocking and sock donners, long-handled reachers, and dressing sticks aid in eliminating the necessity of bending. Other adaptive materials and techniques such as using pieces of Velcro that can be attached to clothing with elastic bands that can then be worn on the client's hands to assist with pulling on and gripping clothing—these also help to make the whole aspect of dressing less stressful. The installation of a floor-to-ceiling pole or a waist-high bar which the client can lean upon aids the client in establishing stability while dressing. If the client is hemiplegic, these items should be installed on his or her nonaffected side.[10,115,127]

The neurodevelopmental treatment (Bobath) approach to donning a shirt with the hemiplegic client and doffing slacks, underwear, and socks/stockings with the hip replacement client has also been previously discussed. An alternative dressing method for the hemiplegic client (or any individual who has dysfunction of one upper extremity [may be due to fractures, burns, peripheral and neuropathic conditions]) will now be described. Generally speaking, it is best to begin with the affected leg or arm first when donning clothing. For doffing clothing the converse is true. That is—the removal of clothing should be initiated with the nonaffected side.[115]

THE DON AND DOFF OF A SHIRT

For donning a shirt the client should first grasp the shirt collar with the nonaffected hand and shake out any twists. Next, the shirt should be positioned on the lap with the inside facing up and the collar toward the chest; the sleeve should be positioned so that the opening is on the affected side and it should be as large and as close to the affected hand as possible. The affected hand should be resting on the lap. Next, the nonaffected hand should place the affected hand in the sleeve opening, and the sleeve should be worked over the affected elbow by pulling on the shirt. The nonaffected arm is then placed into its sleeve and raised up to shake or slide the sleeve into position past the elbow. The nonaffected hand then gathers the shirt up the middle of the back from the hem to the collar, and the shirt is raised over the head. The client then leans forward, ducks his or her head, and passes the shirt over the head. Next, the nonaffected hand adjusts the shirt by leaning forward, then working it down past both shoulders. The client then reaches back and pulls the shirttail down.

The last step is buttoning. The shirt is lined up so that both fronts are equal. All buttoning is begun from the bottom up. The nonaffected hand can button the sleeve cuff of the affected arm. The sleeve cuff of the nonaffected arm may be prebuttoned with a button that has been sewn on with an elastic thread so that it can be easily put on.[115]

Doffing the shirt is much easier than donning it. First the shirt is unbuttoned. Next, the client leans forward. The client then grasps the collar or gathers the material up in the back from the collar to him or her with the nonaffected hand. At this point the client leans forward some more, ducks his or her head, and pulls the shirt over the head. The client then removes the sleeve from the nonaffected arm and, lastly, from the affected arm.[115] There are a number of variations available for one-arm dressing techniques.

THE DON AND DOFF OF SLACKS

The client positions him- or herself in a locked wheelchair or sturdy armchair. Next, the nonaffected leg is positioned in front of the midline of the body and the knee is flexed at 90 degrees. The nonaffected hand then reaches forward and grasps the ankle of the affected leg and then lifts the affected leg over the nonaffected leg so that the affected leg is crossed over the nonaffected leg. The trousers are slipped onto the affected leg so that the foot is completely inside the trouser leg. At this point the client should not pull the trouser above the knee. The affected leg is uncrossed (by grasping the ankle and gently moving it off). The nonaffected leg is then inserted into the trousers and worked onto the hips as far as possible. To prevent the trousers from dropping when pulling the slacks over the hips, the affected hand can be placed in the pocket. If able to do so, the client can then stand and pull the trouser over the hips. If standing balance is good, the client can remain standing to pull up the zipper or button. The client may sit down to button (if balance for standing more than a short period is questionable).

Doffing slacks is much easier than donning. While seated, the client should unfasten the slacks and work down the hips as far as possible. Next, the client can stand and allow the slacks to drop past the hips (or work the slacks down past the hips). The client then removes the slacks from the nonaffected leg. Next the client sits and crosses the affected leg over the normal leg (as described earlier in this discussion). The slacks are then removed from the affected leg, and the leg is then uncrossed.[115]

Chapter 26 in *Occupational Therapy: Practice Skills for Physical Dysfunction* details a variety of don and doff procedures.[115] Chapter 19 of *Willard and Spackman's Occupational Therapy* also provides excellent information regarding self-care activities.[127]

Hygiene and Grooming

The following aids, methods, adaptive equipment, and low technology equipment are useful in this area of self-care skills dealing with hygiene and grooming:

- ✧ Hand-held shower sprays (client can be instructed to hold a finger over the spray to determine sudden temperature changes that might exist in the water) makes washing safer and less energy consuming.
- ✧ Soap-on-a-rope is helpful in preventing bending over in the shower if the soap should slip.
- ✧ Long-handled bath brushes/sponges with a soap insert are useful when trying to reach all parts of the body.
- ✧ Shower chairs, bathtub seats, and transfer benches are helpful in easing the transfer to the tub as well as providing physical support to the client.
- ✧ The installation of grab bars in the shower, in the tub, and near the toilet provides support and promotes safety.
- ✧ Shower and bath doors should be removed and replaced with a shower curtain.
- ✧ Non-skid mats or adhesive strips should be used in the tub or shower bottom to prevent falls. Also, non-skid mats should be placed on the floor of the bathroom as well when using the shower.
- ✧ Installation of indoor-outdoor rugs in the bathroom is another option to promote safety.
- ✧ Long handles on hairbrushes, combs, and toothbrushes (may be constructed from inexpensive dowels, pieces of PVC pipe, or foam tubing which can often be found in hardware stores) are useful when there is limited range of motion.
- ✧ Suction brushes attached to the sink are useful in cleaning fingernails or dentures.
- ✧ Built-up handles or extenders can be applied to faucet handles to promote ease of use and joint protection.
- ✧ Colored contrasting toilet seats can assist individuals who have visual problems.
- ✧ Raised toilet seats with armrests are also helpful for individuals who have difficulty rising. Toilet levators (that fit at the base of the toilet) are devices that can be used to raise the height of the toilet seat (while retaining the normal look of the toilet).
- ✧ For individuals who need a larger door entrance, offset hinges can be used to increase the clearance of a door by 2 inches. These are available at most hardware stores.
- ✧ Razor holders and wash mitts aid in accommodating weak finger dexterity and grip.[115,127]

✧ Electric razors or battery-operated razors are often easier to handle than the traditional nonpowered razor.

Functional Incontinence

Pamela Toto, an independent home care contractor, had some interesting perspectives on home health occupational therapy and functional incontinence. Toto affirms that by identifying and addressing conditions (such as dementia, impaired mobility, low vision, depth perception problems, and limited range of motion), occupational therapists can often resolve or reduce functional incontinence occurrences through compensation for limitations, restoration of abilities, or adaptation of the environment.[128] In her practice (which includes home care and at times nursing home residents), Toto often helps clients diagnosed with stress or urge incontinence to improve mobility so that they are able to reach the bathroom more quickly. Toto encourages her clients to use the bathroom more frequently throughout the day and recommends a bedside commode as needed. Adaptations such as placing a long red tape on the bathroom floor (that measured the exact distance at which a client needed to stop her wheelchair to reach the toilet), along with the modification of added extenders to the wheelchair locking or breaking mechanism, enable late life adults to continue to be independent in self-toileting (at the same time incidences of incontinence can be reduced and the added risk of falls can be prevented).[128] Toto asserts that the "consideration of toileting abilities, continence, and related issues should be an automatic piece of a holistic approach to practice. An understanding of the different causes and interventions for incontinence empowers OT clinicians to effectively assist clients meeting their goals."[128, p. 34]

Self-Feeding

Adaptive equipment and low technology devices that are helpful in assisting late life adults (who have coordination disabilities or grip weakness) feed themselves include the following:[10,115,127]

✧ Plate stabilizers (such as non-skid placements, wet washcloths, or modeling clay placed under the dish as well as the use of suction bases) are helpful in preventing the plate from moving when eating.

✧ Plate guards and scoop dishes are helpful in preventing spillage of food. The plate guard has a portable advantage as it can be carried and used when eating in a restaurant or other people's homes.

✧ When using utensils spills can be eased or eliminated through the use of built-up handles that are weighted. Swivel spoons are also helpful.

✧ Side cutter forks and rocker knives are useful for the individual with only one functioning upper extremity.

✧ Heavy plastic mugs, with a handle that can accommodate four fingers, and filled halfway, can also be helpful in preventing spillage.

✧ Other devices, such as long plastic straws with a straw clip on a cup or glass with a weighted bottom eliminate the need to carry the cup or glass to the mouth and help in avoiding spills. Plastic cups with covers and spouts are also helpful in preventing spills.

✧ Nose cutout plastic glasses enable the user to drink without tilting his or her head backwards.

✧ Flow vacuum cups are available for individuals who need to drink from a supine position.

✧ Palmar clips, wrist supports, and universal cuffs are useful when grip strength is not functional.

✧ When hand-to-mouth action is restricted, extended/angled handles, ball bearing feeders, and offset suspension feeders can be indicated.

✧ Individuals with various visual impairments can best be served by developing a food location system (e.g., foods placed on the plate in a specific manner using a clock identification method, adjusting the food placement so it is in the sight range of the individual, and the use of contrasting colored foods on the plate).

For individuals with dysphagia, please refer to Chapter 14 of this unit.

In order to encourage good eating, food should always be presented in a colorful and pleasant manner. Even with special diets, food should be as "tasty" as possible (e.g., use of a salt substitute when a low sodium diet is being prescribed). The table and chair should be of a comfortable height for the individual, and the chair should be supportive with an armrest. To ensure safe eating, appropriate posture is paramount. The table itself should be pleasantly arranged without clutter.

Affolter developed the intervention technique of guiding as a method that therapists can use to assist clients in perceiving their environment. This is done by physically guiding the clients' hands and bodies in functional activities. This can be very helpful when the caretaker in the home has a significant other who is having difficulty feeding him- or herself and who has had a CVA or other neurological impairment. This method focuses upon the process of cognitive-perceptual development and the relationship that exists between tactile-kinesthetic input and the problem-solving needs that are necessary in maintaining daily living skills. Nonverbal guiding can be taught to the caregiver. Guiding has many different levels. There is maximal assist (heavy guiding), moderate, and minimal (or light) guiding. The client is guided through the task of self-feeding. As the information is processed and assimilated the client is able to take over some aspect of purposeful movement.[129]

An example of the specific facilitation of self-feeding using the Affolter method can occur when the client stabilizes the bowl of the plate with his or her left hand while his or her significant other assists by guiding the right hand. This helps in inhibiting the flexor synergy pattern. As the client is able to process the tactile input, his or her eyes may gaze away and the mouth will open in the expectation of there being food on a utensil.[129]

There is nothing so basic as being able to feed oneself. Instruction in self-feeding, through techniques, low technology equipment, and adaptive devices, is an area in which therapists and assistants can impact on this very important aspect of daily living (in any type of practice setting).

Home Management and Home Adaptations

The therapist needs to carefully assess what homemaking activities can be done safely by the client, what activities can be done safely when adapted and modified, and what activities the client is unable to manage (these activities should be assigned to a caregiver).

The following are adaptations, recommendations, and low technology aids that are useful in home management:

✧ Use easy-open containers (or store food in small plastic containers once opened).

✧ Adapted jar and can openers are available commercially that make opening items easier and less stressful on joints.

✧ Do not lift objects. Instead slide them on counters or floors.

✧ Utilize a wheeled utility cart (for laundry or kitchen usage).

✧ Use stairglides or ramps (when possible).

✧ All stairs should have two banisters (both indoor and outdoor) with adequate lighting at the top and bottom of each landing (motion lighting is useful).

✧ Large button phones, telephone headsets, speaker phones, and telephone clip holders help to make telephone communication easier and less stressful.

✧ Utilize mixing bowls, utensils, pans, and pots that are heavy to improve and increase stability.

✧ Utilize lever-type door handles to make door knobs easier to turn.

✧ Utilize offset hinges on standard door hinges to increase door jam width (by at least 2 inches).

✧ Make use of non-skid mats on work surfaces. Rubber mats at the bottom of the sink are useful in breaking the fall of dishes.

✧ Whenever possible use foods that have been prepared or partially prepared (e.g., peeled carrots, cut cabbage) to eliminate or reduce as many processes as possible (e.g., cutting, chopping, slicing).

✧ Use free-standing appliances (e.g., electric skillet, microwave, countertop mixer, toaster oven) rather than transferring items out of the oven or using a hand-held mixer.

✧ Utilize a milk carton holder with handle to pour milk for ease in handling.

✧ Use a frying basket to cook or steam foods such as vegetables to ensure safe removal and reduce burns.

✧ Utilize graters and pan holders with suction feet for stabilization.

✧ When the client is wheelchair bound and when funds are limited, the removing of cabinet doors for opening and closing operations can eliminate the need for maneuvering around them. Place frequently used items toward the front of cabinets for easy access.

✧ When working with hot items, use long mitts rather than potholders.

✧ Utilize cutting boards with stainless steel nails to stabilize vegetables and meats. To ensure safety—when not in use, the nails should be covered with large corks. These boards should have suction cups on the back to prevent slippage or sliding.

✧ Whenever possible adjust work height of the sink, range, or counter. This is helpful in minimizing leaning, reaching, lifting, and bending.

✧ Utilize tongs to turn food when cooking or serving food as these offer more control and stability than a serving spoon, spatula, or fork.

✧ Promote safety through the use of a serrated knife, as this is less likely to slip than a straight-edged knife. Rocker knives are also helpful in promoting safety and useful with individuals who only have one functioning upper extremity.

✧   Use pots and casserole dishes that have double handles to promote greater stability.

✧   Use dust mitts when dusting.

✧   Utilization of long-handled dustpans and an electric broom are helpful when cleaning.

✧   Use a self-wringing mop to lessen stress on the joints and promote energy efficiency.

✧   Whenever possible, utilize fitted bedsheets to promote energy conservation.

✧   Utilize adjustable closet and cabinet shelves, set an appropriate work height to save energy.

✧   "Lazy susans" and pull-out shelves promote efficiency and energy conservation. At the same time they make items more accessible and promote easy storage.

✧   User rocker light switches and touch operated, motion operated, and sound operated lights to make turning on a lamp easier.

✧   Utilize front-loading washers and dryers with buttons rather than knobs.

✧   Use premeasured detergents, fabric softeners, and bleaches.

✧   Eliminate clutter.

✧   Ensure appropriate illumination in all work areas, bathrooms, hallways, stairs, and sleeping areas.

✧   Eliminate "throw rugs" and encourage the use of low pile carpets.

✧   For the individual in a wheelchair the use of a lapboard may serve as a work surface.

✧   Provide work areas with appropriate seating and strategic places to sit as a way to increase an individual's endurance. Knowledge that there is a place to sit often aids in giving the individual an incentive to walk to participate in home management.

Electronic Aids to Daily Living and the Promotion of Daily Activities

There are many *electronic aids to daily living* (EADLs) that can provide alternative ways to control a variety of electronic devices (e.g., lights, telephones, doors, audiovisual equipment) that can be helpful to older adults who experience dexterity, mobility, cognitive, or sensory limitations as well as security concerns.[130]

When considering dexterity limitations, EADLs allow users to control devices by using a switch or voice control (i.e., instead of struggling to turn the knob on a lamp), touch-activated lamps, table lamps that are foot activated (lamps that are plugged into an adapter that uses a round button, usually 1 inch in diameter, on the floor for foot control), and switch-activated EADLs. These are helpful in ensuring better control of lights and appliances.

Available from:

✧   Home Automation

1-800-SMART-HOME

www.smarthome.com

Common remote control and large-button telephones provide a bigger target and are easier to use than standard telephones. Speakerphones and headsets permit hands-free use. If a client has tried lever handles on doorknobs and is still having difficulty opening and closing a door, a power door opener may be needed.

Available from:

✧ Power Access

1-800-344-0088

www.power-access.com

For late life adults who experience mobility limitations, remote control devices that permit a variety of tasks to be controlled from one location are exceedingly helpful. A universal remote control (using an infrared remote control system for items such as TVs, VCRs, and stereo systems) that reduces several control devices to just one is recommended. These items are available at larger electronic stores. X-10 remote controls are available for turning on and off any light or appliance in the home. These items can be purchase at electronics stores such as Home Automation or Radio Shack (www.radioshack.com). Cellular and cordless telephones, as well as headsets, are available at electronic stores and are very useful for the individual with mobility problems.[130]

If a client experiences difficulty getting to the door, a remote door lock control (that permits visitors to enter on their own) as well as a remote door opener can be utilized. Power Access offers a number of power controls and door openers. Intercoms that permit conversation between different areas of the home without the client having to move are useful to the person with mobility difficulties. Medical supply houses and rehabilitation companies offer a variety of items that encourage independent mobility (not necessarily electronic). These include canes, walkers, and wheelchairs (and power mobile aids as needed). For those persons who experience difficulty arising from a seated position, there are mechanical seat lifts that aid in this activity.[130]

Available from:

✧ Sammons Preston

1-800-323-5547

www.sammonspreston.com

For those older adults who experience cognitive limitations, a VCR and a TV control that utilizes switches with approximately 3-inch diameters (offered at ablenetinc.com) eliminate the need for the late life adult to remember channels, which buttons to push on a remote control, or the sequence necessary to start a movie. Simplified remote controls that offer a limited number of choices (only power, channel up and down, and volume up and down buttons) are also helpful for the memory impaired older adult. Telephones that use memory or speed dial systems eliminate the need to look up or remember a number. Photo phones, in which the user presses a picture of a loved one and that individual's number is automatically dialed, are yet another telephone option.

Available from:

✧ Independent Living Aids

1-800-537-2118

www.independentliving.com

Older individuals who experience sensory deficits and limitations can also be helped by a variety of devices and audiovisual equipment. Some of these include: (1) visually impaired—large phone buttons to increase visibility (some styles offer backlit buttons which can further define them), and (2) hearing limited—phone amplifiers for both the receiver and the ringer. Flashers are also available to alert the individual that the phone is ringing. These items are available at telephone stores and in specialty catalogs such as Independent Living Aids (please see previous paragraph for telephone number and web address). This supplier also offers a light that can be connected to the doorbell that flashes when someone rings it.[130]

Many late life adults live alone and have concerns about their ability to contact others in an emergency situation. Security factors are another consideration that also affect many older adults. There are many options for enhancing security. These include cameras (so the individual can see who is at the door before opening it), motion sensor outdoor lighting and burglar alarms. A wide variety of companies offer these systems. Medical alert companies permit the client to communicate with someone even if she or he is unable to get to a door or a phone.

Available from:

✧   Life Line

    1-800-642-0045

The client wears a pendant and by pushing a button can speak to a service representative. Some companies offer monitoring (e.g., a call is placed to the client at specific times to make certain that all is well).[130]

EADL options help to increase independence and prolong the amount of time that late life clients can live with a minimum of assistance.[130]

The American Occupational Therapy Association also offers materials that focus upon assistive products and technology. These are:

✧   *Applications of technology for persons with disabilities* (video). (1995). The Center for Assistive Technology, State University of New York at Buffalo. Available from the American Occupational Therapy Association, Bethesda, MD. 1-877-404-AOTA

✧   Krantz, G. C., Christenson, M. A., & Lindquist, A. (1998). *Assistive products: An illustrated guide to terminology*. Bethesda, MD: The American Occupational Therapy Association, Inc.

✧   Mann, W. C. & Lane, J. P. *Assistive technology for persons with disabilities: The role of occupational therapy* (2nd Ed.). Bethesda, MD: American Occupational Therapy Association, Inc.

Other helpful and informative assistive technology resources include:

✧   Abledata

    www.abledata.com

    Abledata lists more than 21,000 products involving assistive devices (e.g., wheelchairs, special computer keyboards, devices that support bathing and leisure activities).

✧   RERC Aging products

    Project Link 1-877-770-7303

    http://wings.buffalo.edu/go?rerca/

    Project Link is a direct e-mail service that offers consumers catalogs as well as product literature from companies that supply assistive devices. The RERC also offers case study videos concerning the use of assistive devices and Helpful Products Videos as well as booklets that focus upon the following assistive devices: reachers, wheelchairs, and assistive devices that can be used with passenger vehicles.

✧   State Assistive Technology

    1-800-949-4232

(Part of the Assistive Technology Act of 1998, Public Law 105-394) The mission is to provide (on a statewide basis) consumer-responsive programs of technology and related services for individuals with disabilities at any age. Every state and territory focuses upon a number of basic services. Some of the most prominent are as follows:

1. Referral and information
2. Assistance in being able to obtain devices and services
3. Device demonstration centers
4. Device exchange and recycling programs
5. Training on a variety of topics that can include self-advocacy and funding

Safety Management

Safety is a vital part of any home health evaluation. Safety evaluations, checklists, questionnaires, and safety management recommendations can be found in Chapter 12.

Medical and Health Management

Medical and health management are other aspects of occupational therapy home health. It is a cooperative area in which the nurse has a primary function. However, there is much that occupational therapy has to offer to both the client and the nurse. The occupational therapy evaluation should consider such areas as the client's ability to understand his or her medication usage and its side effects as well as the client's ability to make appropriate medically related judgments (e.g., when to call the physician if a problem arises). The occupational therapist can work with the client to educate him or her on techniques in using efficient telephone procedures as related to health needs (e.g., methods of using the telephone book to find appropriate numbers, establishing a method for keeping needed numbers close at hand, and the procedure for making a medical appointment; including keeping a calendar). Other areas of occupational therapy expertise can include techniques for: measuring liquid medication, the appropriate method for opening medication, and working closely with the nurse to ensure that a client has both the cognitive and perceptual abilities to make judgments concerning drawing insulin out of a bottle, measuring the insulin, and then injecting the insulin.[115] For those clients using a pill form of medication, the occupational therapist can also assess if the client has the ability to swallow and provide techniques (as needed) for safe usage.

Transportation/Community Mobility

Accessibility of community transportation should be considered when working with the home health client. Information needs to be gleaned as to whether the community has door-to-door cab and van services. Questions need to be answered such as:

1. Is the client able to order this type of service (many of these services require a week's notice)?
2. Is the client able to go out the front door and walk to the curb without assistance?
3. Can the client handle money to pay for the service?
4. If using a public bus, can the client read a bus schedule?

The topic of driving will be discussed later in this unit.

Money Management

If it is expected that the client will resume being responsible for financial matters and money management, then cognitive and perceptual evaluations need to be performed to accurately assess these skills. The client may need retraining in activities such as money management, shopping, planning a budget, or balancing a checkbook. If a physical limitation exists, instruction in the use of adaptive writing devices may need to be employed. If the caregiver will be taking over financial matters (and this role is new), the occupational therapist may become involved in training this individual.[115]

Respite

Often occupational therapists are involved in providing information (e.g., body mechanics, energy efficiency) to the caregiver so that he or she will not become exhausted. There is also a great need for periodic relief or respite from caregiving tasks, and therapists can provide information as to community resources (e.g., day care twice a week, respite care weekends in an assisted living facility) to the caregiver and encourage him or her to utilize them. Factors that are poorly tolerated by family caregivers in providing care for their ill elderly family members include sleep disturbances, fecal incontinence, the need for assistance with transfers and toileting, the lack of safety judgment, and the potential for falls. In order to prevent families from becoming quickly overwhelmed (by the amount and type of care that needs to be provided, and the amount of supervision and involvement needed), it is imperative to let the family or significant others understand the importance of relief so that feelings of anger and social isolation do not develop.[125]

Promoting Role Preservation and Life Space Preferences

Susan Bachner affirms that occupational therapists have the training to aid clients in maintaining and preserving a stable home environment and satisfying roles for as long as possible. In home health these are essential attributes that can enhance a client's home setting.

"When entering the life space of a client for professional purposes, understanding the meaning of the setting to the client and the client's significant others is imperative."[131, p. 20]

For any of us, objects that are collected through a lifetime become "treasures." Ego-supportive objects in a client's life space play an important role in helping an elderly client to carry out daily living tasks that may have become a source of pain and frustration due to pain, discomfort, and loss of ability.[131]

In terms of dramaturgical theory, objects have the capacity to become props as they are able to convey information about the individual. This person is viewed as a communicator and props are used as aids in communications.[131]

An example of the use of a prop in promoting a client's improved ability to perform a functional activity can be seen by the following example. Mr. X was a retired interior decorator. For this individual the concept of the necessity of a bedside commode was frightening, as this could be interpreted to mean that his home would become a mini-institution. Offering this client the possibility of acquiring a custom-made reproduction of a Victorian era bedside commode (concealed in what appeared to be a chest of drawers) that was designed for his transfer capabilities and size, allowed him to receive guests in his bedroom without trespassing on his sense of modesty. Thus, the Victorian commode became an example of an ego-supportive prop that permitted Mr.

X to be able to utilize this piece of equipment.[131] Occupational therapists can become more effective in providing intervention when we understand our client's subjective feelings. In this way we are able to learn about their relationships with their life spaces.[131]

An example of role preservation in improving a client's lifestyle outcome and function can be seen by the following example. Mr. Y (a former corporate manager) was recovering from a stroke. Inpatient rehabilitation had focused on restoring his self-care independence. However, sociological issues concerning symbolic value objects, role, and position had not been included. This individual did not feel as pleased with his progress as did professionals working in intervention. First, Mr. Y missed his male camaraderie (the Rotary Club, men's discussion group, golf, and the elimination of leadership positions due to his inability to use former objects to convey being in control). This had led to his self-imposed isolation. Mr. Y provided multiple narratives about his past involvement in a variety of occupations. From the process of analysis (using methods of "the participant-observer"), the occupational therapist realized that this client's role areas had become needlessly limited. Mr. Y's major loss of independence stemmed from his no longer being able to drive due to a right hemianopsia. The automobile, a "prop" that had taken on a role of its own, became a symbol of his self-sufficiency.[131]

During the period when the therapist guided the client through feedback, activities, and exercise, Mr. Y was able to release his grip on the idea that the car alone provided his independence. This helped him to explore other acceptable props and alternatives. In order to restore Mr. Y's "man-in-charge" role, his computer and desk were moved from the lower level of his home to the first floor where he would have greater visibility and easier access. Another important intervention was to help Mr. Y maintain his identity by utilizing male drivers (former friends who were able and willing to take him to his men's activities). Thus, his wife no longer needed to be his chauffeur (which in his mind was a direct advertisement of his weakness), and he could re-establish links with his old friends. This arrangement provided him with his role preservation and a better sense of self.[131]

Resources

The following represent several resources useful in the home health setting:

✧ Emlet, C. A., Crabtree, J. L., Condon, V. A., & Trend, L. A. *In-Home assessment of older adults: An interdisciplinary approach*. Bethesda, MD: Aspen.

  This resource is an interdisciplinary approach to home health assessment (some of the areas of assessment include safety and accessibility, activities of daily living, nutritional needs, social function, and support and disturbances of mood, thought, and memory.

✧ Imaginart

  1-800-828-1376

  Fax: 1-800-737-1376

  Imaginart@compuserve.com

✧ LaFeldt, L. (2001). *The occupational therapist's cognitive ADL workbook*, (2nd Ed.). ADA, MI: Bramley.

  616-682-5555

  This is an instructional book, useful in home health as well as other settings, that deals with the practical applications of everyday living for the cognitively impaired. Intervention involves subjects such as: gathering information, under-standing maps and pavement markings, home management, functional math, and money management (including developing personal banking skills).

✧ Piersol, C. V. & Ehrlich, P. L. (Eds.). *Home health practice: A guide for occupa-tional therapists*. This book includes subjects such as the history of home health, getting started, goal oriented documentation, the practicalities of providing service in the home and discharge planning. It is also available from Imaginart (see previous listing for telephone, fax and internet information).

✧ *Guidelines for Occupational Therapy Practice in Home Health*. This resource presents guidelines useful in occupational therapy home health practice.
   AOTA
   1-877-404-AOTA
   www.aota.org

✧ *Occupational therapy in home health* (a continuing education program). This resource provides a variety of modules such as: the historical aspects and growth of home health care, establishing a frame of reference for home health care practice, referral, assessment, intervention, case studies, reimbursement, managed care, documentation, and personal safety. Available from AOTA.

HOME MODIFICATION

In Unit 1 occupational therapy's participation (regarding wellness in the communi-ty) with planned environments to promote improved functional performance was dis-cussed. The approach in this component is to describe home environmental modifica-tions in which an occupational therapist works with a home modification team (as part of the local area agency on aging). Unlike home health (where there is some focus on home adaptations as well as a variety of other concerns), this type of program focuses solely on adaptive home modification. In essence, it is a specialty area that centers upon clients who have permanent physical disabilities and making these persons' homes more accessible so that they remain in their present community setting.

Evaluation

One such program is the Adaptive Home Modification Program of the Philadelphia Corporation for Aging (an area agency on aging). This agency has a varied model hous-ing program that serves more than 1500 consumers a year. Lois J. Rasage is an occu-pational therapy consultant involved in the Adaptive Home Modification Program. Services are initiated with intake by a social worker to determine a prospective client's eligibility. Once it is determined that the client is eligible, an occupational therapy evaluation, in conjunction with the construction manager (the person who will be responsible for the work and completion of all needed and recommended physical changes to the home), is conducted. The Occupational Therapy Evaluation of the Philadelphia Corporation for Aging Housing Department involves the following areas:[132]

✧ Demographic information (e.g., client's name, address, case manager, phone, anticipated problems serving the household, client's subjective housing needs)

✧ Housebound composition and medical information
✧ Functional deficits resulting from medical problems
✧ Physical activity
✧ Physical transfers
✧ Physical mobility
✧ Activities of daily living and and instrumental activities of daily living status of the client
✧ Home assessment (e.g., front entrance; number of stories; condition of dwelling; whether the doorbell is functioning; whether the bedrooms, kitchen and bathrooms are accessible and safe; the number of steps [inside and outside]; whether the basement is safe; and whether the washer and dryer are accessible and in safe working order)
✧ The kind of equipment that is currently being used by the client
✧ Whether this is an initial request
✧ Problems and comments

With the occupational therapist and the construction manager working side by side, the pragmatic aspects (such as where the studs are and the physical feasibility of construction or modification recommendation in this house setting) of occupational therapy recommendations can be addressed "on the spot." Once the evaluation is completed, the home modification plan is submitted to the agency for approval. When approval is given, construction can begin. After construction is completed, there is a follow-up to assess the effectiveness of the work and ensure quality of service (assess if the adaptations are completed correctly and are useful to the consumer).[132]

Construction and Installation of Modifications

Some of the adaptations under this program have included the construction of ramps (usual ramp pitch is 1 foot for every 10 or 12 feet of length—1:12), and the installation of stairglides (30 inches wide is needed on a set of stairs), the installation of telecabs (elevators) that go up one story (also has a phone in it with room for a wheelchair and an attendant). At times there is a need to have a ceiling tract on the second floor so that a client can be transported to a bedroom area. Outdoor lifts are used when a ramp is not possible for access from the outside to the inside of the home. Frequently city housing is attached (known as row housing if the attachment covers a large area), and there is little space for ramps. Installation of hand-held shower sprays, slide bars, and bath chairs is needed. Construction of stall showers, installation of grab bars, offset hinges, bidets, and side faucets in the bathroom or kitchen where the client has limited room may help. Also helpful are the installation of continuous countertops and the construction of pullout shelves and cutting boards (which can act as a work station in the kitchen).[132]

Resources

Recommended resources in the home modification area include:
✧ Center for Universal Design
School of Design
North Carolina State University
P.O. Box 8613

Raleigh, NC 27695-8613

1-800-647-6777, 919-515-3082

cud@ncsu.edu

✧ Philadelphia Consumers

Philadelphia Corporation for the Aging

Adaptive Modification Program

642 N. Broad St.

Philadelphia, PA 19130-3409

215-895-5692 (HCDI), 215-895-5609 (TDD)

✧ Growing Older in Your Home: Modification for Your Changing Needs—Kitchen Modifications, Bedroom Modifications, Bathroom Modifications (useful with consumers)

Available from:

AOTA

1-877-404-AOTA

www.aota.org

✧ University Design at Buffalo

School of Architecture and Planning

SUNY/Buffalo

www.ap.buffalo.edu/rercud

✧ University of Southern California

Online Certification Program in Home Modifications

In conjunction with the University of Southern California's Ethel Percy Andrus Gerontology Center and the National Resource Center on Supportive Housing and Home Modification.

Maria Henke

213-740-1364

mhenke@usc.edu

www.homemod.org

Home modification is a growing area of practice for occupational therapists that is rewarding both to the consumer and the therapist. Providing opportunities, through home adaptations and modifications, so that elderly persons are able to remain in their community has important ramifications for us all. First, in terms of taxes, it is a wise investment that allows older adults to remain in their homes as long as possible. Thus, costly institutional care can be avoided. Second, psychologically and socially it enables late life adults to continue with their current roles and occupations. Third, it promotes a "well" mode rather than a "sick" mode. Fourth, it provides an improved quality of life to elderly persons (e.g., ensures greater accessibility to function as independently as possible with daily routines and activities). Finally, it promotes a marvelous venue for occupational therapists to execute their expert knowledge and skills in occupations, disabilities, abilities, medical knowledge, and adaptive environments.

Summary

Occupational therapy service in the home health setting is a very rewarding area of practice. One is always challenged by a variety of conditions and diagnoses (including all aspects of physical disabilities, mental health diagnoses, and developmentally delayed late life adults), family dynamics, multicultural and varied social environments, and the home setting as the clinic. The occupational therapist is an integral part of the home health team who works with a multiprofessional staff. The practitioner must be ready to problem solve and act as a resource the moment he or she enters the client's home. Flexibility, awareness of the current occupational therapy knowledge base, responsibility, the ability to interact and communicate with others, creativity, good organizational skills, the ability to keep meaningful records, and the willingness to face challenges are all part of the occupational therapy picture in home health. It is an exciting and meaningful area of practice.

DRIVING AND THE OLDER ADULT

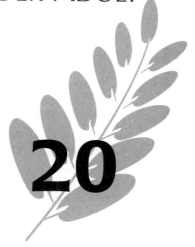

20

DEMOGRAPHICS

Mobility in the community is an essential aspect of everyday living. Most individuals consider driving an automobile to be necessary in modern day society. Indeed, it is a specialized part of activities of daily living.

As the elderly population increases, so too does the number of late life drivers. In 1997, in the United States, there were 17.7 million older licensed drivers. This represents a 45% increase from the number in 1987.[133] Many late life drivers will self-restrict their driving habits (e.g., limiting the number of miles they drive, avoiding driving at night, driving slowly, avoiding driving in inclement weather, and avoiding highways that have limited access). Despite these attempts to avoid highway risk driving conditions, late life drivers' crash rates slowly begin rising at age 60. In 1997, accidental deaths from automobile crashes for those persons aged 65 to 85 were the leading cause of all accidental deaths.

Older adults have a disproportionate rate of crashes involving the following problems: (1) failure to yield, (2) making improper left turns, and (3) failure to heed traffic signs.[134,135] Although age by itself is not an indicator of one's driving ability, there are a number of factors associated with aging that can compromise safe driving. "Occupational therapy can make a unique contribution and provide indispensable information to assist in identifying older drivers who are at risk and, if appropriate, assist in remediating skills."[135, p. E-1]

Driving is one of the most complex daily living activities that individuals of any age can pursue. It is performed with virtually little thought of the skills that are involved in moving and handling a vehicle in a continually changing traffic environment. Driving, an overlearned task, involves skills and areas that can be significantly affected by aging itself. There are a number of skills used in driving performance such as sensorimotor (visual processing, visual perception, vision, and physical) capacities and psychosocial and cognitive abilities. Driving involves the process of making decisions that are dependent upon judgments and perceptions. Age-related impairments that can prevent an individual from operating an automobile safely include the following conditions:

1. Age-associated diseases (e.g., arthritis, CVA, dementia, chronic obstructive pulmonary disease, diabetes type 2, Parkinson's disease, retinal disorders such as macular degeneration, diabetic retinopathy, glaucoma, and cataracts).

2. Physiological changes occurring in late life (hearing loss, slowing of physical functioning that can affect reaction time, loss of range of motion and strength which can prevent the individual from operating the automobile safety).

3. A decline in cognitive functioning that can result in slowed concentration and poor judgment. This may result in poor insight into problem areas which can be very dangerous as the driver may be unaware that he or she is making mistakes.

4. Polypharmacy (many late life adults take multiple medications. Some of these medications can be a causative factor in inhibiting an individual's physical or mental ability to drive carefully).[135,136]

The Clinical Assessment/Evaluation

Many occupational therapists interested in driver education for those with disabilities have elected to further their education in this area by becoming certified driving rehabilitation specialists (CDRS). For those settings looking for individuals with CDRS, the following organization will provide a list:

❖ Association of Driver Education for the Disabled ADED

    109 West St.

    Edgertown, WI 53534

    608-884-8833

The following organization will provide driver education courses for therapists:[137]

❖ Adaptive Mobility Services, Inc.

    Susan Pierce, OTR, CDRS

    407-855-8050, fax 407-855-9953

Because driving is an activity of daily living, the occupational therapist is the most logical member of the team to ensure that this issue is addressed (whether the therapist works for a home health agency, a temporary residential care facility, a continued care life community, or a rehabilitation center).

Evaluation of Physical Functioning

When addressing physical functioning, the following areas need to be evaluated:

❖ *Range of motion*—Reduction in range of motion can compromise the ability to operate the gas and brake pedals, fasten a seat belt, operate secondary controls, (gear selector, directional lights, headlights, and parking brake), and safely control the steering wheel (primary control). If there is a loss of motion in the neck, the individual's ability to turn the head (to check for traffic at intersections, when changing lanes, when backing up, and when merging in lanes) can become impaired.

❖ *Muscle strength*—Limited lower and upper extremity strength as well as hand strength can impair steering skills (especially that of parking and turning around). If lower extremity strength becomes limited, the ability to apply and maintain pressure on the brake pedals and the accelerator may become diminished. Power steering and power brakes can be useful for those individuals with limited strength.[135-137] Head and trunk balance are other important factors involving strength and as such these capabilities also need to be assessed.[115]

❖ *Endurance*—This is an area that affects how long and when a person is able to drive. There are some medical conditions that affect endurance at specific times of the day. This may result in the need to schedule driving when one's endurance levels are the highest.

❖ *Coordination*—Decreases in coordination can affect how efficiently and quickly the feet and hands can be synchronized for a variety of tasks (e.g., pressing the accelerator, braking the pedals, or steering).

❖ *Reaction time*—This is defined as the speed at which a driver can move his or her feet from the gas pedal to the brake pedal. For most elderly persons, reaction time increases with age. When this happens it means that the distance that is required to stop a vehicle also increases. This reaction time distance also increases as the speed increases. To ensure safety older drivers need to maintain a greater following distance.[135-137]

❖ *Sensation*—A decline in sensation (particularly lower extremity kinesthesia and proprioception) can significantly decrease one's ability to locate and maintain control of the brake and accelerator pedals. Hand controls offer an option to late life adults who are no longer able to safely operate the brake and accelerator pedals with lower limbs.[135-137]

❖ *Hand dexterity*—Limited hand dexterity compromises many needed aspects of driving such as the ability to grasp and manipulate the steering wheel, manage secondary control (e.g., lights, heater, defroster windshield wipers), and operate the ignition.[135-137]

❖ *Positioning and transfer ability*—Many late life adults experience difficulty getting into and out of small vehicles that have low seat heights or higher vehicles that require a step up. Once the older adult is inside the vehicle it is important to ensure an appropriate sitting height so that there is a good line of view. In many instances the older person sits too low in the seat, which can impair the driver's ability to see out of the middle of the windshield and above the steering wheel.[135-137]

❖ *Mobility aids*—Limitations in physical functioning can often be improved through the use of factory selected vehicle adaptive equipment and vehicle options (e.g., power brakes and steering mechanism, additional mirrors, automatic transmissions, built up levers and switches, turning knobs, hand controls, or a left foot accelerator). Appropriate training in the use of these driving devices and aids is critical to ensure and promote safety. Another factor, when discussing mobility aids, is developing ways in which older adults can bring their mobility equipment (such as canes, walkers, wheelchairs, and scooters) with them into their vehicles as they travel into the community. Canes and walkers can usually be stored in a standard automobile. For the larger items, such as a scooter or a wheelchair, a loading device is significantly helpful.[135-137]

Perceptual and Visual Functioning

The next area for assessment is an evaluation of perceptual and visual functioning. This includes the following components:

✧ *Visual acuity*—Dynamic visual acuity involves the ability to see moving objects. Limitations in dynamic acuity can cause delays or misinterpretations in recognizing signs; responding to the environment, or estimating speeds. Generally, most states accept vision that is 20/40 to 2/50 as a cutoff before prescription lenses are required.[115,135]

✧ *Contrast sensitivity*—This is the ability to perceive and detect objects in relationship to the background of their environment. Poor contrast vision can result in difficulties identifying dangers in specific environments (e.g., objects at dawn or dusk, dark vehicles approaching from a shaded street, pedestrians on a dark or cloudy day).[115,135]

✧ *Night vision*—Many late life adults experience difficulty with night vision. Older adults' pupils decrease in size as they age. Consequently, greater illumination is needed in order to see. This results in increased difficulty in being able to see on roads or streets that are not well lit (such as are found in some residential and rural areas).[115,135]

✧ *Glare recovery*—Sensitivity to glare increases as one ages. This causes increased time for glare recovery from ongoing headlights. Avoiding night driving is a common strategy used by older adults in combatting this problem.[135] Amber tinted lenses can also be used to lessen this problem.

✧ *Peripheral vision*—In driving, the purpose of adequate peripheral awareness is to draw one's attention to peripheral objects (although not in focus, movement and light can alert the driver that "something" is present). The two major components of peripheral awareness are that an adequate visual field is present as well as a measure of alertness. With all drivers, when there is an increase in speed, there is a reduction in peripheral vision. For late life adults with a peripheral field loss, the ability to compensate by turning the head and a reduction in speed is essential. The Useful Field of View Test (measures how drivers process visual information) has demonstrated some predictive value in being able to identify at-risk drivers.[135]

This can be found in the following resource:

✧ Owsley, C., Ball, K., McGuin, G., Sloan, M., Roenker, D., White, M., et al. (1998). Visual processing impairment and risk of motor vehicle crash among older adults. *JAMA, 279*, 1083-1088.

The Useful Field of View (UFOV), another resource offering, is a computer-administrative and computer scored test of visual attention for adults. This test determines (in approximately 15 minutes) the visual field area over which a driver can process rapidly presented visual information.

✧ Ball, K., & Roenker, D. *Useful Field of View* (UFOV) Software

Therapy Skill Builders

1-800-211-8378

www.tpcweb.com

✧ *Depth perception*—Depth perception is the ability to judge distances. This ability decreases with age. It is used in judging stopped distance, following distance, merging, parking, gap acceptance when pulling into traffic, and the timing of turns. Depth perception is more difficult to judge when one is moving than when stationary. Depth perception encompasses the ability to estimate the speed of other vehicles and the amount of time that is necessary to safely interact with them. All of these factors become compromised where there is a decrease in depth perception.

✧ *Visual perception*—Visual perception involves constancy of shape, position in space, visual memory, figure ground, spatial relations, unilateral neglect, visual search and scanning, directionality, visual organization, and topographical orientation.[115,135] Driving places a high demand on visual-perceptual functioning because there is a large amount of visual information that needs to be processed in a limited amount of time. The Motor Free Visual Perceptual Test (MVPT) is often used by driver rehabilitation specialists to assess visual perception.[115,135]

✧ *Color vision*—Color vision involves the ability to determine the color of an object or an item. It is important in driving to determine the meaning of various signs and traffic signals. The aging process can lead to diminished color recognition. For instance, the color red does not usually appear as bright to an older person's eyes. This may result in an older driver taking twice as long as a younger driver to detect and react to the brake and tail lights.[135]

Cognitive Functioning Awareness

Even with moderate cognitive dysfunction the physical act of driving may remain intact. That is because driving is based upon *procedural memory* (which is associated with everyday tasks that have become automatic). However, cognitive changes that occur in late life may definitely affect safe driving procedures (e.g., problems with obeying traffic signals, signs, and the ability to interact in a safe manner with traffic). Cognitive problems associated with aging that directly affect driving include diminished selective and divided attention. Reaction in selective attention can compromise one's ability to attend to relevant information while driving in complex traffic situations such as heavy traffic. Driving with a reduction in divided attention can affect the way that one responds simultaneously to multiple tasks such as maintaining an appropriate road position while attending to signs, traffic, and signals, and navigating in an unfamiliar area or turning the head to check blind spots. Reduced scanning and searching abilities (directly affecting selective attention); increased difficulty ignoring irrelevant stimuli; reduced quick processing (slower retrieval and processing of information) which directly affects the quick decision making that is needed for safe driving; reduced safety judgment; diminished abilities to plan ahead and an inability to understand one's disability or diminished driving status directly affects driving safety.[115,135]

It is important for therapists working in driver rehabilitation programs to become fully aware of their clients' cognitive deficits. If these should impede safe driving practices, then no further assessments or driver training is warranted.

Stationary Assessment

This component evaluates the equipment set up and the predriving tasks in the static position. The vehicle for evaluation must be chosen first because of the many variations in the driver station (e.g., gas/brake pedal angle, size and resistance, steering resistance, seating, and general layout). A checklist of the stationary assessment is helpful to ensure that all basic elements of the driving task are routinely included.

Predriving tasks include mobility to the vehicle (inserting and turning the door key or use of keyless entry; opening and closing the door; loading and unloading mobility devices such as a cane, wheelchair, or walker; entering and exiting the vehicle; adjusting the driver's seat and the mirrors; fastening the seat belt or chest strap when needed). There are numerous devices that are available to facilitate independence in predriving tasks such as loops for lower extremity management, special key holders, a wheelchair strap to extend the reach for wheelchair loading, and any modifications for independent seatbelt retrieval. Mechanical devices are also available that can enable some clients to independently manage mobility equipment and continue to use their own vehicle without expensive modifications.[115]

The first step in assessment of primary control is to achieve optimal positioning of the driver. This is important for optimal upper extremity safety and function. Securement devices (e.g., chest straps, seat belts) should be in place before initiating a primary control assessment (as these devices alter substitution pattern or inhibit the reach of the client). The primary controls are those devices that are involved in controlling the steering, acceleration, and braking in a vehicle. The assessment of the primary controls follows the following order: assess the steering controls first and then the gas and brake controls. The secondary controls such as the horn, the headlights, the windshield wiper, the dimmer switch, and the turn signals are assessed after the primary control assessment is concluded.[115]

Steering options are varied. The main goal in steering is to promote smooth, controlled steering. A driver may use two-handed steering techniques (e.g., shuffling, hand-over-hand, or feeding the wheel) to fulfill this goal or one-handed steering with a steering device (e.g., spinner knob, tripin, V-grip, palmar cuff, or amputee ring) which allows constant control of the steering wheel as well as fosters the ability to make turns efficiently, quickly, and effectively. Other modifications can include smaller diameter steering wheels as well as reduced levels of steering resistance. Both of these modifications need meticulous evaluations for safety.[115,135]

The next modifications include the accelerator and brake controls. To compensate for limited reach, a pedal extension can be installed on both of these controls. For individuals with significant right hemiplegia, a left-sided accelerator pedal can be placed to the left of the standard gas pedal. The left foot can also operate the gas and the brakes safely. Hand controls can be used if the individual lacks adequate lower motor control. A device termed a "hand control" permits the operation of the accelerator and the brake pedal with an upper extremity. Hand controls can use push/pull, push/pull down, side-to-side, or rotary motions to apply the appropriate pressure to the accelerator and the brake. However, the occupational therapist must be aware if a specific hand motion might be detrimental to an individual's medical condition. For instance, if an older adult has severe arthritis in the hand, the rotary style hand control could cause an exacerbation of the symptoms. High-tech gas and brake controls that are operated by vacuum, computer, or pneumatics permit the older disabled driver to drive a vehicle with less range of motion than ever before.

VEHICLE SELECTION

A car is considered appropriate if the older adult can independently enter and exit the vehicle and load mobility equipment devices independently. There are a number of transfer methods that can be employed. These include the stand pivot, the sliding board, the bent pivot, and upper extremity depression. An individual using the upper extremity depression method or the sliding board needs to be able to transfer up inclines (transferring from a car to a wheelchair is usually in an upward direction). If manual loading is not feasible, a mechanical device can be used to perform this task. In general, compact and subcompact automobiles are usually too small to accommodate most mechanical-loading aids.[115]

The standard car that is recommended is a two-door vehicle with power brakes, power steering, automatic transmission, and bench seats for easy transfer. These types of seats are becoming harder to find. If possible, one should avoid gear shift levers that are positioned in a central console between the driver and the passenger. This interferes with transfers and the dexterity that is needed to depress the gear shift release button (needed to shift gears). Individuals with hand impairments will most likely perform better with a gear shift lever that is mounted on the steering column.

VAN SELECTION

Drivers of vans must choose between full-size or minivans. Those individuals who choose to drive from their wheelchairs require more complex evaluations and greater skills because of a variety of increased variables that affect equipment selection and driving performance.[115]

Entry into a van requires a mechanical lift for those who use a scooter or a wheelchair. There are basically two types of categories—rotary (also known as "swing-in-style") lifts and platform lifts. Minivans can also have fully automatic mechanical ramps that promote independent entry and exit. The practitioner and the client need to find a compatible and safe match between parking needs, lift choice, and lifestyle.[115]

OTHER SCREENING TOOLS

Pierce recommends two resources that can be used as predriving screening tools.

The Elemental Driving Assessment Simulator evaluates cognitive abilities that are critical for driving (mental processing efficiency, impulse control, simultaneous information processing, and perceptual motor skills). It makes use of a steering wheel, turn signal, and gas pedal. A 386 or better computer with 16 megabytes of RAM, VGA graphics, and 2 megabytes of hard drive space are required. This tool is available from:

✧ The Elemental Driving System

Life Science Associates

Bayport, NY 11704

516-472-2111

The Doron Driving Simulator, a more costly machine, uses real driving scenes and has face validity components as well. This tool is available from:

✧ Doron Precision Systems

P.O. Box 400

Binghamton, NY

607-772-1610[136,137]

BEHIND-THE-WHEEL ASSESSMENT

This aspect of the driving assessment is often termed the behind-the-wheel or on-the-road component. "Although clinical assessments are of great value in identifying potential problem areas, a functional assessment of actual driving skills is necessary to more fully determine skills and safety."[135, p. CE-5]

The first aspect of the functional assessment is to obtain information concerning the older driver's driving history, habits, and records. Much of this information can be discussed and utilized. Most older drivers (especially men who may have been driving some 70 years) learned to drive without formalized instruction. Many of their driving behaviors may be the result of lack of knowledge rather than declining skills. This lack of knowledge may be demonstrated when the individual improperly uses shared left-turn lanes, stops on the entrance ramp to a highway, brakes for green lights, or does not check for blind spots. Driving records can also be helpful in identifying problem areas. For instance, an individual who is frequently involved in rear-end collisions may be stopping unexpectedly. Another person who is frequently involved in "fender bender" accidents in parking lots may have difficulty with visual observations that occur to the rear or the sides of the car.[135]

Before the actual road test, it is important that the most appropriate equipment setups are used. Sometimes several setups are needed to ensure the right combination of aids for safe driving.[115]

The road test is considered to be the optimal measure of driving competence. Lillie recommends that the moving vehicle portions of a driver evaluation include the driver educator/instructor who sits in the front passenger seat (can be an occupational therapist with specialized training or a state licensed instructor) and the driving evaluator (most often an occupational therapist) who sits in the back. The instructor informs the client where to drive, maintains vehicle control by intervening as needed, instructs in the use of adaptive equipment and, in general, maintains the safety of the vehicle occupants by adhering to the laws and rules of the road. It is the evaluator's job to observe the task of driving. In doing so he or she takes written notes and, in many instances, completes a scoring sheet.[115]

The behind-the-wheel assessment should progress from basic maneuvers to those of increased complexity. The initial phase is the operation of vehicle controls. This part can be assessed on a parking lot or driving range. Observations need to be conducted on positioning (e.g., adjusting the seat height, airbag, and distance from the pedals; managing the seat belt; adjusting the mirror; operating the ignition; using the appropriate gear selector; operating the windshield wipers, lights, and turn signals). There are a number of common errors found with older drivers in this phase of the evaluation. Some of these include sitting too low in the seat, inappropriate use of the seat belt (for instance, placing the shoulder harness under the arm), not applying the brake before shifting the vehicle's gear, and confusing the pedals or depressing both pedals at the same time. After this part of the assessment is conducted the actual driving experience can be initiated.[135]

The driving route should include a sampling of road conditions and traffic patterns. In residential areas observations of vehicle control skills at slow speeds, use of directions, proper road position before turning, appropriate speed adjustments when making turns, or coming to a complete stop are essential. During light and heavy situations the following skills can be observed: adequate following and stopping distance, proper speed adjustment, yielding the right of way, attentiveness to signals and signs, safe lane changes, safe gap utilization, and general attentiveness to potential hazards and other traffic. In highway driving the evaluator can assess merging speed control and proper use of acceleration and deceleration lanes.[135]

The final aspects of the functional (road test) evaluation is parking. Most older drivers do not parallel park. However, perpendicular parking is a necessity. The parking lot requires a very high level of attention to pedestrians and other vehicles. It involves being able to observe behind the vehicle as well as safely maneuvering between two vehicles.[135]

In 1997, the New York State Office for Aging conducted a survey among families who were concerned about unsafe older drivers. This survey indicated that many of these concerns included a variety of driving problems that late life drivers manifest, such as driving too slowly, not paying attention to road hazards or to other drivers, slow reaction time, delayed acceleration and braking, not reacting to emerging situations, not staying in lane, not yielding the right of way, stopping inappropriately, following too closely, not obeying traffic signals, not signaling, being overly cautious, exhibiting confusion and getting lost, making short or excessively wide turns, and misjudging.[138]

In general, the driving route should be graded and allow the client ample time to become familiar with any adaptive equipment that he or she will be using. Driving performance scores should focus upon the client's ability to use the adaptive equipment, adherence to the rules and laws concerned with driving, and sound physical management of the vehicle.[115,135]

RECOMMENDATIONS TO THE CLIENT

Following the functional assessment, the driving team reviews the results with the driver. By asking the client for feedback first, the evaluator may be provided with a valuable perspective on the client's insight. The results of the team's and/or the evaluator's recommendations for driving are discussed with the client. It is at this point that the driver's demonstration of safe driving was in evidence or if additional training might be needed. Training is indicated if the deficits were caused by bad habits, or if compensatory strategies or specific adaptive equipment could be used. For training to be successful, drivers must be able to be insightful into their problem areas and be receptive to being able to change their driving habits and behaviors. These changes may include limitations such as no night driving, limited use of access roadways or highways with speeds that are in excess of a specified speed limit, and no driving permitted in unfamiliar areas. If the problems were due to conditions that cannot be changed (such as slow processing, poor judgment, or impaired visual-perceptual functioning), then training would not be indicated.

When one is discussing the results with a client who does not demonstrate good driving skills, it is important to be aware if the client is attempting to resume driving too soon after a change in medical status (such as a CVA or an exacerbation of a chronic condition). If this is the case, then additional intervention might be recommended before reevaluating the client's driving abilities.[135]

Safe Driving Prevention Programs

The Elder Mobility Project in Boca Raton, FL, is an example of a prevention program in which occupational therapists play a pivotal role. The program includes three major areas of focus:

1. There is an education campaign to raise awareness among community agencies, members, and health care providers about elder mobility issues.

2. The program is involved in a voluntary community-based driver assessment for well elders. This assessment includes cognition, vision, motor performance, reaction time, and driver vehicle fit. After the evaluation, the driver receives feedback on his or her driving skills, and strategies are offered to encourage safer driving.

3. The last part of the project is to provide counseling for those who can no longer drive and to help them connect with alternative resources for transportation needs.[139]

The Elder Mobility Project conducted its first assessment on November 27, 2000. By April 25, 2001, it had served 254 clients.[139]

Surrendering the License

One of the most sensitive and difficult discussions for a driver rehabilitation evaluator is to inform the client and his or her family that their family member is no longer a safe driver, and that a complete cessation of driving is recommended. However, before this step actually occurs, Pierce recommends these following steps:

✧ The individual closest to the driver should have a frank discussion as to why it is not safe for him or her to continue driving.

✧ The older person should be encouraged to have his or her driving skills evaluated.

✧ Counseling should be available to make the transition easier.

✧ Alternative transportation should be arranged and provided. Family members, volunteers, and friends can drive the older adult to appointments, social functions, and errands. Information regarding available senior transportation services should be presented, and local bus, train, and trolley routes should be made accessible.[136,137]

The driving laws within each state are varied. Most driving programs will report the information to the referring physician so that he or she can determine the best course of action.[135]

Resources

An excellent resource concerning driving for older adults is available from the American Occupational Therapy Association:

✧ *Able Driving is Safe Driving*

   1-877-404-AOTA

This brochure delineates the ways in which occupational therapists can assist older drivers in coping with their changing abilities that may affect their driving skills.

Programs designed to retrain older drivers are also discussed. The brochure is displayed in enlarged type and bright color, which makes for easier reading.

The American Association for Retired Persons (AARP) offers a self-rating questionnaire booklet entitled "Older Driver Skill Assessment and Resource Guide," which also includes remedial advice (e.g., use a route plan that avoids left turns at busy intersections), as well as enabling mature drivers to recognize their limitations and unsafe practices. Available from:

✧   AARP

601 E St., N.W.

Washington, DC 20049

Since 1979, AARP has sponsored driver refresher courses (55 Alive/Mature Driving) that are available in most states.

With our "unique skills and background, as well as the increased attention being paid to the issue of impaired drivers by the medical community and the demand for more specialized programs, there is increased opportunity for occupational therapists to pursue this exciting and needed area of specialization."[135, p. CE-6]

Summary

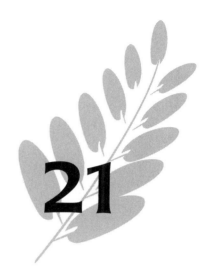

21

We have seen how far our profession has developed—from the early days of occupational therapy at the close of World War I—into a multifaceted profession interested in promoting enhanced performance in all areas of life skills as well as improving environmental concerns that affect function.

In our rehabilitation and wellness procedures we "see" the whole person (not an arm, not an eye, not a hand) who has physical, psychosocial, economic, cognitive, cultural, and role needs. During the curative process, we address each one of these concerns in collaboration with the client, the family, significant others, and the therapeutic team.

Working with late life adults has many rewards and challenges. This age group represents a growing segment of our population who will have much need for our expertise in order to live productive lives within the community as long as possible. Because our knowledge base and training is diverse, we have become especially aware of the many facets involved in providing care to both the ill and well elderly. We are problem solvers with a health science background who use our specific training to achieve pragmatic short- and long-term goals. In most instances the basic aim is to provide service that will enhance each client's functioning capacity to its fullest potential (while at the same time being sensitive and aware of spiritual, social, cultural, ethnic, and economic considerations).

The need for our services is great. The challenge lies ahead of us. The 21st century beckons us to play a major role in the provision of meaningful intervention options to late life adults.

UNIT 3 REFERENCES

1. Tigges, K. N., & Marcil, W. M. (1996). Palliative medicine and rehabilitation: Assessment and treatment in hospice care. In K. O. Larson, R. G. Stevens-Ratchford, L. Pedretti, & J. L. Crabtree (Eds.), *The role of occupational therapy with the elderly* (2nd Ed., pp. 743-763). Bethesda, MD: The American Occupational Therapy Association, Inc.

2. Freda, M. (1998). Facility-based practice settings. In M. E. Neistadt, & E. G. Crepeau (Eds.), *Willard and Spackman's occupational therapy* (9th Ed., pp. 803-814). Philadelphia: Lippincott-Raven.

3. Granger, C. V., Ottenbacher, K. J., & Fiedler, R. C. (1995). The uniform data system for medical rehabilitation. *American Journal of Physical Medicine and Rehabilitation, 74,* 62-66.

4. Aitken, M. J., & Lohman, H. (1996). Health care systems: Changing positions. In K. O. Larson, R. G. Stevens-Ratchford, L. Pedretti, & J. L. Crabtree (Eds.), *The role of occupational therapy with the elderly* (2nd Ed., pp. 56-91). Bethesda, MD: The American Occupational Therapy Association, Inc.

5. JCAHO. (1995). *1995 survey protocol for subacute programs.* Oakbrook Terrace, IL: Author.

6. Hasselkus, B. R., & Brown, M. (1983). Respite care for the community elderly. *Am J of Occup Ther, 2*(37), 83-88.

7. Stevens-Ratchford, R. G. (1996). Occupational therapy sources within the rehabilitation health care system. In K. O. Larson, R. G. Stevens-Ratchford, L. Pedretti, & J. L. Crabtree (Eds.), *The role of occupational therapy with the elderly* (2nd Ed., pp. 307-320). Bethesda, MD: The American Occupational Therapy Association, Inc.

8. Neistadt, M. E., & Crepeau, E. B. (1998). Introduction to occupational therapy. In M. E. Neistadt, & E. B. Crepeau (Eds.), *Willard and Spackman's occupational therapy* (9th Ed., pp. 10-11). Philadelphia: Lippincott-Raven.

9. Anonymous. (1999, February 4). Effective January 1, 1999. *OT Week, 9.*

10. Lewis, S. L. (1989). *Elder care in occupational therapy.* Thorofare, NJ: SLACK Incorporated.

11. Stanciff, B. L. (1997). Developing a marketing mindset. *OT Practice, 11*(2), 32-36.

12. Lyons, A. (2000). Cultural competence in occupational therapy practice. *Home and Community Health: Special Interest Section Quarterly, 3*(7), 1,2.

13. Taugher, M. (2000). Persons with limited English proficiency: A challenge for home and community practitioners. *Home and Community Health: Special Interest Section Quarterly, 3*(7), 3, 4.

14. Perinchief, J. M. (1998). Management of occupational therapy services. In M. E. Neistadt, & E. G. Crepeau (Eds.), *Willard and Spackman's occupational therapy* (9th Ed., pp. 783-787). Philadelphia: Lippincott-Raven.

15. Warchol, K. (2000). The challenge of dementia care: Focusing on remaining abilities, not deficits, creates a positive foundation for treatment. *OT Practice, 22*(5), 15-19.

16. Levy, L. L. (1996). Section 2: Cognitive integration and cognitive components. In K. O. Larson, R. G. Stevens-Ratchford, L. Pedretti, & J. L. Crabtree (Eds.), *The role of occupational therapy with the elderly* (2nd Ed., pp. 573-595). Bethesda, MD: The American Occupational Therapy Association, Inc.

17. Copeland, C. (2000). Dementia: Using the ACL with individuals with dementia. *Advance for Occupational Therapy Practitioners, 22*(16), 34.

18. Reisberg, B., Ferris, S. H., Leon, M. J., & Cook, T. (1982). The global deterioration scale for the assessment of primary degenerative dementia. *Am J Psych, 139,* 1136-1139.

19. Hladik, P. (1985). *Once I have had my tea: A guide to understanding and caring for the memory-impaired elderly* (2nd Ed., pp. 1-35). Jacksonville, FL: Author.

20. Birnesser, L. R. (1997). Treating dementia: Practical strategies for long-term-care residents. *OT Practice, 6*(2), 16-21.

21. Hellen, C. R. (1992). *Alzheimer's disease: Activity focused care* (pp. 60-77). Boston: Andover Medical Publishers/Butterworth-Heinemann.

22. Szekais, B. (1991). Treatment approaches for patients with dementing illness. In J. M. Kiernat (Ed.), *Occupational therapy and the older adult: A clinical manual* (pp. 192-214). Gaithersberg, MD: Aspen.

23. Christenson, M. A. (1996). Environmental design, modification, and adaptation. In K. O. Larson, R. G. Stevens-Ratchford, L. Pedretti, & J. L. Crabtree (Eds.), *The role of occupational therapy with the elderly* (2nd Ed., pp. 384-415). Bethesda, MD: The American Occupational Therapy Association, Inc.

24. Painter, J. (1998). Enhancing function for persons with Alzheimer's disease. *OT Practice, 1*(3), 24-29.

25. Wingert, P., Grossman, K. N., Weingarten, T., & Raymond, J. (2000, Jan 31). Coping with the darkness. *Newsweek,* 52-54.

26. Skolaski-Pellitteri, T. (1983). Environmental adaptations which compensate for dementia. *Physical and Occupational Therapy in Geriatrics, 1*(3), 31-44.

27. Daniel, M. S., & Strickland, L. R. (1992). *Occupational therapy protocol management in adult physical dysfunction* (pp. 1-106,139-159,195-261). Gaithersberg, MD: Aspen.

28. Wheatley, C. J. (1996). Evaluation and treatment of cognitive dysfunction. In L. W. Pedretti (Ed.), *Occupational therapy: Practice skills for physical dysfunction* (Rev. 4th Ed., pp. 241-252). New York: Mosby.

29. Zoltan, B., Siev, E., & Freishtat, B. (1986). *The adult stroke patient: A manual for evaluation and treatment of perceptual and cognitive dysfunction* (2nd Ed., pp. 3-174). Thorofare, NJ: SLACK Incorporated.

30. Zoltan, B. (1996). *Vision, perception and cognition: A manual for the evaluation and treatment of the neurologically impaired adult* (3rd Ed.). Thorofare, NJ: SLACK Incorporated.

31. Golisz, K. M. & Toglia, J. P. (1998). Section 2: Evaluation of perception and cognition. In M. E. Neistadt, & E. B. Crepeau (Eds.), *Willard and Spackman's occupational therapy* (9th Ed., pp. 260-278). Philadelphia: Lippincott-Raven.

32. Ludwig, F. M. (1991). Cognitive impairments in older adults. In J. M. Kiernat (Ed.), *Occupational therapy and the older adult: A clinical manual* (pp. 156-174). Gaithersberg, MD: Aspen.

33. Butin, D. N. (1996). Section 4: Psychosocial and psychological components. In K. O. Larson, R. G. Stevens-Ratchford, L. Pedretti, & J. L. Crabtree (Eds.), *The role of occupational therapy with the elderly* (2nd Ed., pp. 610-629). Bethesda, MD: The American Occupational Therapy Association, Inc.

34. Moore, S. D. (1986). Older adult day care. In L. J. Davis, & M. Kirkland (Eds.), The role of occupational therapy with the elderly (1st Ed., pp. 171-177). Rockville, MD: The American Occupational Therapy Association.

35. Wolfe, F. D., & Paulson, C. P. (1991). Day treatment for behavioral health needs. In J. M. Kiernat (Ed.), *Occupational therapy and the older adult: A clinical manual* (pp. 175-191). Gaithersberg, MD: Aspen.

36. Earle, G. K. (1999). OT's role in mental health home care. *OT Practice, 1*(4), 16-19.

37. Allen, C. K. (1985). *Occupational therapy for psychiatric diseases: Measurement and management of cognitive disabilities.* Boston: Little, Brown and Company.

38. Richman, L. (1969). Sensory training for geriatric patients. *Am J Occup Ther, 3*(23), 244-245.

39. Paire, J. A., & Karney, R. J. (1984). The effectiveness of sensory stimulation for geropsychiatric inpatients. *Am J Occup Ther, 8*(38), 505-509.

40. Ross, M. (1997). *Integrative group therapy: Mobilizing coping abilities with the five-stage group.* Bethesda, MD: The American Occupational Therapy Association, Inc.

41. Ayres, A. J., & Heskitt, W. M. (1972). Sensory-integrative dysfunction in a young schizophrenic girl. *Journal of Autism of Child Schizophrenia, 2,* 174-181.

42. Balinski, C. (1988, June 6). Social skills on center stage. *OT Advance, 6,* 6-7.

43. Paire, J., Zigon, J., & Lichtenwalner, D. (1987). Activities used in teaching social skills to psychiatric patients. *An occupation therapy department inservice.* Norristown, PA: Norristown State Hospital.

44. Butler, R. N. (1964). The life review: An interpretation of reminiscence in the aged. In R. Kastenbaum (Ed.), *New thoughts on old age* (p. 266). New York: Springer Publishing Co.

45. Amado, A.N., Lakin, K.C., & Menke, J. M. (1990). *Services for people with developmental disabilities.* Minneapolis, MN: The University of Minnesota Center for Residential and Community Services.

46. Smith, G. C. (1997). Aging families of adults with mental retardation: Patterns and correlates of service use, need, and knowledge. *Am J Ment Retard, 1*(14), 59-77.

47. University of Minnesota Research and Training Center on Community Integration (UAP). (1999). *College of Education and Human Development: MR/DD data brief.* Minneapolis, MN: Author.

48. Herge, E. A., & Campbell, J. E. (2000). Occupational therapy for adults with developmental disabilities. *OT Practice, 13*(5), 18-23.

49. Crocker, A. (1992). Expansion of the health care delivery system. In L. Rowitz (Ed.). *Mental retardation in the year 2000.* New York: Springer-Verlag.

50. Martin, B. A. (1997). Primary care of adults with mental retardation living in the community. *Am Fam Physician, 56,* 485-495.

51. Warren, M. (1996). Evaluation and treatment of visual deficits. In L. W. Pedretti (Ed.), *Occupational therapy: Practice skills for physical dysfunction* (4th Ed., pp. 193-212). St. Louis, MO: CV Mosby.

52. Sullivan, K. M. (1997). The occupational therapist and the low-vision specialist: Working together. *OT Practice, 11*(2), 37-39.

53. Collins, L. F. (1996). Understanding visual impairments. *OT Practice, 1*(1), 22-29.

54. Thamb, K., Borell, L., & Anders, G. (2000). The discovery of disability: A phenomenological study of unilateral neglect. *Am J Occup Ther, 4*(54), 398-405.

55. Watson, G. R. (1996). Older adults with low vision. In A. L. Corn, & A. Koenig (Eds.), *Foundations of low vision: Clinical and functional perspectives.* New York: AFB.

56. Toth-Riddering, A. (1998). Living with age-related macular degeneration. *OT Practice, 1*(3), 18-23.

57. Schuchard, R., & Fletcher, D. (1994). Preferred retinal locus: A review with applications in low vision rehabilitation. *Low Vision Rehabilitation, 7,* 243-256.

58. Toglia, J. B. (1998). Section 6: Cognitive perceptual retraining and rehabilitation. In M. E. Neistadt, & E. B. Crepeau (Eds.), *Willard and Spackman's occupational therapy* (9th Ed., pp. 428-432). Philadelphia: Lippincott-Raven.

59. Pedretti, L. W., Zoltan, B., & Wheatley, C. J. (1996). Evaluation and treatment of perceptual and perceptual-motor defects. In L. W. Pedretti (Ed.), *Occupational therapy: Practice skills for physical dysfunction* (4th Ed., pp. 231-239). St. Louis, MO: CV Mosby-Year Book Inc.

60. Eggers, O. (1984). *Occupational therapy in the treatment of adult hemiplegia.* Rockville, MD: Aspen.

61. National Center for Health Statistics. (1995). *Trends in the health of older Americans 1994. National Center for Health Statistics (DHHS Pub No [PH595]-1414).* Washington, DC: US Government Printing Office.

62. Aquaviva, J. (1996). *Occupational therapy practice guidelines for adults with stroke.* Bethesda, MD: The American Occupational Therapy Association, Inc.

63. Pulaski, K. H. (1998). Adult neurological dysfunction. In M. E. Neistadt, & E. B. Crepeau (Eds.), *Willard and Spackman's occupational therapy* (9th Ed., pp. 660-680). Philadelphia: Lippincott-Raven.

64. Gresham, G. E. (1995). *Post stroke rehabilitation. Clinical practice guideline, Number 16.* Rockville, MD: US Department of Health and Human Services.

65. Kohlmeger, K. (1998). Evaluation of sensory and neuromuscular performance components. In M. E. Neistadt, & E. B. Crepeau (Eds.), *Willard and Spackman's occupational therapy* (9th Ed., pp. 223-290). Philadelphia: Lippincott-Raven.

66. Pedretti, L. W. (1996). Evaluation of sensation and treatment of sensory dysfunction. In L. W. Pedretti (Ed.), *Occupational therapy: Practice skills for physical dysfunction* (4th Ed., pp. 213-230). St. Louis, MO: CV Mosby-Year Book.

67. Nelson, K. Dysphagia: Evaluation and treatment. In L. W. Pedretti (Ed.), *Occupational therapy: Practice skills for physical dysfunction* (4th Ed., pp. 165-191). St. Louis, MO: CV Mosby-Year Book Inc.

68. Avery-Smith, W. (1998). An occupational therapist-coordinated dysphagia program. *OT Practice, 3*(10), 20-23.

69. Pedretti, L. W., Smith, J. A., & Pendleton, H. M. (1996). Cerebral vascular accident. In L. W. Pedretti (Ed.), *Occupational therapy: Practice skills for physical dysfunction* (4th Ed., pp. 785-805). St. Louis, MO: CV Mosby-Year Book Inc.

70. Pedretti, L. W. (1996). Movement therapy: The Brunnstrom approach to treatment of hemiplegia. In L. W. Pedretti (Ed.), *Occupational therapy: Practice skills for physical dysfunction* (4th Ed., pp. 401-416). St. Louis, MO: CV Mosby-Year Book Inc.

71. Davis, J. Z. (1996). Neurodevelopmental treatment of adult hemiplegia: The Bobath approach. In L. W. Pedretti (Ed.), *Occupational therapy: Practice skills for physical dysfunction* (4th Ed., pp. 435-450). St. Louis, MO: CV Mosby-Year Book Inc.

72. Pope-Davis, S. (1996). The proprioceptive neuromuscular facilitation approach. In L. W. Pedretti (Ed.), *Occupational therapy: Practice skills for physical dysfunction* (4th Ed., pp. 417-432). St. Louis, MO: CV Mosby-Year Book Inc.

73. McCormack, G. I. (1996). The Rood approach to treatment of neuromuscular dysfunction. In L. W. Pedretti (Ed.), *Occupational therapy: Practice skills for physical dysfunction* (4th Ed., pp. 377-399). St. Louis, MO: CV Mosby-Year Book Inc.

74. Blakeslee, S. (2000, June 2). Study offers hope for use of limbs disabled by stroke: Therapy is found to work in 2 to 3 weeks. *The New York Times (The National Report),* A12.

75. Stump, J. R. (1999). Treating chronic pulmonary disease. *OT Practice, 6*(4), 28-32.

76. Ferraro, R. (1998). Cardiopulmonary dysfunction in adults. In M. E. Neistadt, & E. B. Crepeau (Eds.), *Willard and Spackman's occupational therapy* (9th Ed., pp. 693-704). Philadelphia: Lippincott-Raven.

77. Trump, S. M., & Jessamine, L. (1999). Pulmonary rehabilitation in home health care. *Home and Community Health Special Interest Section Quarterly, 3*(6), 1-3.

78. Ford, J., & Weaver, F. H. (2000). Breathing retraining and relaxation techniques for clients with pulmonary disease. *OT Practice, 13*(5), 33-34.

79. Matthews, M. M., Foderaro, D., & O'Leary, S. (1996). Cardiac dysfunction. In L. W. Pedretti (Ed.), *Occupational therapy: Practice skills for physical dysfunction* (4th Ed., pp. 693-714). St. Louis, MO: CV Mosby-Year Book Inc.

80. Miller, M. A., & Kirchman, M. M. (1991). Geriatric rehabilitation programs. In J. M. Kiernat (Ed.), *Occupational therapy and the older adult: A clinical manual* (pp. 99-122). Gaithersburg, MD: Aspen Publishers.

81. Hooks, M. L. (1996). Parkinson's disease. In L. W. Pedretti (Ed.), *Occupational therapy: Practice skills for physical dysfunction* (4th Ed., pp. 845-851). St. Louis, MO: CV Mosby-Year Book Inc.

82. Pomerov, V. (1990). Development of an ADL oriented assessment-of-mobility scale suited for use with elderly people with dementia. *Physiotherapy, 8*(76), 446-448.

83. Friedman, J., & Friedman, H. (1989). Fatigue in Parkinson's disease. *Neurology, 43,* 2016.

84. Schenkman, M., et al. (1989). Management of individuals with Parkinson's disease. *Phys Ther, 69,* 947.

85. Pizzi, M., & Burkhardt, A. (1998). Occupational therapy for adults with immunological diseases. In M. E. Neistadt, & E. B. Crepeau (Eds.), *Willard and Spackman's occupational therapy* (9th Ed., pp. 703-715). Philadelphia: Lippincott-Raven.

86. Adler, J., & Kalb, C. (2000, Sept 4). An American epidemic: Diabetes. *Newsweek,* 40-47.

87. Herbert-Green, C. (1986). Developing exercise programs for the elderly person with diabetes. *Gerontology Special Interest Section Newsletter of the American Occupational Association, 4*(9), 2,3.

88. Melvin, J. L. (1995). *Osteoarthritis: Caring for your hands.* Bethesda, MD: American Occupational Therapy Association, Inc.

89. Melvin, J. (1981). Occupational therapy: Restoring independence. *Perspective on Aging, 3*(X), 24-25.

90. Fischer, M. S, Kvatz, A., Jimenec, B. Watson, C., Spence, C., & Sandford, T., et al. (2001). Aquatic therapy: An occupational perspective. *OT Practice, 3*(6), 14-16.

91. Cook, A., & Miller, P. A. (1996). Section 2: Prevention of falls in the elderly. In K. O. Larson, R. G. Stevens-Ratchford, L. Pedretti, & J. L. Crabtree (Eds.), *The role of occupational therapy with the elderly* (2nd Ed., pp. 653-668). Bethesda, MD: American Occupational Therapy Association, Inc.

92. Kalb, C. (2000, Dec 11). The meaning of falling. *Newsweek,* 63-64.

93. American College of Emergency Physicians. (1998). *Spotlight on safety: Help the elderly cope with falls.* Irving, TX: Author.

94. Baraff, L. J., Penna, R. D., Williams, N., & Sanders, A. (1997). Practice guideline for the ED management of falls in community-dwelling elderly persons. *Ann Emerg Medi, 30,* 480-492.

95. Walls, B. S. (1999). A dangerous secret: "I had a fall." *OT Practice, 11*(4), 12-16.

96. Kiernat, J. M. (1991). Preventing falls in the hospital and the home. In J. M. Kiernat (Ed.), *Occupational therapy and the older adult: A clinical manual* (pp. 123-136). Gaithersburg, MD: Aspen Publishers.

97. Johansson, C. (2001). Fitness implicated in falls. *OT Practice, 3*(6), 7.

98. Herring, C. L. (1991). Maintaining fitness in later life. In J. M. Kiernat (Ed.), *Occupational therapy and the older adult: A clinical manual* (pp. 43-59). Gaithersburg, MD: Aspen.

99. Stonecypher, D. D. Jr. (1974). *Getting older and staying young.* New York: WW Norton Inc.

100. Borgurd-Krenik, M. (1988). OT teaching exercise class to help elderly stay fit. *OT Week, 11*(2), 2.

101. Tinetti, M. E. (1986). Performance-oriented assessment of mobility problems in elderly patients. *J Am Geriatr Soc, 34*(3), 119-126.

102. Morawski, D. M., Pitbladdo, K., Biandi, E. M., Lieberman, S. C., Novic, J. P., & Bobrove, H. (1996). Hip fractures and total hip replacement. In L. W. Pedretti (Ed.), *Occupational therapy: Practice skills for physical dysfunction* (4th Ed., pp. 735-745). St. Louis, MO: CV Mosby-Year Book Inc.

103. Platt, J. V., Hahn, R., Kessler, S., & McCarthy, D. Q. (1994). *Daily activities after your hip surgery* (6th Ed.). Bethesda, MD: American Occupational Therapy Association, Inc.

104. Aaron, D. H., Stegin, K., & Jansen, C. W. (2000). Hand rehabilitation: Matching patient priorities and performance with pathology and tissue healing. *OT Practice, 6*(5), 10-15.

105. Swedberg, L. M. (1996). Splinting the difficult hand. *Gerontology Special Interest Section Newsletter, 2*(19), 1-3.

106. Stinnett, K. (1999). Geriatric seating intervention in the skilled nursing facility. *OT Practice, 6*(4), 40-42.

107. Perr, A. (1998). Elements of seating and wheeled mobility intervention. *OT Practice, 6*(3), 16-24.

108. Mayall, J. K., & Desharnais, G. (1990). *Positioning in a wheelchair: A guide for professional care givers of the disabled adult.* Thorofare, NJ: SLACK Incorporated.

109. Lange, M. L. (2000). Seating systems. *OT Practice, 22*(5), 23-24.

110. Swedberg, L. M. (1998). Low-tech adaptations for seating and positioning. *OT Practice, 9*(3), 26-31.

111. Foti, D. (1996). Evaluations and interventions for the performance areas. Section 1: Evaluation and interventions for the performance area of self-maintenance. In K. O. Larson, R. G. Stevens-Ratchford, L. Pedretti, & J. L. Crabtree (Eds.), *The role of occupational therapy with the elderly* (2nd Ed., pp. 631-649). Bethesda, MD: American Occupational Therapy Association, Inc.

112. Snell, M. A. (1999). Guidelines for safety transporting wheelchair users. *OT Practice, 6*(4), 35-38.

113. Crepeau, E. B. (1998). Activity analysis: A way of thinking about occupational performance. In M. E. Neistadt, & E. B. Crepeau (Eds.), *Willard and Spackman's occupational therapy* (9th Ed., pp. 135-146). Philadelphia: Lippincott-Raven.

114. Knox, S. H. (1998). Evaluation of play and leisure. In M. E. Neistadt, & E. B. Crepeau (Eds.), *Willard and Spackman's occupational therapy* (9th Ed., pp. 213-222). Philadelphia: Lippincott-Raven.

115. Foti, D., Pedretti, L. W., & Lillie, S. (1996). Activities of daily living. In L. W. Pedretti (Ed.), *Occupational therapy: Practice skills for physical dysfunction* (4th Ed., pp. 463-506). St. Louis, MO: CV Mosby-Year Book Inc.

116. Matsutsuyu, J. S. (1969). The interest checklist. *Am J Occup Ther, 23*, 323-334.

117. Rogers, J., Weinstein, J., & Fignon, J. (1978). The interest checklist. *Am J Occup Ther, 32*, 628-630.

118. Nystrom, E. P. (1974). Activity patterns and leisure concepts among the elderly. *Am J Occup Ther, 28*, 337-345.

119. Gregory, M. D. (1983). Occupational behavior and life satisfaction among retirees. *Am J Occup Ther, 37*, 548-553.

120. Howe, C. (1988). Using qualitative structured interviews in leisure research: Illustrations from one case study. *Journal of Leisure Research, 20*, 305-324.

121. Cynkin, S., & Robinson, A. M. (1990). *Occupational therapy and activities health: Toward health through activities.* Boston: Little, Brown, and Co.

122. Watanabe, S. (1968). *Activities configuration: Regional institute on the evaluation process. Final Rep. RSA-123-T-68.* New York: American Occupational Therapy Association.

123. Glantz, C. H., & Richman, N. (1996). Evaluation and intervention for leisure activities. In K. O. Larson, R. G. Stevens-Ratchford, L. Pedretti, & J. L. Crabtree (Eds.), *The role of occupational therapy with the elderly* (2nd Ed., pp. 729-741). Bethesda, MD: American Occupational Therapy Association, Inc.

124. Zahoransky, M. (1998). Teamwork in home care: Fundamental to survival. *OT Practice, 11*(3), 29-31.

125. Paulson, C. P. (1991). Home care programs. In J. M. Kiernat (Ed.), *Occupational therapy and the older adult: A clinical manual* (pp. 220-240). Gaithersburg, MD: Aspen Publishers.

126. Park, S. (1996). Restoring occupational performance: Rehabilitation services for older adults. In K. O. Larson, R. G. Stevens-Ratchford, L. Pedretti, & J. L. Crabtree (Eds.), *The role of occupational therapy with the elderly* (2nd Ed., pp. 366-382). Bethesda, MD: American Occupational Therapy Association, Inc.

127. Holm, M. B., Rogers, J. C., & James, A. B. (1998). Treatment of occupational performance areas. Section 1: Treatment of activities of daily living. In M. E. Neistadt, & E. B. Crepeau (Eds.), *Willard and Spackman's occupational therapy* (9th Ed., pp. 323-364). Philadelphia: Lippincott-Raven.

128. Diffendal, J. (2001). Staying dry: OTs should help patients get the right treatment for urinary continence problems. *Advance, 6*(17), 33-34.

129. Bonfils, K. B. (1996). The Affolter approach to treatment: A perceptual-cognitive perspective of function. In L. W. Pedretti (Ed.), *Occupational therapy: Practice skills for physical dysfunction* (4th Ed., pp. 451-461). St. Louis, MO: CV Mosby-Year Book.

130. Lange, M. L. (2001). EADLs and aging clients. *OT Practice, 14*(6), 16-18.

131. Bachner, S. (2000). Objects, physical environment, and self: Implications for home interventions. *OT Practice, 4*(5), 19-22.

132. Rosage, L. J., & Klein, S. I. Home modifications: Occupational therapy and the Philadelphia Corporation for Aging. Philadelphia: American Occupational Therapy Association 81st Annual Conference and Exposition, April 19, 2001.

133. US Department of Transportation National Highway Traffic Safety Administration. (1999). *Traffic safety facts: 1998 older population.* Washington, DC: Author. Retrieved April 18, 2000, from the http://www.nhtsa.dot.gov.

134. Centers for Disease Control and Prevention. (2000). *10 leading causes of death in the United States 1997, all races, both sexes.* Atlanta, GA: Author. Retrieved April 18, 2000, from http://www.cuc.gov/ncipc/osp/states/101c97.html.

135. Stressel, D. L. (2000). Driving issues of the older adult. *OT Practice, 14*(5), CE1-CE7.

136. Pierce, S. (1996). Section 3: Transportation. In K. O. Larson, R. G. Stevens-Ratchford, L. Pedretti, & J. L. Crabtree (Eds.), *The role of occupational therapy with the elderly* (2nd Ed., pp. 669-678). Bethesda, MD: American Occupational Therapy Association, Inc.

137. Pierce, S. (1998). On the road again? OT and the older driver. *OT Practice, 1*(3), 30-32.

138. Le Pore, P. (1997). *1997 survey of families and caregivers concerned about the safety of an older driver. Unpublished survey of the older driver family assistance project.* Albany, NY: New York State Office for Aging.

139. Diffendal, J. (2001, May 14). Stop signs. *Advance for Occupational Therapy Practitioners, 10*(17), 8-9.

CASE STUDIES

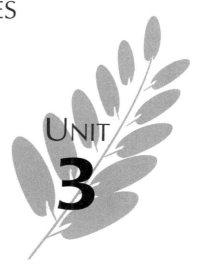

UNIT
3

CASE STUDY 5

The Process of Building Client Compliance Toward an Occupational Therapy Remediation Program in a Home Health Setting

Mr. M was an 86-year-old male recovering from a recent hospitalization. His primary diagnosis was bronchial pneumonia. Other diagnoses included cardiac artery disease, osteoarthritis of the knees, type 2 diabetes, and hypertension.

Mr. M was a widower who lived alone in a two-story home. Before his retirement, Mr. M had worked for more than 30 years in the maintenance department of a moderately sized suburban school district. Avocational interests included all types of electronics (radios, computers, and most recently robots). Prior to this hospitalization Mr. M was completely independent for his needs and was able to dress, bathe, cook, and clean in an efficient and effective manner. He had not experienced fatigue from these daily activities.

Nursing and physical therapy had reported to this therapist that Mr. M often did not comply with suggested intervention regimens.

At the initial occupational therapy evaluation, Mr. M was apprehensive at first and stated, "You therapists always ask the same questions." However, he became absolutely enthusiastic and expansive when discussing his avocational interests. Mr. M was proud to demonstrate his latest invention—two robots in the formative stages. One robot walked and shook hands. A second robot was programmed to answer questions such as "What did you have for breakfast?"

As soon as Mr. M realized that the therapist was genuinely concerned about him as a "whole person," he became very interested in collaboratively working on a plan for his occupational therapy intervention program. Taking time to view his robots in action had made the difference in this man's perception that therapy could be tailored to his own needs.

The occupational therapy evaluation revealed that Mr. M was not able to bathe, dress, or prepare food efficiently and effectively. He experienced shortness of breath whenever he had to climb stairs to the second floor. Because the only bathroom and his bedroom were on the second floor, this was a real challenge to his endurance. He stated that he felt exhausted by the time he reached the top of the stairs.

Upon mutually discussing his needs and interests, it was determined that Mr. M would benefit from training in energy conservation techniques as associated with activities of daily living (e.g., sliding pots on the counter in the kitchen instead of lifting them or dressing and bathing with rest periods in between stages to prevent exhaustion), instruction in appropriate upper body therapeutic exercise to strengthen endurance in the chest and arms to improve performance in activities of daily living, instruction in pursed breathing techniques to decrease shortness of breath, and the appropriate rearrangement of kitchen items (with the most used items in the kitchen arranged at eye level for ease of reaching) to promote endurance in the kitchen.

Mr. M readily understood the importance of the program and was most willing to participate. After the physician in charge was apprised of the occupational therapy findings and recommendations, he was in full agreement with the care plan. Mr. M would be seen by occupational therapy two times weekly for 4 weeks with the utilization of the modalities that have been previously described.

By the end of the 4 weeks Mr. M was no longer out of breath. He practiced his upper body therapeutic exercises three times daily. He was able to dress, bathe, and prepare food in a more timely and efficient manner and no longer became fatigued when performing activities of daily living or climbing the stairs to the second floor of his home. Mr. M stated that he intended to "keep up his exercises" after occupational therapy concluded.

There was no doubt in the therapist's mind that without demonstrating an initial interest in the client as a "whole person," this effective program would never have been established and utilized.

CASE STUDY 6

The Use of the Life Review and Professional Advocacy Within the Realm of Occupational Therapy in a Mental Health Setting

Miss W was a very frail elderly female client of more than 80 years, who had been hospitalized in a large mental health facility for schizophrenia for most of her adult life.

During her long hospitalization Miss W maintained her skill as an oil painter (mostly of nature or flowers). During that time Miss W's lifetime friend, Mrs. G, would visit her regularly and bring in specialized art materials. Occupational therapy had provided a special area in which Miss W could paint, standard art supplies, support, and encouragement.

Mrs. G's health was also becoming frail, and she desperately wanted to provide her friend with an opportunity to view her life's work as she had kept Miss W's artwork in her home during Miss W's long hospitalization. Mrs. G arranged for the art supply store (where she had for so long purchased Miss W's supplies) to display Miss W's artwork in their storefront. The store was in the center of a large city (involving a 40-mile commute).

Miss W asked the occupational therapist to "plead her case" before the intervention team. Miss W knew she was physically weak and stated, "This is the most important moment of my life—please help me see my show." After much discussion the therapist pointed out to the team that this was Miss W's wish and that no matter the outcome, she should be enabled to make use of this opportunity to see her art show and review her life's work. The team agreed.

It was an exceedingly hot day when Miss W, the social worker, and the occupational therapist set out by automobile to see the art show. Despite the heat, Miss W insisted on a "proper" hat and white gloves, stating, "A lady always wears a hat and gloves when going out." On viewing her displayed work, Miss W turned to the occupational therapist and said, "You know it's not bad, not bad at all. In fact, it's quite good."

On the ride back Miss W spoke of having experienced an inner peace and that she was "now ready to meet her maker." From then on until her death, whenever she saw the occupational therapist, she never forgot to mention how much seeing her art show had meant to her.[1]

CASE STUDY 7

Home Modification in Preparation for Discharge From a Rehabilitation Facility

Linda Burgess, OTR/L very aptly describes the home modification process in the July/August 1999 issue of *OT Practice*.

Ms. A was a 77-year-old female recovering from a left CVA. This client had a mild right hemiparesis, and she also exhibited weakness in all four extremities. Ms. A also manifested a moderate-to-severe kyphosis. Her fine motor coordination skills were also limited. Ms. A was also beginning to develop a bilateral foot drop, despite the fact that she had active hip, knee, and ankle flexion and extension. Perceptually, this individual exhibited a moderate visual neglect and decreased right-left discrimination. There was no indication of agnosia, spatial relations deficits, or apraxia. Initiation, concentration, and short-term memory were problematic due to accompanying conditions of depression and anxiety. Although Ms. A had an expressive aphasia, she was able to make her needs known. This included her desire to return to her home upon discharge. It was expected that Ms. A would receive 24-hour assistance from caregivers.

A home evaluation (focused upon street and outside access, safety and security features, indoor mobility, and caregiver support) was conducted by the occupational and physical therapists. Ms. A was interested in updating the kitchen and bathroom facilities (to ease caregiver burden), with the prescription of durable medical equipment, as necessary.

Ms. A's residence was a three-story town house. The first floor housed a dining/living area, a kitchen, and a powder room with an attached laundry room. The second floor housed a formal living room, and the third floor included two bedrooms and a full bathroom. All three floors were connected by a spiral staircase.

The garden and patio entrance (the front and back entrances had multiple steps and landings. Also the front could not be modified due to historical restrictions and a common street entrance shared by two other town houses) became the focus of indoor/outdoor access.

The major considerations for renovation (after discussion with Ms. A, her financial power of attorney, her personal caregiver and close friends—there were no spouse or children) included converting/modifying the combination powder and laundry room to include bathing facilities. The living/dining area could also be modified to function as a bed/sitting room. An outdoor access to the back yard was available via the patio door. The living space in this area could also be extended by enclosing it with glass, and a chair lift could be installed to provide access to the garden level.

In collaboration with the architect and contractor, only the most important elements affecting function and safety were addressed. These included the following:

✧   Removing all nonessential items and clutter

✧   Installing grounded outlets and new electrical wiring and additional lighting on the first level

✧   Renovating the bathroom to include a wheelchair-accessible shower stall, a grab bar, a nonskid floor surface and widening the doorways for wheelchair clearance

✧   Installing low-pile carpeting in the dining/living room and hallway

✧   Installing new drywall in the bathroom area

✧   Applying paint in the new sitting/bedroom area

✧   Providing durable medical equipment to include a bedside commode, a hoyer lift, a hospital bed, and a custom manual wheelchair.

This whole process required the occupational therapist to provide information about services, equipment, vendors, contractors, and architects to the client and significant others so that all became informed in ensuring an independent and safe environment based on the desires of the client. In this way an individual is empowered to make informed choices.[2]

CASE STUDY 8

Using Motivational Strategies to Promote and Facilitate Improved Health Status Via a Home Health Occupational Therapy Setting

In a recent text, Sorensen aptly discusses the use of motivational strategies and techniques as playing a vital part of the intervention process in home health occupational therapy.

Dr. Y is a 67-year-old semiretired male who has never been married. Although he has no living relatives, he has many friends who visit. He lives in a one-bedroom apartment in a large city. Dr. Y suffered a right CVA while undergoing *cardiac bypass surgery* (CABG). Other diagnoses included hypertension and arthritis in the left shoulder. At the initial occupational therapy interview he reported that his left shoulder pain was tolerable. Dr. Y's left upper extremity passive range of motion was intact without flexion synergy. He exhibited some active motion in all of his joints of the left arm and hand, and his sensation was intact.

Dr. Y had received intensive rehabilitation in a center for 3 weeks after his hospitalization. Upon discharge his home health intervention program included occupational therapy one to three times per week.

Dr. Y was a tenured professor with an expertise of political science (specifically Latin American). Avocational interests included playing the piano, bookbinding, and collecting furniture and artifacts.

Dr. Y's occupational therapy short-term goals were to increase the range of motion of his left upper extremity, increase its strength, decrease pain in his left shoulder, and to prepare a cold meal. Long-term goals were for his left upper extremity to become a good functional assist, for him to independently prepare meals, and to manage his own shoulder pain.

However, Dr. Y's anger and depression had become motivational issues. During his home occupational therapy sessions he spent most of the time complaining about his bad luck and would not follow (or forgot) his home exercise plan. Dr. Y had gone into surgery expecting to have a good outcome. Instead, he became disabled and experienced a great deal of difficulty resolving this issue.

Before Dr. Y would be able to actually participate in his physical program, it became necessary to treat his depression so that his anger and lack of concentration would diminish.

The most effective way to engage Dr. Y with his occupational therapy program was to verbally interact with him about his interests (e.g., What had he been teaching? What was his favorite of the topics that he taught?) and to ask him about the interesting craft and art pieces that he displayed in his apartment. By encouraging discussion, Dr. Y had an opportunity to regain his composure.

The first specific therapeutic activity was to involve Dr. Y in "faux stained glass" such as a sun catcher. The color and design had to complement his décor and be of his choosing. During the fabrication Dr. Y learned to use his left hand as a good assist. This activity provided a successful experience within his new physical reality, and it proved to be emotionally stabilizing.

Once Dr. Y became engaged in this activity, he was introduced to his home exercise program. Each exercise was explained as to how it would help his physiology. In this way Dr. Y would become more accepting and involved in his home occupational therapy and his occupational therapy prognosis in achieving stated goals was good.[3]

CASE STUDY 9

Promoting Positive Behavior by Means of Occupational Therapy Intervention Within a Psychiatric Institutional Setting

In a recent monogram, Hengel deftly describes occupational therapy intervention within the psychiatric institutional setting.

Miss ME was a 72-year-old female with long-standing diagnosis of schizophrenia. Miss ME had been hospitalized in a state psychiatric institution in her late teens and had remained institutionalized for some 50 years. Her institutional behaviors made it difficult for her to be discharged to another type of setting. She annoyed staff, visitors, and other clients by waiting by the door for someone to enter the unit. As soon as an individual would appear at the door, she would typically barrage him or her with questions and follow him or her wherever he or she went. For this behavior she received attention (mostly negative and at times punitive). She was often told to leave people alone and go sit down. Through the years Miss ME had attended numerous social and interpersonal development programs. However, these programs were unable to make a difference in these institutional-type behaviors.

Since Miss ME had behaved so long in this manner, it became accepted that little could be done except for her to learn to leave others alone. As a consequence, the staff focused upon controlling her behavior rather than changing it. This led to a conflict with Miss ME and reinforced her client role of having little control over her own existence.

A group of occupational therapy students, assigned to Miss ME's unit, were given the mission to take a fresh needed look at what could be done to improve the discharge potential and quality of life for these clients.

In Miss ME's case they decided to change her negative behavior into a positive one—a virtual asset. She became the "unit greeter." A good part of this role was already in the client's repertoire and did not require new learning. It was a role, valued by others, that was viewed as helpful rather than annoying.

Miss ME's greeting behavior, then, became a positive source of feedback rather than a negative source. Miss ME's role of unit greeter supported her sense of autonomy, self-worth, and control over some aspects of her life. No longer was she regarded exclusively as a client and "the unit annoyer." She now had a specific job or role to perform that was respected. She performed her new role eagerly and well. Later, when she was transferred to another setting, she continued in this role in a positive and respected manner.[4]

CASE STUDY 10

Occupational Therapy Intervention in a Skilled Nursing Rehabilitation Setting Involving Transfer Back to the Client's Home

Mrs. B was a 75-year-old widow who had formerly lived in a one-bedroom apartment. There she was able to attend to her own cooking, bathing, and light housekeeping (dusting, making her bed). Her daughter performed heavier chores such as washing the floors, laundry, vacuuming, and washing the bathroom facilities. Once weekly Mrs. B and her daughter went food shopping together. Mrs. B's daughter helped to bring in the grocery bags.

Mrs. B tripped and fell in her apartment, which resulted in a left hip fracture. This required a total hip replacement. Mrs. B's medical history included hypertension, coronary artery disease, and osteoporosis. After a brief period in the hospital (approximately 1 week) where she received bedside instruction in physical and occupational therapy, she was later placed in a skilled nursing facility.

Mrs. B was well motivated and determined to eventually return to her apartment. The occupational therapy evaluation revealed that Mrs. B was not able to dress and bathe her lower body. She was on full hip precautions and could only stand for 2 to 3 minutes with walker support. Mrs. B collaborated with the occupational therapist in her intervention plan. The therapist apprised the physician of the occupational therapy findings and intervention recommendations. These were met with full agreement by the physician involved in the case.

Mrs. B received occupational therapy five times weekly for 6 weeks. During that time she was instructed in safe management techniques (e.g., precautions in regard to body movement when performing activities of daily living—entrance and exit of shower/tub using a transfer bench and leg lifter); introduction and instruction in the use of adaptive equipment such as a long-handled reacher, a sock/stocking donner, a long-handled shoe horn, and a leg lifter to enable efficiency and safety when performing activities of daily living, and therapeutic activities to strengthen endurance for standing and movement while performing homemaking tasks (such as cooking). A walker bag was purchased and attached to the walker so that Mrs. B could bring her belongings with her as she moved. Mrs. B was also instructed in energy conservation techniques when involving activities of daily living (e.g., sliding a pot across a counter instead of lifting the pot).

Within the 6 week period Mrs. B was able to dress and bathe herself and perform light cooking tasks on an independent level (using adaptive equipment as needed). A home visit by the therapist determined that she would benefit from the purchase of a raised toilet seat with armrests as well as a transfer tub bench. This Mrs. B was most willing to do. During her occupational therapy training in the nursing home, Mrs. B also purchased a variety of adaptive equipment (such as a leg lifter, a long-handled reacher, a sock donner, a long-handled sponge, and a long-handled shoe horn). The therapist suggested to Mrs. B and her daughter that they move the most frequently used items (in the bedroom, bathroom, and kitchen) to eye level so that reaching items would be safer and more readily at hand.

Mrs. B returned to her apartment (her daughter would resume her former duties such as food shopping and heavy cleaning as well as laundry) and was able to live independently as she formerly had done. Mrs. B was most pleased with her progress and wrote the occupational therapy department a "thank you note" in which she expressed how much she had benefited from her occupational therapy experience.

CASE STUDY 11

Providing Occupational Therapy Via a Home Health Agency to Promote Independence and Ultimate Transfer from Home-Based Services to Outpatient Occupational Therapy

Mrs. S was a 76-year-old widow who lived independently in a ranch-style home (with a basement) in a residential section of a large city.

Mrs. S suffered a fracture of her left proximal humerus. She was treated with a left shoulder arthroplasty and a brief stay in a general hospital.

Previous to this fracture, Mrs. S was independent in all activities of daily living activities of daily living and had full range of motion of her left shoulder. Other long-standing diagnoses included hypertension, cataract extraction, and degenerative joint disease.

Mrs. S had supportive neighbors and a daughter who lived nearby. Mrs. S was well motivated and felt very positive about participating in an occupational therapy program.

The occupational therapy evaluation revealed that Mrs. S's left shoulder strength was 2+/5. Her shoulder range of motion was also extremely limited. For instance, her left shoulder flexion was 0 to 1 degrees and left shoulder abduction was 0 to 30 degrees. Dressing was minimum (24%) assistance and showering was moderate (50%) assistance (with plastic protection on operated area). Homemaking (making the bed, laundry, dusting, shopping for food) was dependent, and all these chores were performed by her daughter. Meal preparation was minimum assistance (with daughter or neighbors providing some meals). Physician's orders required that Mrs. S wear an immobilizer at all times (except when washing or when performing therapeutic exercises).

The intervention plan recommended by occupational therapy (and with collaboration of the client) involved occupational therapy intervention sessions two times weekly for 6 weeks, instruction in activities of daily living techniques (including use of the public bus), education in energy conservation techniques as associated with activities of daily living instruction in adaptive devices (e.g., long-handled reacher, long-handled sponge, long-handled dressing stick, long-handled shoe horn, buttonhole device, sock/stocking donner), instruction in activities of daily living performance using one-handed techniques, and instruction in left upper extremity exercise to improve range of motion and strength to enhance activities of daily living performance (initiating with exercise such as the pendulum and gradually increasing to a home pulley exercise program).

Long-term goals included achieving independence in dressing, bathing, food preparation, and in improving range of motion and strength of the left upper extremity with eventual transfer to outpatient occupational therapy. The physician in charge of the case was apprised of the findings and the occupational therapy intervention recommendations, and he was in full agreement.

By the end of the 6 weeks Mrs. S no longer required the immobilizer. She was independent in dressing, independent in the shower with safe entry and exit, independent for food preparation tasks, and able to perform light housekeeping (e.g., "straightening up" her bed, performing full dusting, washing dishes, performing light laundry loads, and accompanying her daughter for food shopping). Mrs. S had also been instructed by occupational therapy in the safe use of the public bus, and she was now able to perform this task independently. Her left shoulder range of motion and strength had also improved. Specifically, left shoulder strength was 3/5, left shoulder flexion was 0 to 85 degrees, and left shoulder abduction was 0 to 90 degrees. It was apparent that Mrs. S was ready for outpatient occupational therapy and no longer needed homebound services. The physician was apprised, and arrangements were made for Mrs. S to begin outpatient occupational therapy.

Mrs. S had been extremely pleased with her home occupational therapy program, and she telephoned the therapist and said "Without home-based occupational therapy, I would still be homebound."

CASE STUDY 12

Occupational Therapy Intervention Involving Skilled Nursing Rehabilitation of a Late Life Client With Developmental Delay

The reader is advised to review the Chapter 14, under "Occupational Therapy

Intervention Involving Skilled Nursing Rehabilitation of a Late Life Client With Developmental Delay."

REFERENCES

1. Lewis, S. C. (1989). *Elder care in occupational therapy* (p. 48). Thorofare, NJ: SLACK Incorporated.

2. Burgess, L. (1999, July/August). Home modification: Bridging the gap between inpatient and community practice. *OT Practice, 6* (38-42).

3. Sorensen, J. (1997). CVA in surgery: Can he bounce back? In M. S. Rosenfield (Ed.), *Motivational strategies in geriatric occupational therapy* (pp. 60-61). Bethesda, MD: American Occupational Therapy Association, Inc.

4. Hengel, J. (1997). Motivational strategies in geriatric rehabilitation. In M. S. Rosenfeld (Ed.), *Motivational strategies in geriatric rehabilitation* (pp 109-110). Bethesda, MD: American Occupational Therapy Association, Inc.

Reimbursement Issues (Including PPS) in the United States

Appendix A

Social Security

Social Security is a federal intergenerational transfer program that enables workers to have a certain level of income during retirement. It is not a pension program in that present day workers pay for those who are retired and future generations will pay for them. This program was first initiated in 1935 during President Franklin Roosevelt's administration. Benefits are paid through trust funds that are supported by contributions from workers and employers. Benefits vary according to the annual earnings of the individual worker (and years worked before retirement). Widows, widowers, and dependent children also qualify for survivors' benefits upon the death of the worker. Later, Congress added disability insurance to the Social Security program. This allowed disabled workers (under the age of 65) to qualify for benefits. In 1972, Congress established cost of living adjustments (known as COLAs) as part of Social Security benefits. One-third of older adults receive virtually all of their income from Social Security. Another third of late life adults receive more than half of their income from this source.[1]

Social Security has an uncertain future. A disturbing issue is that as the "baby boomer generation" comes of retirement age, there will be an increasingly smaller labor pool to support a relatively larger number of retirees. Just how to solve this problem has been a matter of great debate.

Supplemental Security Income

Supplemental Security Income (SSI), initiated by Congress in 1972, was designed to protect the blind, the aged, and the disabled from total destitution. However, SSI supplies only a national minimum income that may actually be lower than federal poverty guidelines.[2]

RETIREMENT EQUITY ACT

The Retirement Equity Act (REACT), passed in 1984, gives a spouse some minimum share of the partner's income after the partner's death. This has been of great significance to large numbers of widows who formerly received nothing.[2]

THE OLDER AMERICANS ACT

This act, first established on July 14, 1965 (PL 89-73), has been amended numerous times. It was reauthorized in November 2000.[3,4] Areas of specific interest have traditionally included the declaration of objectives, the establishment and continued development of the Administration on Aging, grants for community and state programs on aging research and training, national older American volunteer programs, multipurpose senior centers, nutrition programs, and amendments to other acts that are designed to enrich the intellectual pursuits of older adults. Mobile programs have been designed to increase job opportunities and training for older adults to help achieve community service employment.[2]

Area agencies on aging (part of the Older Americans Act) provide services on a local basis. Some of these involve helping adults or caregivers find necessary programs and services—such as the following:[3-5]

- ✧ Adult day care
- ✧ Available senior discounts
- ✧ Chore services
- ✧ Assistance with Medicare paperwork
- ✧ Homemaker's aides
- ✧ Home health aides
- ✧ Hospice services
- ✧ Hotline numbers
- ✧ Legal assistance
- ✧ Friendly visitors
- ✧ Meal services (e.g., meals on wheels)
- ✧ Medical equipment and supplies
- ✧ Support groups and counseling

Other aspects of the Older Americans Act reauthorization include such important issues as:

1. Allowing the municipalities and states greater flexibility in administering programs based on their respective priorities and needs
2. Enhancing and balancing the availability of services to vulnerable segments of the late life population (especially to those living in rural areas and low income minorities)[3,4]
3. Providing for new legislation (Senior Community Service Employment Program) under Title V that establishes procedures to ensure greater accountability, strong but reasonable placement and performance standards, introduces constructive competition into the program, establishes clear administrative cost definitions, affirms the importance of the legal assistance and ombudsman program, and

supports consumer grievance procedures as well as provides access to public hearings (without imposing an array of burdensome federal mandates).[3] The community services section of the reauthorized Older Americans Act makes possible about 60,000 part-time minimum-wage jobs for low-income people 55 and older.[4]

On November 13, 2000, Congress passed (H.R. 782) and President Clinton signed into law the National Family Caregiver Program. The funds are distributed to the states to provide counseling, caregiver training, respite care, and peer support as well as other assistance. These services will be available to younger individuals caring for older relatives as well as for older individuals providing care to younger disabled relatives.[4]

THE NATIONAL INSTITUTE ON AGING

The National Institute on Aging's purpose is to support and conduct social biomedical and behavioral aspects of training and research as related to disease of the elderly, special problems of older Americans, and the aging process.

MEDICARE

Medicare, a nationwide health insurance program for Social Security or railroad retirement beneficiaries and their spouses, was first established in 1965. It is also available to workers who are on disability (after an established waiting period).

Medicare now offers a number of health care options such as:[6]

1. Health maintenance organizations (HMOs). In this type of option consumers pay a specific fee to the HMO to cover services and then receive those services from providers of that HMO.

2. Preferred provider organizations (PPOs) are a form of managed care in which there are networks of providers who compete to provide services to the consumers of the PPO.

3. The newly established (in 2001) private fee-for-service plans. These services are only available in some areas of the United States. In this type of program the private insurance company provides health care to individuals (with Medicare) who join the plan. The consumer pays, and the insurance company pays a fee for each physician service or visit. It is the insurance company that decides how much it will pay and how much the consumer will pay. To receive service, hospitals and physicians (as well as other services) must accept the plan.

Within all these optional plans, private companies can decide if a plan will be available to everyone within the state or open only in certain counties. The company may also choose to offer more than one plan in an area with different costs and benefits.[6]

In general, the federal government provides a certain set amount of funds for private companies to provide health services (such as those just described). It has been this writer's experience that under Medicare managed care plans therapists often need to call the insurance company for weekly updates and permission for continued service.

The original Medicare plan is also known as fee-for-service. However, it is federally funded (not a part of a private insurance company) and is offered nationwide. In this plan the consumer is charged for each health care service or supply.[6]

Medicare is divided into two parts—"A" and "B." In all Medicare health plans the following applies: the consumer pays the monthly Medicare Part B premium. There is no monthly fee for Part A. The Part B fee is usually deducted from the monthly Social Security, railroad retirement, or civil service retirement payment.[6]

If a consumer has Medicare and qualifies for Medicaid (a joint federal and state program that helps to pay medical costs for some individuals with limited resources and low incomes who meet Medicaid guidelines), health care payments (including services such as nursing home care and outpatient prescription drugs that are not presently covered by Medicare) can be provided by Medicaid.[6]

If a client has questions regarding Medicare or Social Security the following resource telephone numbers are helpful:

- ✧ Medicare

  1-800-633-4227

  1-877-486-2048 (hearing and speech impaired)

- ✧ Social Security

  1-800-772-1213

  www.medicare.gov

The remainder of this appendix will include a description of the health services offered under Part A and Part B of the federal medicare program.

Part A provides for a variety of services such as inhospitalization (both acute and rehabilitation hospitals), skilled nursing facility (SNF) care, hospice, and home health.

Inhospital—Part A

If an individual requires medically necessary hospital care, he or she is entitled to 90 days per benefit period. There are also 60 additional hospital lifetime reserve days (not replenishable). No premium is required, but there are deductible and co-payments (varies in accordance to a specific payment schedule and is dependent upon the number of days hospitalized).[6]

Specifically, hospital stays usually cover a semi-private room, meals, general nursing, and other hospital services. The beneficiary pays a deductible during each benefit period. Occupational therapy is covered under Part A of the Medicare prospective payment system (which utilizes a present unit of payment known as diagnostic related groups [DRGs]. There are 470 DRGs and five major variables (age, diagnosis, sex, intervention procedure, and discharge status). In the hospital setting occupational therapy is considered to be a medically prescribed intervention that is concerned with improving or restoring functions that have been impaired by injury or illness.[6]

Inpatient mental health coverage in a psychiatric facility consists of 190 lifetime benefit days.[6]

Therapists need to keep current regarding any medical changes that Congress enacts throughout each year. The Balanced Budget Act of 1997 (Public Law 105-33) changed the type and the way coverage is utilized for SNFs, home health agencies, and rehabilitation hospitals. Formerly all these services were funded through a cost-based system with routine limits.

Rehabilitation Hospitals (Part A—Inpatient and Distinct Part Rehabilitation Units)

Under the prospective payment system for inpatient rehabilitation (RPPS) payments are based on national cost averages. These payments are directly proportional to the costs for "like" clients. Payments are higher for those individuals who are more costly to care for.[7]

The RPPS payment system is based upon an episode of care (per discharge). There is also a case mix classification system that defines client discharges by functional-related groups (know as FRGs). Categories such as client age, impairment, cognitive score, comorbidities, and functional capacity are used to differentiate clients.[7,8]

Each case mix group has a relative weight representative of the resources required to provide appropriate rehabilitation. As an example, an "average client" has a relative weight of 1.0. Clients with greater needs may have a relative weight greater than 1.0, while clients who require fewer resources may have a relative weight of less than 1.0. Payments are based upon the relative weight of the case mix group (CMG).[7]

CMGs are determined by the completion of a new assessment tool, the MDS-PAC (post-acute care). This is sometimes referred to as the client assessment instrument. Initially each client is placed into a rehab impairment category (RIC). Some of these examples include: traumatic brain injury, cardiovascular accident, hip fracture, neurological injury, orthopedic injury, amputation, cardiac, pulmonary, and osteoarthritis. Initially, there were 92 CMG payment groups. An example of how the payment system works can be considered by the following discussion. A client may be classified in the "stroke" impairment category and then is further subclassified into 11 different CMGs based on age and functional scores in the areas of mobility and activities of daily living.[7] Facility payments are then determined by a "wage index adjustment," a "rural hospital adjustment," and adjustments to hospitals who care for a disproportionate share of low-income clients. The RPPS encourages the completion of a full rehabilitation program (with discharge to the home).[7]

As we go to press, additional information has now been included regarding inpatient rehabilitation facilities.

✧   Roberts, P. (2002, July 8). Navigating the inpatient rehabilitation facility prospective payment system (IRF PPS). *OT Practice. (7)*12, CE-1-CE-8.

On August 7, 2001, the final rule for IRF PPS was published. All inpatient rehabilitation hospitals and units are now required to send medical payment information to the Centers for Medicare and Medicaid Services (CMS) as of January 1, 2002 (for clients in the facility on that date or admitted after that date). An IRF clinician (any clinician who assesses the client—may include the occupational therapist) must inform the client of his or her rights before assessment. This includes:

✧   The right to be informed of the purpose of the client assessment data collection

✧   The right to have client assessment information to remain secure and confidential

✧   The right to be informed that the client assessment information will not be disclosed to others (except for legitimate purposes that are permitted by federal or state regulations and the Federal Privacy Act of 1974)

✧   The right to see, review, or request changes on the assessment tool

✧   The right to refuse to answer client assessment data questions

The client assessment tool (IRF PA1) is used at admission and at discharge. This tool includes a function modifier (The Functional Independence Measure [FIM] instrument, (see resource on page 350) as developed and discussed by Hamilton, Granger, Sherwin, Zielenzy, and Tashman—1987) and mandatory and optional areas. Voluntary areas include medical needs such as determining if a person is delirious, comatose, dehydrated, or having swallowing difficulties. Another voluntary section addresses the quality of life indicators such as: pain, respiratory status, pressure and ulcer, and safety concerns such as balance and falls. Function modifiers such as bladder level of assistance, the frequency of bladder accidents, bowel level of assistance, the frequency of bowel accidents, shower transfer, tub transfer, distance walked, and distance traveled in a wheelchair are FIM items. This tool must be completed by the fourth day of admission and on discharge for all Medicare Part A clients. The lowest score on the functional modifiers and the FIM is evaluated on the first 3 days of admission and the last 3 days before discharge.

There are now 21 diagnostic categories that are used to determine the appropriate impairment code. *Comorbidities* (specific client conditions that are secondary to the client's etiological diagnoses) are also used to determine if a client can qualify for additional payment. These are divided into three tiers. If there are multiple comorbidities, the one under the highest cost tier is selected. There are now 95 clinical CMGs used in a typical case and five non-clinical CMGs (one for short stay and four for clients who expire while at the rehabilitation facility). *Cost outliers* (clients whose estimate cost exceeds the Medicare CMG payment plus a threshold amount); short stays; expired cases; and program interruptions are now considered special cases, with each category receiving specific payment guidelines.

Besides complying with the new PPS, rehabilitation hospitals and units must have a Medicare provider agreement and are required to provide rehabilitation nursing, occupational therapy, physical therapy, and/or speech-language pathology 3 hours daily, 5 to 6 days a week. Social work and psychosocial intervention as well as prosthetic and orthotic services must be available as needed. These facilities must also demonstrate that they serve an inpatient population of whom at least 75% require intensive rehabilitation services of intervention of at least one or more of the following 10 diagnostic categories:

1. Spinal cord injury
2. Congenital deformity
3. Stroke
4. Amputation
5. Major multiple trauma
6. Brain injury
7. Fracture of the femur
8. Polyarthritis
9. Burns
10. Neurological disorders

Many believe that this 75% rule (developed in 1984) needs to be amended, as it is thought that significant problems for Medicare beneficiaries who seek rehabilitation services may arise. Currently, the recommendation for Center for Medicare and Medicaid Services to adopt a policy whereby if 75% of an IRF's Medicare clients fall into 20% of the 21 RICs, the inpatient rehabilitation facility would be presumed to comply with the 75% rule.

Medicare changes, as demonstrated by PPS in IRFs, have been enormous. The only way to stay current is to consistently monitor changes that the federal government makes on a timely basis (via sources such as the Federal Register).

Skilled Nursing Homes—Part A Medicare

The PPS in the skilled nursing home setting depends upon accurate classification of the residents into resource utilization groups (RUG III or RUGs). The Health Care Financing Administration (now known as the Center for Medicare and Medicaid Services or CMS) uses 44 RUGs that are based upon the level of the resident's functional status. This includes categories such as activities of daily living performance, the need for therapies, the presence of depression, and the need for nursing rehabilitation. The per diem rate to a specific facility for each resident is based upon the established reimbursement for the RUG into which that particular resident is categorized.[9]

Residents are classified into a RUG using assessments from the minimum data set (MDS). The current MDS 2.0 uses 20 main sections (e.g., assessments of cognitive patterns, psychosocial, communication, disease diagnosis, structural problems, oral/nutritional problems, special procedures and interventions, and activity pursuit patterns). The assessments in each area are based on the most care a resident needs across a 7-day time frame and must be performed at a minimum on the following days: days 5, 14, 30, 60, and 90 of each resident's SNF stay.[9] The 5-day assessment is accomplished by reviewing the first 5 consecutive days of therapy a resident receives in the first 7 days of his or her SNF stay.[9] The activities of daily living category, which is found in section G, is one of the most often addressed for rehabilitation by occupational therapy. The section includes such activities as toileting, dressing, bed mobility, transfers, eating, and locomotion. However, these activities are also addressed by nursing caregivers during their daily care of the resident. Therefore, the assistance needed by a resident to perform an activities of daily living task needs to be seen by both a therapist and a nursing assistant's viewpoint.[9] It is exceedingly important that all team members (e.g., speech-language pathologists, occupational therapists, physical therapists, social workers, nurses, and physicians) work together in assessing residents.[9]

In Part A, skilled nursing homes utilize case mix requirements. The case mix is a system that measures the intensity of care and services required for each resident. This is then translated into a payment level. There are five rehabilitation subcategories for the MEDPAR (Medicare Provider Analysis and Review) Analogy. These are as follows:

- ✧ *Low rehabilitation*. Residents in this category receive at least 45 minutes of rehabilitative therapy services a minimum of three times a week.
- ✧ *Medium rehabilitation*. Requirements for this group provide residents with 150 minutes of therapy (in any combination of disciplines) for a minimum of 5 days (five 30-minute sessions) a week.
- ✧ *High rehabilitation*. High rehabilitation requires that residents receive a minimum of 325 minutes of therapy (one of the rehabilitation disciplines must be provided daily) at least 5 days per week.
- ✧ *Very high rehabilitation*. Residents in this category must be seen by therapy 500 minutes per week and must be receiving at least one of the disciplines for 5 days a week.
- ✧ *Ultra high rehabilitation*. This category is intended to apply to the most complex of rehabilitation therapy cases. In this subgroup two of the three therapy disci-

plines must provide services at least 720 minutes per week. One discipline provides services five times a week, and the second discipline provides services 3 days a week.

Categories medium to ultra high may also involve specified group sessions.[10]

The Federal Register (Medicare program, PPS, and consolidated billing for skilled nursing facilities—update final rule and notice) states that up to 25% of the intervention minutes that are recorded on the MDS can be conducted in a group setting (of no more than four participants) for each discipline involved.

    ✧   Federal Register (Health Care Financing Administration). (1999, July 30). Federal Register. 64(146): 41643-41668.

For example, occupational therapy might conduct a homemaking group. An OT or an OTA must run the group. Group intervention is an effective and efficient way to provide quality occupational therapy, and it also provides a means of achieving RUGS levels.[10,11]

To qualify for skilled nursing care services under Medicare A, an individual must have had a hospital stay of 3 consecutive calendar days. The beneficiary must be referred by a physician and require skilled nursing or skilled rehabilitation services for which they were treated while they were in the hospital. Beneficiaries are entitled to a semi-private room, meals, and skilled nursing and rehabilitative services, as well as other services and supplies.[6]

Restorative Nursing in Long-Term Care (and Prospective Payment System)

Through restorative care, residents maintain their highest functioning level. They enter restorative care after being discharged from skilled therapy services or when the nursing staff believes that the resident would benefit from this program (e.g., when a resident demonstrates increased tone, when a resident needs better positioning in a wheelchair or bed, and if there is a decline in activities of daily living functioning—particularly as it relates to toileting or transfers). Certified nursing assistants (CNAs) can provide opportunities in which residents may experience optimal independence in one or more of the following: performing general hygiene, self-feeding with verbal cues at the restorative dining table or in the restorative dining room, being led in exercises with graded resistance, having splints applied to a resident as to a specific wearing schedule to maintain or increase range of motion, and positioning in a bed or wheelchair.[12]

The Balanced Budget Act of 1997 and the PPS increased the need for quality restorative care in the nursing home setting. The low level of the RUGs requires residents to receive restorative care services and therapy simultaneously. The restorative program also plays an important role in promoting a successful state survey because it demonstrates follow-through after discharge from skilled therapy as well as maximizing functional independence. In many states there may also be a higher medical reimbursement for those Medicaid residents needing restorative care.[12]

The key to a successful restorative program is a well-trained and committed restorative CNA and a team effort between the nursing and therapy staff members. Therapy needs to be involved in CNA training (educating CNAs in the following areas such as ambulation, splinting, feeding, range of motion, transfers, activities of daily living, body mechanics and safety, prosthesis management, bed mobility, positioning, documentation [including daily and weekly documentation], and the PPS) so that the CNAs are aware of and can utilize methods, procedures, and documentation.[12]

Therapists as Managers Under Skilled Nursing Facilities and Prospective Payment Systems

Under the new PPS in SNFs, therapy managers will need to expand their role by adapting to a business model of rehabilitation. Within the PPS structure there are 14 rehabilitation categories. The rehabilitation category that a client falls into is determined by the number of days and minutes per week that therapy is provided. Thus, the higher the number of therapy minutes, the higher the daily rate. However, when one factors in the cost of providing the highest intensity therapy, the lower intensity rehabilitation levels (such as the low rehabilitation category) can, at times, actually prove to be more profitable for the facility. The Balanced Budget Refinement Act, recently enacted, provides some PPS relief to long-term care facilities by allowing them to opt for federal rates immediately rather than waiting 3 full years. On April 1, 2000, facilities began receiving a 20% rate increase in 15 RUG categories.[13]

There is a great deal of importance attached to timing utilization decisions. The MDS is filled out five times during the first 100 days of therapy. The facilities category and daily rate are based on the data that is recorded on the MDS for each of the five time periods. The MDS is the classification and payment tool. Therefore, programming decisions need to be coordinated with the MDS schedule so that any changes in program intensity are considered in light of facility resource advantage and client need. It is important to always meet therapy qualifiers. A mistake in this area could place a client into the default rate (the lowest rate category) and could be exceedingly costly to the facility. The five qualifiers must be managed efficiently and effectively in order to ensure proper entry time on the MDS.[13]

The therapy manager must continuously analyze the nursing documentation, the therapy documentation, and the MDS to ensure that the therapy program can be supported appropriately. For instance: *Section B: Cognitive Patterns* (memory, cognitive skills for decision making, and indicators of disordered thinking/awareness) are important areas and have implications whether a client is appropriate to receive skilled rehabilitation.[13]

Marilyn Rosee, MS, OTR (co-owner of Therapeutic Resources, a New York City-based rehabilitation staffing and management company) includes a sample Case Management Tracking Sheet and an MDS Schedule/Length of Stay Progress Note Tracking Calendar in her excellent article, "The Therapist as a Fiscal Manager: Surviving the SNF PPS and Beyond."[13] These resources are helpful tools for enabling clinicians to keep appropriate time tracking and client status on the MDS. This article explains the basics of effective therapy management under the new SNF PPS regulations.

On final thoughts regarding managing denials Rosee points out three high-risk areas found on the MDS:[13]

1. High utilization of rehabilitation without an appropriate diagnosis documented in the "I" section

2. Technical errors in the recording of day and time qualifications in the "P" section

3. Any MDS items that contradict the need for highly intense skilled rehabilitation.

For facilities to successfully capture shrinking rehabilitation dollars, therapists need to demonstrate that they are effective and efficient. Rosee suggests the FIM where outcomes can be measured against a national database.[13]

This is available from the following resource:
✧   Functional Independence Measure (1993)
      Uniform Data System for Medical Rehabilitation
      232 Parker Hall
      State University of New York at Buffalo
      3435 Main St.
      Buffalo, NY 14214

Rosee affirms that clinician managers can guarantee our profession a prominent position in the long-term care setting by developing strategies that pair quality care and functional outcomes for our clients with financial health for facilities that we serve.[13]

Hospice—Part A

Regulations for certification of Medicare providers became effective on November 1, 1983. The five basic tenets of hospice care are: symptom and pain control, diagnostic honesty, maintaining a high quality of life (as much as is possible), around-the-clock care (all disciplines are on call and must be available 24 hours a day as needed), and bereavement care.[14]

Hospice may be provided in a number of settings, such as free standing, institution based, home-based, a consortium, or respite care. A full array of services must be provided as needed. These include nursing care, occupational therapy, physical therapy, speech and language pathology, medical social services, physician services, home health aide and homemaker services, counseling (including spiritual, social, and mental health services), medical supplies (such as medication, dressings), and durable medical equipment (e.g., hospital beds, oxygen, walkers, and wheelchair).[6,14]

Hospices receive reimbursement through Medicare A, most private insurers, and most medical assistance plans. Reimbursement includes a per diem rate with a rate cap. This varies from provider to provider (based upon location, current guidelines, and the agency).[15] Inpatient respite care is provided to the caregiver (in a home situation) and available up to 5 days at a time. Beneficiaries are entitled to two 90-day periods, one 30-day period, and, in some instances, an extension period of indefinite duration.

Under the Medicare hospice benefit, the client is required to meet three major conditions. First, the individual must have a medical prognosis of 6 months or less to live. Second, the client cannot undergo curative intervention—all intervention must be palliative in nature. Third and lastly, the client and/or family members must be aware of the prognosis, or at least be able to understand the difference between palliative and curative care. In some cases, however, Medicare benefits may cover standard Medicare benefits. For instance, if an individual with end-stage renal disease falls and fractures a hip, the medical expenses can be billed to his or her standard Medicare plan. In this case, hospice will continue to provide services that are related to the end-stage renal condition.[15]

Medicare Home Health Services (May Be Under Medicare Part A or B)

Medicare Part A is redefined as a post-institutional home health benefit. It requires a 3-day hospital or SNF stay as an eligibility requirement. The client must also be certified as homebound, be under a physician's care, and be in need of part-time skilled nursing care or physical therapy and speech-language therapy. Home health agencies are responsible for other services such as: occupational therapy, social services, home health aide services, supplies, and other related services. Agencies are not responsible for providing durable hospital beds, walkers, and oxygen; these are provided by billing Medicare directly.[16]

New regulations and guidelines for reimbursement were established October 1, 2000. These include a variety of changes using a prospective payment approach. The PPS for home health agencies can be found in Subpart E under part 484 of the Conditions of Participation (HCFA, July 3, 2000).[17] The home health agency PPS final rule does not change the role of occupational therapy practitioners in performing the initial and comprehensive client assessment, known as the Outcome and Information Set (OASIS). At present time an occupational therapist cannot complete the initial OASIS assessments but can conduct the follow-up, transfer, and discharge assessments. This is due to the fact that occupational therapy is not recognized (under the Social Security Act) as an initial qualifying service under the Medicare home health benefit. The American Occupational Therapy Association is currently working to change this barrier. Although occupational therapy is not a qualifying service to initiate care, once occupational therapy is involved in the case, it may remain in (even after other qualifying services leave the case) as long as Medicare guidelines are followed.[16]

Under PPS 8 hours of therapy is measured by 10 visits and is inclusive of any visit ordered for any rehabilitation discipline.[17]

With the PPS, a home health agency receives a fixed payment from an episode of care which is based upon the client's characteristics and health status. This episode of care is a 60-day period that will coincide under a 60-day certification period. Clients may be recertified for an unlimited number of certifications/episodes as long as the client needs and qualifies for home health care services. Each episode is paid on the basis of the status of the client at the beginning of each episode. Four clinical scoring categories, four services utilization categories, and five functional status scoring categories are involved in determining 80 case mix categories.[18]

There are also provisions for a number of atypical episodes. One such category is the low utilization payment adjustment (LUPA) in which four or fewer visits are provided to a beneficiary. In this case payments will be received on the number of visits rather than episodic care.[18]

Another atypical episode is the significant change in condition (SCIC) in which the client's status changes significantly (either improvement or deterioration) in the 60-day episode. This change must be dramatic enough to reassign the client to another case mix grouping (HHRG).[18]

The partial episode payment (PEP) involves either the client's election to transfer to another home health care agency or the client is discharged from a home health agency and then is readmitted to the same agency within 60 days of the original start-of-care. There are stipulated payments to cover each situation.[18]

Outlier payment is a term that refers to cases in which the cost of resources utilized to meet a client's needs far exceeds the set payment. This loss is to be shared by CMS (Health Care Financing Administration, now termed the Centers for Medicare and Medicaid Services) and the agency.[18]

If a client continues to need and qualify for home health care after the 60-day period, the OASIS data collected during the final 5 days of certification will determine the HHRG for the next 60-day episode. The HHRG payment is for all visits and supplies that a particular home care agency provides. Visits and supplies are billed through the agency (consolidated billing).[18]

It is clear that the home health PPS system recognizes a client's functional status and therapy utilization as indicators of the kinds of intervention/resources the client needs and as such provides an opportunity for occupational therapy intervention.[18] In another article Siebert continues to discuss as follows: "Accurate assessment means payment will be appropriate for client care needs. Effective intervention means clients will achieve functional outcomes. OTs have expertise to share in both areas."[19, p. 13] By sharing strategies for accurate assessment and by demonstrating that occupational services enhance outcomes, occupational therapy can demonstrate that our services will benefit not only the client, but our agencies as well.[19]

PRIVATE PRACTICE—PART B (ALSO KNOWN AS OCCUPATIONAL THERAPY IN PRIVATE PRACTICE)

How to Qualify to Become a Medicare Provider

Occupational therapy is a Medicare provider. Occupational therapists are given a provider number and can directly bill Medicare for services rendered in a SNF, the office, the home, or any other appropriate setting. There have been payment limits (caps) in the past. However, Congress has declared a moratorium on Medicare Part B for outpatient caps during 2000, 2001, and 2002. For that period of time there will not be a dollar limit.

In a recent article, Clark very aptly describes how therapists can establish a private practice. Besides Medicare, a therapist may be directly reimbursed by other third-party payers or an individual.[20]

To obtain Medicare certification information as a private practitioner, one can tap into the CMS web site at www.cms.gov. There, one may find a state-by-state listing of intermediaries and carriers. Medicare certification permits a private practitioner to bill for services provided under Part B, or the outpatient benefit. Next, it is important to contact the Provider Enrollment Office to request HCFA Form 855, the Application for the Provider. A practice may be established as an "individual practitioner," a "corporation," or a "partnership." To become fully Medicare certified as an individual practitioner, a Federal Employee Identification Number for one's business must be submitted with HCFA Form 855 to the regional Medicare carrier for approval.[20]

Medicaid certification may be available, but it varies state by state, and restrictions on age may apply. Each state has different regulations for Medicaid.

Information concerning Medicaid may be obtained from the web page www.lcfa.gov/medicaid/mcaidpti.htm. This web page provides program information (including eligibility criteria and direct links to individual state Medicaid agencies). It may be easier to receive Medicaid certification if one has already received a Medicare provider number.[20]

Medicare guidelines require a physician to sign for recertification of the intervention plan every 30 days and that the physician actually see the chart every 30 days to allow for therapy reimbursement. Family nurse practitioners, clinical nurse specialists, physi-

Medicare and Occupational Therapy Coverage				
Area/Title of Service	*Provision for OT*		*Part*	
	Yes	No	A	B
Skilled nursing facility	X		X	X
Occupational therapy private practice (OTPP)	X			X
Comprehensive outpatient rehabilitation facilities (CORFs)	X			X
Hospital outpatient services	X			X
Physician's office or physician-directed clinic	X			X
Medicare managed options (Medicare & Choice): Health maintenance organization (HMO); Preferred provider organization (PPO); Competitive medical plan (CMP)	X		X	X
Home health	X		X	X
Hospital inpatient (including rehabilitation hospitals)	X		X	

cian assistants, and physicians may sign plans of intervention that therapists have established.[18]

Diagnosis must be accurate. For each intervention visit, current procedural terminology (CPT) coding of intervention procedures must match actual services. Each regional Medicare carrier publishes lists of International Classification of Diseases (ICD) codes that the carrier believes link appropriately to CPT codes for therapy modalities and procedures.[20] Current CPT codes can be obtained from the American Medical Association by calling 1-800-621-8335.

Occupational therapists are paid according to the physician's fee schedule that is published by CMS each year. Medicare pays 80% of Part B approved charges, and the secondary insurance carrier or client pays the remaining 20%. Each procedure that is identified by a CPT code is paid according to a formula that is adjusted by a geographical area.[20]

Occupational Therapy Private Practice—Understanding Terms

As of January 1, 1999, occupational therapy private practice (OTPP) bears the following description. An OTPP is an individual who meets all local and state licensing laws as an unincorporated partnership or unincorporated sole practitioner. An OTPP may also be defined as an individual who practices therapy as an employee of an unincorporated professional corporation, an unincorporated practice, or other incorporated therapy practice.[21]

Therapy services must be provided in the therapist's office or the client's home. An office is officially described as "the location(s) where the practice is operated in the state(s) where the therapist (and practice, if applicable) is legally authorized to furnish services, during the hours that the therapist engages in practice at that location."[21, p. 9] The OTPP must meet all state regulatory licensing requirements. Each therapist in a group must enroll "as an individual" with the appropriate carrier. Aides and assistants must be personally supervised by the therapist and employed by either the practice to which the therapist belongs or by the therapist directly.[21]

Other Part B Medicare Services

Other Part B Medicare services that occupational therapists may participate in include hospital outpatient services, SNFs rehabilitation services, physician offices (including physician-directed clinics), and comprehensive outpatient rehabilitation facilities (CORFs). Annual cap limits had been set in the past for Part B SNF rehabilitation services, but at this writing, there is a moratorium. However, Congress reserves the right to vote on this each year.

Occupational therapists who work for physicians and whose services are billed as "incident to physician's services" are now able to have their evaluations or re-evaluation services billed to Medicare B (even if the occupational therapy evaluative services take place on the same day that the physician bills a management code and evaluation [E and M] code for the client). Accordingly, the new modification of the CPT codes permits a physician's office to bill Medicare Part B as either 97004 or 97003 and an E & M code using the –25 modifier when the client is seen by the physician and the occupational therapist on the very same day.[22]

The policy affects only bills that physicians' offices submit to carriers. Billing by occupational therapists for Medicare B in private practice, SNF, CORFs, hospitals, and rehabilitation agencies were not affected by the original edits.[22]

Part B—Hospital Outpatient

As of August 1, 2000, the hospital outpatient setting uses the *hospital prospective payment system* (HOPPS) and *Correct Coding Initiative* (CCI). HOPPS changes the way all hospital outpatient services are paid and alters the Medicare reimbursement and billing for occupational therapy services that is provided in *partial hospitalization programs* (PHPs). HOPPS does not apply to occupational therapy services that are provided through hospital outpatient departments. These services are still paid under the Medicare Physician Fee Schedule. Billing for occupational therapy services that are provided in PHPs under hospital outpatient services, hospitals, and Medicare-certified community mental health centers (CMHCs) require the use of the HCPCS code G0129, revenue code 43X and condition code 41 on the HCFA-1450 claim. Under the HOPPS, a unit of service for a PHP is 1 day. There is only one HCPCS code that describes occupational therapy services in a PHP. The mix of services that are provided to PHP clients is determined by the CMHC or hospital. The Medicare program does not restrict the types of occupational therapy services provided in a PHP.[16]

Occupational therapy clinicians and practitioners in hospital outpatient departments must be aware of the current CCI edits when they bill Medicare for their services. New CCI edits are issued in January, April, July, and October of each year. The CCI manual specifics for Medicare carriers Mutually Exclusive Procedures, or those that cannot be performed during the same session. Comprehensive and Component Procedures are code combinations that will not be reimbursed when performed on the same date of service. These edits serve as "red flags" for insurance carriers when determining service reimbursement. The American Occupational Therapy Association works with the American Medical Association's Correct Coding Policy Committee in reviewing these code pairs and in recommending deletions or changes of code pairs that do not reflect CPT present practice patterns or rules.[16,23] Current copies of the CCI Manual can be ordered by calling the National Technical Information Service at 703-605-6000 and requesting Chapter 11, "Medicare, Evaluation, and Management Services."

APPEALS, DENIALS, CODES, AND WRITING FOR REIMBURSEMENT

The Medicare review is based upon diagnosis, ICD9 codes (e.g., contracture of the hand 718.44; abnormal posture 781.9; feeding difficulties 783.3; late effects of cerebrovascular disease [include conditions specified such as sequelae, which may occur at any time after the onset of causal condition] 438; hemiplegia; unspecified 342.9), number of visits, and duration of service.

Appeals

Medicare does allow for an appeal process. The following questions need to be asked and answered appropriately to ensure successful reimbursement.[24,25]

✧ Is the client eligible for Medicare benefits?

✧ Is the facility that the therapist is working in certified by Medicare?

✧ Is the therapist providing services that are appropriate for the diagnosis, and are those services covered under the law?

✧ Is there a physician's prescription/order?

✧ Does all documentation follow Medicare guidelines?

✧ Are qualified occupational therapy personnel providing skilled services?

✧ Are the occupational therapy services necessary and reasonable in meeting the client's intervention needs?

✧ Are the services being duplicated?

✧ Has the client been overtreated?[24]

✧ Is there expectation that the condition of the client will improve in a significant manner and within a reasonable time frame based on the client's rehabilitation potential?

Documentation that is appropriate is extremely important in addressing any appeal. First there must be evidence that skilled service was performed. Terminology such as "instruction and training in activities of daily living was provided by this occupational therapist" indicates what the therapist did for the client. Comparison data such as "previously the client was at maximum assist when standing at sink, has progressed to minimum assistance when standing at the sink" allows the reviewer and other medical personnel to conclude that there is a definite improvement in skill level. Functional outcome also needs to be addressed. Hence, the note should include the fact that the client was able to achieve sit-to-stand at minimum assistance which enabled him or her to transfer from the wheelchair to wash at the sink. A positive expectation of improvement must also be indicated. Achievement of goals and indications for new ongoing goals need to be employed (if intervention is to continue and be reimbursed). Indications of modifying or adjusting an intervention program based on the client's reaction to the intervention program can also be utilized to demonstrate that skilled intervention was carried out.[25]

CPT and Other Related Codes

CPT codes (a trademark of the American Medical Association Current Procedural Terminology [CPT] five-digit codes, two-digit codes, modifiers, and descriptions) are also a vital part of appropriate documentation. Providers must use the Health Care Financing Administration's (now the Centers for Medicare and Medicaid Services or CMS) Common Procedure Coding System. This represents the American Medical Association's CPT, and the CMS alphanumeric codes and local codes created by Medicare and other carriers to be used on an as-needed basis. Edits and modifiers are ongoing, and the CMS plans to issue a new manual every 3 months (January 1, April 1, July 1, and October 1). It is wise for every department, agency, facility, and practitioner to have access of these updates on a regular basis (through the CCI manual described earlier in this appendix). The CPT code book changes every January 1. The American Medical Association's annual update is usually available in October (edits, codes, modifiers) and can be ordered by calling 1-800-621-8335.[23]

In 1987, through legislation, Congress expanded Medicare coverage for occupational therapy as a Part B benefit in all outpatient settings. It recognized independent occupational therapists for direct billing. In 1992, payment for occupational therapy services was incorporated into the Medicare physician's resource-based relative value scale (known as the RBRVS) fee schedule. Under this system the CMS must pay for services in an office-based practice that is based upon the resources that are necessary to provide them. The formula that is utilized for computing this fee schedule rate divides each service into the components of work (approximately 54%), practice expense (41%), and malpractice or professional liability. The relative values for each of these components is adjusted by means of a geographic factor and multiplied by a dollar conversion factor. This was $38.2581 for the year 2001. This information is published in the Federal Register.[26]

Health care providers, when billing Medicare Part B, must use the current CPT codes. This means that occupational therapy and certified occupational therapy assistants providing services in work settings such as outpatient hospital services, SNFs (Part B), comprehensive outpatient rehabilitation agencies, outpatient rehabilitation agencies/services, and outpatient occupation therapy providers must be keenly aware of current terminology edits and modifiers. As an example of a change in CPT codes in 2001 the following is noted. Formerly reported as 97770 in the physical medicine and rehabilitation section, the American Occupational Therapy Association has worked with CMS and the American Medical Association to separate the following services for separate billing:

- ✧ *97532*: Development of cognitive skills to improve attention, memory, problem solving (includes compensatory training); direct (one-on-one) client contact by the provider, each 15 minutes.[26]

❖ *97533*: Sensory integrative techniques to enhance sensory processing and promote adaptive responses to environmental demands; direct (one-on-one) client
contact by the provider, for each 15 minutes.[26]

New Medicare Coverage—A Policy Change

An article in *The New York Times* (front page, Sunday edition, March 31, 2002) stated that Medicare coverage would now be allowed for older adults diagnosed with
Alzheimer's disease.[27] Under this policy Medicare will pay for more therapy (such as
occupational, physical, respiratory, and speech therapy; pharmacological services; and
psychotherapy). In regard to this new view of coverage, Kim A. Marchol (an occupational therapist from Itasca, Il) remarked, "People with Alzheimer's will be able to live
at home much longer and avoid institutionalization."[27] Christina A. Metzler (Director
of Federal Affairs at the American Occupation Therapy Association) also commented in
this article that the new policy was tremendously significant for clients. "In the past a
diagnosis of Alzheimer's could prevent a client from getting Medicare coverage for
therapy to treat other conditions—a broken hip, a broken wrist, or a stroke."[27] This new
policy signals that Medicare beneficiaries can no longer be denied reimbursement of
hospice care, home health care, or mental health care simply because they have an
Alzheimer's diagnosis.

Previously, individuals with this condition were often being denied medically necessary services due to the belief that these persons could not benefit or improve. It is
now believed, based on new studies, that individuals with Alzheimer's (especially in
the early stages) can often benefit from these formerly denied services. Most of the
companies that review claims for the federal government (under federal contracts) had
programmed their computers to reject claims for individuals with dementia (including
dementia of the Alzheimer's type). The new policy bans such computer software
instructions.[27]

This new interpretation of coverage indicates that occupational therapy personnel
will have added responsibilities and will be able to provide expanded services to those
late life individuals with a dementia diagnosis.

The Appeals Process: Handling Denials

There are four basic steps to the Medicare appeals process Part A and five to Part B.
❖ *Step 1: Reconsideration by the intermediary.* The following information should
be submitted: client identification, diagnosis (including the ICD9 Code), duration, the number of visits, the date intervention was initiated, and the billing
period.[24, 25] This process is also know as the *request for information.*

❖ *Step 2: Letter of recommendation.* Items that may trigger this level of review can
involve: The claim may have the limits that are set in the edits, the ICD9 code
that was previously submitted is not listed in the edits, the reviewer might feel
that a specific claim requires an intensified review (due to cyclical trends in
billing, such as a volume of claims increase on a quarterly basis), an extremely
high bill was submitted, overuse, or the claim was randomly selected for
review.[24, 25] The intermediary usually sends "a request for information letter." A

billing form (usually a HCFA1500) is then prepared by the provider that indicates the beneficiary's name, HICN, provider name and number, number of visits, duration and charges, service dates, itemization of all charges, history and physical examination, the discharge summary, previous history of therapy, the physician's orders/recertification/referral, process, evaluation notes and documentation, intervention logs and therapy records, initial evaluation with the intervention plan and intervention notes, diagnostic studies and screening, nurse's notes, the MDS form (used in SNFs and ICFs), and M23s or UB92s forms (when applicable). Documentation should indicate positive expectation of progress, need for skilled occupational therapy intervention, and progress achieved toward functional goals. There are 60 days for the provider to submit the letter of reconsideration. Other causes for denial at this level may involve the fact that one discipline that is unrelated to nursing or occupation therapy has written a statement that contradicts the results that have been documented by therapy and/or nursing.[24, 25]

✧ *Step 3*: If the Letter of Reconsideration is denied, then this information is presented at a hearing before an administrative law judge. The provider has 60 days to submit this appeal.

✧ Part B has an extra step from Part A. In Part B this step is known as a *fair hearing*. It comes before the hearing before an administrative law judge. In the fair hearing step the provider has 6 months in which to submit an appeal.[24, 25]

✧ *Step 4*: Finally, there is review by the United States District Court (Federal Court).

Steps 2 through 3 require minimal fees.[24, 25]

MEDICAL ASSISTANCE PROGRAM (UNDER TITLE XIX)—KNOWN AS MEDICAID

Under Medicaid, grants are given to each state to provide comprehensive health care to low-income people. Eligibility can vary from state to state because each state is permitted to develop its own criteria (within federal guidelines) based upon income, family composition, and resources. States are obligated to cover all persons who receive cash assistance (the aged, the disabled, and those receiving SSI are some of the categories affecting the elderly). These obligated services consist of inpatient hospital care, outpatient hospital care, rural health clinic services, SNFs, laboratory and x-ray services, home health care for those entitled to SNF services, and physician services.[24]

THE POLITICAL PROCESS: WHERE TO GET INFORMATION

Because the acts and laws governing federal funding of health care services are set by Congress, they will (most likely) be constantly changing. Therefore, it is important to know where to look for ongoing governmental changes. Three of the most important resources include:

✧   U.S. Statutes at Large
    U.S. Government Printing Office
    P.O. Box 371954
    Pittsburgh, PA 15250-7950
    202-512-1800
    fax: 202-512-2250
    At the end of each session of Congress this publication arranges laws in chrono-
    logical order by the date they were enacted.

✧   The Federal Register
    U.S. Government Printing Office
    Agencies (like CMS) publish finalized rules and regulations concerning admin-
    istrative law in the Federal Register.

✧   Reimbursement page of American Occupational Therapy Association's web site
    at www.aota.org.

Regarding federal funding and occupational coverage, there is much to consider.

Another important issue in governmental funding is that many health care providers do not choose to "run" for political/legislative offices. Therefore, many lawmakers may not fully understand the health care needs of their citizens. A partial answer to this is for health care professional providers to become part of the political process and run for office.

Rosee aptly affirms the need for occupational therapists to demonstrate their skills in improving functional outcomes in their clients with the following statement. "We need to integrate all of the reimbursement and compliance variables into a program design that demonstrates to third-party payers our value in the rehabilitation process and demonstrates to our facilities our contributions as revenue generators."[11, p. 21]

REFERENCES

1. Sloan, A. (2000, July 3). The Social Security crack up. *Newsweek*, 18-24.

2. Sykes, J. T. (Chairperson Public Policy Committee et al.). (1986, March/April). Public Policy Agenda 1986-1987. *Perspective on Aging—National Council on the Aging, 7,* 9-11, 33-37.

3. Deets, H. (2000, December). The Older American Act: A crowning achievement. *AARP Bulletin,* 20.

4. Deets, H. (2000, December). Hill deadlock stalls key bills. *AARP Bulletin,* 21.

5. Richman, N. & Glantz, C. H. (1996). *Section 5 Transition to home after hospitalization or reha-bilitation program.* In K. O. Larson, R. G. Stevens-Ratchford, L. Pedretti, & J. L. Crabtree (Eds.), *The role of occupational therapy with the elderly* (2nd Ed., p. 697). Bethesda, MD: The American Occupational Therapy Association, Inc.

6. Shalala, D. E. & De Parle, N. A. (2000, September). *Medicare and you 2001.* (Publication NO-HFA-10050). Washington, DC: US Department of Health and Human Services Health Care Financing Administration.

7. Lambert, A. S. (2001, March 5). Understanding inpatient PPPS. *Advance for Occupational Therapy Practitioners, 17*(5), 35.

8. Thomas, J. (2000, February 14). Payment changes on the horizon, *OT Practice, 5*(4), 13.

9. Bishop, S. E. & Thomas-George, R. (2000, June 5). Interdisciplinary teamwork and the prospec-tive payment system. *OT Practice, 5*(12), 11-14.

10. Colmar, M. (1998, June 22).: Terms and definitions under BBA. *Advance for Occupational Therapy Practitioners, 6,* 27-29.

11. Rosee, M. (2000, April 24). The Therapist as a Fiscal Manager: Surviving the SNF PPS and beyond. *OT Practice, 5*(9), 20-26.

12. Jain, M. N. & Wilson, L. (2000, August 14). Making restorative nursing work in long-term care. *OT Practice, 5*(16), 16-18.

13. Rosee, M. (2000, April 24). The Therapist as a fiscal manager: Surviving the SNF PPS and beyond. *OT Practice, 5*(9), 20-26.

14. Tigges, K. N. & Maral, W. M. (1996). Palliative Medicare and rehabilitation: Assessment and treatment in hospice care. In K. O. Larson, R. G. Stevens-Ratchford, L. Pedretti, & J. L. Crabtree (Eds.), *The role of occupational therapy with the elderly* (2nd Ed., p. 747). Bethseda, MD: The American Occupational Therapy Association, Inc.

15. Trump, S. M. (2000, June). The role of occupational therapy in hospice. *Home and Community Health—Special Interest Section Quarterly, 7*(2), 1-4.

16. (2000, September 25). AOTA's Reimbursement and Regulatory Policy Department: Capital briefing: Medicare News…The saga continues. *OT Practice, 5*(19), 10.

17. Johnson, K. V. (2000, September 11). Home health PPS: The new payment methodology. *OT Practice, 5*(18), CE-1-CE-8.

18. Siebert, C. (2000, March). An overview of the PPS for home health care. *Home and Community Health Special Interest Section Quarterly 7*(1), 3-4.

19. Diffendal, J. (2001, July 9). You can make it a happy ending: PPS in home health can actually benefit OTS. *Advance for Occupational Therapists, 17*(14), 12-13.

20. Clark, D. H. (2000, March). Considerations for the new private practitioner in occupational therapy. *Home and Community Health—Special Interest Section Quarterly, 7*(1), 1-2.

21. AOTA's Reimbursement & Regulatory Policy Department: Effective January 1, 1999. (1999, February 4). *OT Week,* 9.

22. AOTA's Reimbursement and Regulatory Policy Department. (2001, October 1). Medicare Potpourri. *OT Practice,6*(8), 5.

23. Hostetler, H., Stein, L., & Thomas, J. (2000, August 14). Capital briefing: Take responsibility for appropriate coding. *OT Practice, 5*(16), 9.

24. Lewis, S. (1989). *Elder care in occupational therapy* (pp. 33, 35, 204, 205, 242, 245, 250). Thorofare, NJ: SLACK Incorporated.

25. Lopes, M. & Slominski, T. J. (Eds.). (2000). *Medicare guidelines explained for the occupational therapist: A practical resource guide for occupational therapy service delivery.* Gaylord, MI: National Rehabilitation Services.

26. Thomas, J. Lloyd, L., & Hostetler, H. (2001, February 5). Capital briefing: New 2001 CPT codes. *OT Practice, 6*(3), 8.

27. Pear, R. (2002, March 31). Medicare is now covering treatment for Alzheimer's: New policy forbids denial of reimbursement. *The New York Times,* 1, 24-Section A

SUGGESTED READING

Benemerito, T. (2000, April 24). Capital briefing: Why you need to know your practice act. *OT Practice, 5*(9), 10.

Bishop, S. E. & Thomas-George, R. (2000, June 5). Interdisciplinary teamwork and the prospective payment system. *OT Practice, 5*(12), 11-14.

Fleischman, L. M. & Messick, B. W. (2000, November 20). Capital briefing: Occupational therapists in private practice: No simple answer. Part 1. *OT Practice, 5*(23), 8.

Fleischman, L. M. & Messick, B. W. (2000, December 4, 18). Capital briefing: Occupational therapists in private practice: No simple answer (Part 2). *OT Practice, 5*(24), 8.

Gourley, M. (2001, May 7). Choosing partners in private practice. *OT Practice 6*(9), 17-19.

Kass, J. E. (2001, March 19). Capital briefing: Understanding Stark and OT (Part 1 of 2). *OT Practice, 6*(6), 7.

Kass, J. E. (2001, April 2). Capital briefing: Understanding Stark and OT (Part 2 of 2). *OT Practice 6*(7), 8.

Toto, P., & Hill, M. (2001, June). OT/OTA Team building in the SNF environment: Meeting the challenge. *Gerontology Special Interest Section Quarterly, 24*(2), 1-4

Trump, S. M. (2001, November 5). Occupational therapy and hospice: A natural fit. *OT Practice, 6*(20), 7-11.

PACE: The Program of All-Inclusive Care for the Elderly (United States)

Appendix

B

The Program of All-inclusive Care for the Elderly (PACE) is a new Medicaid/Medicare benefit that provides social and medical services to frail older adults who would otherwise be eligible for nursing home care. PACE agencies/organizations employ a multi disciplinary team. This includes occupational therapy services that can be provided in the participants' homes, inpatient facilities, and in adult day health centers.[1] "Sections of the PACE regulation, published in November 1999, imply that occupational therapists have the requisite skills for not only the clinical, but also administrative positions with PACE organizations."[2, p. 13] This program is derived from a model of acute and long-term social and medical services that were offered by On Lok Senior Health Services in the 1970s.[2] In 1986, the Health Care Financing Administration (now termed the Center for Medicare and Medicaid Services) began approving demonstration project sites.[2] In 1997, the Balanced Budget Act established permanent benefits for PACE within the Medicare program. States were permitted to provide PACE services as a State Medicaid option.[3] At present there are 25 PACE organizations in 13 states (operating with dual coverage). The 25 PACE sites receive a per participant (per month) capitated payment from Medicaid and Medicare. There are eight sites that operate PACE programs under Medicaid-only capitation. Forty-one organizations are exploring the prospect of developing PACE centers to provide services to their community's seniors.[4]

An example of a PACE center is the Johns Hopkins Bay View Medical Center's Hopkins Elder Plus Program (Baltimore, MD). In 1996, this program began a 3-year PACE demonstration project.[2] Today this PACE program has 95 participants, and plans are underway for a second PACE center. The Hopkins Elder Plus Facility has 40 staff members (termed a *multidisciplinary care team*). This team collaborates closely with each participant. Every elder in the program has a primary care coordination team whose members are knowledgeable about his or her social and medical history. Comprehensive wellness, social, and medical services are provided at the PACE facility as well as in the elder's home. When needed, in-home personal care and skilled nursing services are arranged by the care coordination team. These services are provided by means of preselected contracting agencies.[2] Two meals are provided each day in the PACE facility. These consist of a continental breakfast in the morning and a hot, nutritious lunch. These meals are served in a large community room. Throughout the day a number of activities are held, such as nursing services (e.g., medications), restorative activities (including reviewing of and instructing in activities) that promote range of motion exercise to maintain upper and lower extremity/body movement, social activities such as a community bingo game; grooming (e.g., manicures), and scheduled appointments with other professionals.[2]

"The objective of PACE is to provide integrative preventive, acute, and long-term quality health care while maximizing state and federal reimbursement. By having a central facility with medical and social services, participants are encouraged to remain as healthy and independent as possible and to remain active members of society."[2, p. 21] The PACE organization is responsible for utilizing the present Medicare and medical prospective capitation payments. Because of this type of payment the organization needs to provide quality service and at the same time responsively manage costs. "Keeping participants healthy for as long as possible is the focus of care versus simply treating the illness or disease."[2, p. 21]

Participant enrollment is voluntary. Elder participants can stay as long as they like and can disenroll at any time. Occupational therapy is one of the core descriptives involved in evaluation, assessment, and reassessment. Occupational therapists can work directly with clients at PACE centers. They can also work in private agencies that have contracts with the PACE program organizations.[2]

According to a report from Abt Associates, Inc., the effect of costs that are associated with PACE and PACE's impact on Medicare indicate that there is evidence suggesting that the PACE program is responsible for the following:

PACE sites are able to operate a "modest surplus" (by keeping nursing home stays and the number of inpatient hospitalizations low).

Although the results were inconclusive, the participation in the PACE program suggests that there is an increase of satisfaction in health care and lowered mortality rates.

Funding from various sources (Medicare, Medicaid, grants, nonprofit agencies, and private insurance) creates a diverse revenue pool to make use of when a determination concerning a participant's health care service needs to be made (as itemizations and reporting to each funding source is not required).[5]

A number of cities in the United States have more than one PACE organization. Programs that have been successful throughout the demonstration period have done so because of their ability to establish standards of care that promote the importance of preventive care and cost-effective practices.[6]

Occupational therapists adapt, prevent, alter, restore, and establish new venues for performing daily activities. The goals, created with a client, are specific as to that individual's needs at a given time. "As a required PACE team member, occupational therapists assist in providing vital person-based and function-designed information that no other discipline offers."[2, p. 22] As the move toward wellness and community-based services affects reimbursement practices in state and federal regulation, the skills that occupational therapy has traditionally offered will become increasingly more meaningful and indispensable.[2]

REFERENCES

1. Thomas, J. (2000, February 14). Capital briefing: Payment changes on the horizon. *OT Practice, 5*(4), 13.

2. Alexander, T. C. (2000, July 17, 31). Setting the pace: The innovative program of all-inclusive care for the elderly—(PACE) offers a perfect fit for occupational therapists. *OT Practice, 5*(15), 20-22.

3. Balanced Budget Act of 1997. Pub. L. 105-33, 111 Stat 251.

4. Anonymous. (1999, May). *What is PACE? Locations and Links.* National PACE Association. Retrieved in May 1999 from www.natlpaceassn.org/overview/pace/locations.shtml.

5. White, A. J. (2000). The effect of PACE on costs to Medicare: A comparison of Medicare capitation rates to projected costs in the absence of PACE. (HCFA Contract No. 500-01-0027). Cambridge, MA: Abt Associates.

6. Rollins, G. (1999, June). Customer focus: Newly recognized PACE Programs benefit patients, providers, payers. *Executive Solutions for Healthcare Management, 7,* 13-16.

EVALUATION AND ASSESSMENT RESOURCES IN GERONTIC OCCUPATIONAL THERAPY

The most frequently used resources by occupational therapists:

ACTIVITIES/INTERESTS

✧ *Activity Assessment*

Crepeau, E. L. (1986). *Activity programming for the elderly* (pp. 39-41). Boston: Little, Brown.

✧ *Activities Configuration Tool* (gathers data concerning a client's education, work history, values, and other plans and interests).

Cynkin, S. & Robinson, A. M. (1990). *Occupational therapy and activities health: Toward health through activities*. Boston: Little, Brown.

✧ *Interest Checklist*

Matsutsuyu, J. S. (1969). The interest checklist. *Am J Occup Ther, 23,* 323-334.

Later revised to include factor analysis:

Nystrom, E. P. (1974). Activity patterns and leisure concepts among the elderly. *Am J Occup Ther, 28,* 337-345.

Later revised to include life satisfaction and the meaning of activities:

Gregory, M. D. (1983). Occupational behavior and life satisfaction among retirees. *Am J Occup Ther, 37,* 548-592.

A measure of occupation of older adults (instrumental, leisure, and social activities are evaluated)

✧ *The Washington University Activity Card Sort* (Baum, C. M., Edwards, D. F.)

Washington University

Program in Occupational Therapy

Campus Box 8505

4444 Forest Park Ave.

St. Louis, MO 63108

Fax: 314-285-1601

logsdonb@msnotes.wustl.edu

✧   Components of task-focused activity analysis

Crepeau, E. D. (1998). Activity analysis: A way of thinking about occupational performance. In M. E. Neistadt & E. B. Crepeau (Eds.), *Willard and Spackman's occupational therapy* (9th Ed., pp. 135-146). Philadelphia: Lippincott-Raven.

BEHAVIOR

Assessment that uses caregiver reports to obtain client information (with dementia clients):

✧   *The Functional Behavior Profile*

Baum, C. M., Edwards, D. F., & Morrow-Howell, N. (1993). Identification and measurement of productive behaviors in senile dementia of the Alzheimer's type. *Gerontologist, 33,* 403-408.

Assessment of *general behavior* (e.g., appearance, expression, reality orientation, nonproductive behavior); *interpersonal behavior* (e.g., cooperative, self-assertion, attention-getting behavior); and *task behavior* (e.g., engagement, concentration, coordination, ability to follow directions):

✧   *The Comprehensive Occupational Therapy Evaluation Scale* (COTE)

Brayman, S. J., Kirby, T. F., Misenheimer, A. M., & Short, M. J. (1976). Comprehensive Occupational Therapy Evaluation. *Am J Occup Ther, 30*(2), 94-100.

COGNITION (INCLUDING MEMORY AND FUNCTION)

Cognitive performance as related to functional status:

✧   *Allen Cognitive Level Test* (A Standardized Leather Lacing Task)

✧   *Large Allen Cognitive Level Test* (used specifically with geriatric patients who manifest cognitive disabilities and physical limitations)

✧   *The Routine Task Inventory* (pragmatic observational measure of performance)

✧   *The Cognitive Performance Test* (Standardized ADL-based tool for assessing the client's functional level in Alzheimer's disease)

Allen, K. A., Kehrberg, K.,& Burns, T. (1992). Evaluation instruments. In K. A. Allen, C. A. Earhart, & T. Blue (Eds.), *Occupational therapy treatment goals for the physically and cognitively disabled* (pp. 31-84). Bethesda, MD: The American Occupational Therapy Association, Inc.

1-877-404-AOTA

www.aota.org

Memory and Orientation:

✧ *The Galveston Orientation and Amnesia Test* (GOAT)

Levin, H. S.

Division of Neurosurgery, Department of Surgery

University of Texas Medical Branch

Galveston, TX

Levin, O-Donnell, Rossman, 1979

Daniel, M. S. & Strickland, L. P. (1992). *Occupational therapy protocol management in adult physical dysfunction* (pp. 62-63). Gaithersberg, MD: Aspen.

Cognitive abilities:

✧ *The Cognitive Assessment of Minnesota*

Rustad, R. and Associates

Therapy Skill Builders

555 Academic Court

San Antonio, TX 78204

1-800-211-8378

www.tpcweb.com

Memory:

✧ *The Contextual Memory Test*

Toglia, J. P.

Therapy Skill Builders

555 Academic Court

San Antonio, TX 78204

1-800-211-8378

www.tpcweb.com

Functional assessment for persons with Alzheimer's disease:

✧ *The Daily Activities Questionnaire: A Functional Assessment for People with Alzheimer's Disease*

Oakley, F., Sunderlan, T., Hill, J. L., Phillips, S. L., Makuhon, R., & Ebner, J. P. (1992). The Daily Activities Questionnaire: A functional assessment for people with Alzheimer's disease. *Physical and Occupational Therapy in Geriatrics, 10,* 67-81.

Mental status/cognitive performance:

✧ *The Global Deterioration Scale for Assessment of Primary Degenerative Dementia*

Reisberg, B., Ferris, S. H., Leon, M.J., & Crook, T. (1982). *Am J Psychiatry, 139,* 1136-1139.

✧ Mini-Mental State

Folstein, M. F., Folstein, S. E., & McHugh, P. R. (1975). Mini-Mental State: A practical method for grading the cognitive state of patients for the clinician. *J Psychiatr Res, 12,* 180-198.

Cognitive functioning (multi context—cognitive attention):

✧ *Assessment of the Components of Attention*

Golisz, S. M. & Toglia, J. P. (1998). Section 2: Evaluation of Perception and Cognition. In M. E. Neistadt & E. B. Crepeau (Eds.), *Willard and Spackman's occupational therapy* (9th Ed., p. 267). Philadelphia: Lippincott-Raven.

CANCER

Cancer evaluation components:
✧   Cancer Evaluation Process

Pizzi, M., & Burkhardt, A. (1998). Occupational therapy for adults with immunological diseases. In M. Neistadt & E. P. Crepeau (Eds.), *Willard and Spackman's occupational therapy* (9th Ed., pp. 703-715). Philadelphia: Lippincott-Raven.

✧   Lymphedema: Aspects of evaluation and treatment

Botten, L. (2001, September 17). Lymphedema management: An emerging practice area. *OT Practice, 6*(17), 13-15.

CHRONIC OBSTRUCTIVE PULMONARY DISEASE

Chronic obstructive pulmonary disease (COPD) evaluation components:

Stump, J. R. (1999, July/August). Treating chronic pulmonary disease. *OT Practice, 4*(6), 28-31.

CARDIAC

Cardiac evaluation components:
✧   The Cardiac Evaluation Process

Ferraro, R. (1998). Cardiopulmonary dysfunction in adults. In M. E. Neistadt & E. B. Crepeau (Eds.), *Willard and Spackman's occupational therapy* (9th Ed., pp. 693-696). Philadelphia: Lippincott-Raven.

DEPRESSION

Depression:
✧   *The Geriatric Depression Scale*

Gallo, J., Reichel, W., & Anderson, L. (1988). *Handbook of geriatric assessment*. Rockville, MD: Aspen.

Also found in:

Butin, D. N. (1996). Section 4: Psychosocial and Psychological Components. In K. O. Larson, R. G. Stevens-Ratchford, L. Pedretti, & J. L. Crabtree (Eds.), *The role of occupation therapy with the elderly* (2nd Ed., p. 616). Bethesda, MD: The American Occupational Therapy Association, Inc.

✧   *The Beck Depression Inventory*

Gallagher, D. (1986). The Beck Depression Inventory and older adults: Review of its development and utility. In T. L. Brink (Ed.), *Clinical gerontology: A guide to assessment and intervention,* (pp. 149-163). New York: Haworth.

✧   *The Short-Care* (assess dementia, functional disability, and depression)
Gurland, B. & Wilder, D. (1984). The Care Interview Revisited: Development of an efficient system of clinical assessment. *J Gerontol, 39,* 129-137.

DIABETES

Diabetes mellitus Type 2 evaluation components:

✧   Diabetes Mellitus Type 2 Evaluation Process
Daniel, M. S. & Strickland, L. R. (1992). *Occupational therapy protocol management in adult physical dysfunction.* Gaithersberg, MD: Aspen.

DEVELOPMENTAL DISABILITIES

Assessment of older adults with DD who may be experiencing dementia (focuses upon identifying dementia with late life adults who are already diagnosed with developmental delay):

✧   *The Ruocco Geriatric Assessment*
Ruocco, L. E. (2000, February). *Geriatric Assessment of Individuals with Intellectual Disabilities—A Four Part Rating Scale.* Paper presented at the Office of Mental Retardation, "Everyday Lives Conference": Hershey, PA.

DRIVING

✧   *The Useful Field of View Test* (Measures how drivers process visual information)
Owsley, C., Ball, K., McGuin, G., Sloan, M., Roenker, D., White, M., et al. (1998). Visual processing impairment and risk of motor vehicle crash among older adults. *JAMA, 279,* 1083-1088.

✧   *The Useful Field of View* (UFOV) (a computer-administrative and computer scored test of visual attention for adults)
Ball, K., Roenker, D.
Useful Field of View (UFOV) Software
Therapy Skill Builders
1-800-211-8378
www.tpcweb.com

DYSPHAGIA

Dysphagia evaluation components:

✧   *Dysphagia Evaluation Form*
Nelson, K. (1996). Dysphagia evaluation and treatment. In L. W. Pedretti (Ed.), *Occupational therapy: Practice skills for physical dysfunction* (4th Ed., pp. 178-179). St. Louis, MO: CV Mosby Year Books.

✧   *Dysphagia Evaluation Protocol*
      Avery-Smith, W., Rosen, A. B., & Dellarouse, D.
      Therapy Skill Builders
      The Psychological Corporation
      555 Academic Court
      San Antonio, TX 78204
      1-800-211-8378

FALLS

Assessing the fear of falling:
✧   *Fall Efficacy Scale*
      Tinetti, M., Richman, D., & Powel, L. (1900). Falls efficacy as a measure of fear
      of falling. *J Gerontol, 45,* 239-240.

Fall hazards:
✧   *Falls Interview Schedule* (FIS) (Falls History)
      Cook, A. & Miller, P. A. (1996). Section 2: Prevention of Falls in the elderly
      (Appendix A). In K. O. Larson, R. G. Stevens-Ratchford, L. Pedretti, & J. L.
      Crabtree (Eds.), *The role of occupational therapy with the elderly* (2nd Ed., pp.
      662-663). Bethesda, MD: The American Occupational Therapy Association,
      Inc.

FUNCTIONAL EVALUATIONS/ASSESSMENTS

Functional evaluations and assessments:
✧   *The Barthel Index* or *Barthel Self-Care Index*
      Mahoney, F. S. & Barthel, D. W. (1965). Functional Evaluation: The Barthel
      Index. *MD State Medical Journal, 14,* 61-68.
✧   *The Functional Independence Measure* (FIM)
      Uniform Data System for Medical Rehabilitation
      Center for Functional Assessment Research
      State University of New York at Buffalo
      3435 Main St.
      Buffalo, NY 14214

Practical measure of cognitive functioning using a demonstrated task:
✧   *The Kitchen Task Assessment*
      Baum, C. & Edward, D. F. (1993). Cognitive performance in senile dementia
      of the Alzheimer's type: The Kitchen Task Assessment. *Am J Occup Ther, 47,*
      431-435.

Meal preparation/Kitchen evaluation:
✧   *Rabideau Kitchen Evaluation — Revised* (RKE-R)
      Neistadt, M. E. (1994). A meal preparation treatment protocol for adults with
      brain injury. *Am J Occup Ther, 48,* 437.

Neistadt, M. E. & Crepeau, E. B. (Eds.). (1998). *Willard and Spackman's occupational therapy* (9th Ed., pp. 318-319). Philadelphia: Lippincott-Raven.

Living skills:

❖ *Kohlman Evaluation of Living Skills* (KELS) (3rd Ed.)

The American Occupational Therapy Association, Inc.

1-877-404-AOTA

www.aota.org

HOME HEALTH/ HOME ASSESSMENT/HOME MANAGEMENT

❖ *Structured Observational Test of Function* (SOTOF)

Laver, A. J. (1994). The Structured Observational Test of Function (SOTOF). AOTA *Gerontology Special Interest Section Newsletter, 1*(17), 1-3.

Laver, A. J. & Powel, G. E. (1995). *The structured observation test of function (SOTOF): Test manual.* Windsor: NFER-Nelson.

Analysis of functional activities to identify cognitive skill deficit areas:

❖ *The Arnadottir OT-ADL Neuro Behavioral Evaluation* (A-One)

Arnadottir, G. (1990). *The brain and behavior: Assessing cortical dysfunction through activities of daily living.* St. Louis: CV Mosby.

General geriatric occupational therapy evaluation (useful in a number of therapeutic settings in which rehabilitation has taken place and the consumer is in his or her home or plans to return to his or her home):

❖ *The General Occupational Therapy Evaluation for Geriatric Clients*

Lewis, S. C. (2003). *Elder care in occupational therapy* (2nd Ed.). Thorofare, NJ: SLACK Incorporated.

Areas of concern when observing and evaluating home and self-care tasks:

❖ *Table 15-1: Functional Mobility, Personal Care and Home Management Tasks Included in Evaluation Tools*

Rogers, J. C. & Holm, B. M. B. (1998). Evaluation of occupational performance areas. In M. E. Neistadt & E. B. Crepeau (Eds.), *Willard and Spackman's occupational therapy* (9th Ed., p. 189). Philadelphia: Lippincott-Raven.

Home health management:

❖ *The Home Assessment Checklist for Fall Hazards*

Cook, A. & Miller, P. A. (1996). Section 2: Prevention of falls in the elderly. In K. O. Larson, R. G. Stevens-Ratchford, L. Pedretti, & J. L. Crabtree (Eds.), *The role of occupational therapy with the elderly* (2nd Ed., pp. 664-666). Bethesda, MD: American Occupational Therapy Association, Inc.

Home Health:

❖ *Activities of Daily Living Evaluation* (Adapted from the Activities of Daily Living Evaluation Form 461-1, Hartford, CT: The Hartford Easter Seal Rehabilitation Center)

Foti, D., Pedretti, L. W., & Lillie, S. (1996). Activities of daily living. In L. W. Pedretti (Ed.), *Occupational therapy: practice skills for physical dysfunction* (4th Ed., p. 487). St. Louis, MO: CV Mosby Year Books.

✧ *Occupational therapy department activities home management form* (adapted from Activities Home Management Form, Occupational Therapy Department, University Hospital, Ohio State University at Columbus).

> Foti, D., Pedretti, L. W. &, Lillie, S. (1996). Activities of daily living. In L. W. Pedretti (Ed.), *Occupational therapy: Practice skills for physical dysfunction* (4th Ed., p. 463). St. Louis, MO: CV Mosby Year Book.

Home assessment activities competency (client-oriented functional assessment):
✧ *The Home Activities Check List*

> Trombly, C. A. (1997). *Occupational therapy for physical dysfunction*. New York: Lippincott, Williams and Wilkins.

Adaptive home management:
✧ *Occupational Therapy Evaluation of the Philadelphia Corporation for Aging Housing Department*

> Rosage, L. J. & Klein, S. I. (2001, April 19). *Home modifications: Occupational therapy and the Philadelphia Corporation for Aging*. Philadelphia: American Occupational Therapy Association 81st Annual Conference.

HOSPICE AND BEREAVEMENT

✧ *Locus of Control*

> Reid, D. W. & Ziegler, M. (1981). The desired control measure and adjustment among the elderly. In H. Lefcourt (Ed.), *Research with the Locus of Construct* (Vol.1). New York: Academic Press.

✧ *Occupational History—Occupational Inquiries* (K.N. Tigges)

> Larson, K. O., Stevens-Ratchford, R. G., Pedretti, L., & Crabtree, J. L. (1996). *The role of occupational therapy and the elderly* (2nd Ed., pp. 127-159). Bethesda, MD: American Occupational Therapy Association, Inc.

> Tigges, K. N. (1993). Occupational therapy. In D. Doyle, G. Hanks, & N. MacDonald, (Eds.), *Occupational textbook of palliative medicine*. Oxford: Oxford University.

✧ *Role Adaptation Bereavement Inventory* (for clients grieving the death of a primary life partner who experience difficulty adapting to new roles as a result of depression or atypical grief reactions).

> Larson, K. O. (1992). *Initial study for internal reliability of the Role Adaptation Bereavement Inventory*. Unpublished Master's Thesis, New York University.

INTEGRATIVE ABILITIES

✧ *The Smaga and Ross Integrative Battery* (SARIB)

> Ross, M. (1997). *Integrative group therapy: Mobilizing coping abilities with the five-stage group*. Bethesda, MD: American Occupational Therapy Association, Inc.

Sensory integration inventory:
✧ *The Sensory Integration Inventory* (identifies possible patterns of S.I. dysfunction)

Reisman, J. & Hanschu, B. (1992). *Sensory integrative inventory—Revised for individuals with developmental disabilities.* Hugo, MN: PDP.

MUSCLES/MANUAL MUSCLE TESTING/ FUNCTIONAL MOVEMENT

Manual muscle testing/Joint range measures:

✧ *Rehabilitation Institute of Chicago Occupational Therapy Department— Functional Skills/Motor Function*

Neistadt, M. E. & Crepeau, E. B. (Eds.). (1998). *Willard and Spackman's occupational therapy* (9th Ed., pp. 244-245). Philadelphia: Lippincott-Raven.

Functional balance and movement:

✧ *The Gait and Balance Test* (performance based mobility evaluation)

Tinetti, M. E. (1986). Performance-oriented assessment of mobility problems in elderly patients. *J Am Geriatr Soc, 34,* 119-126.

Hip Fracture:

✧ Baseline evaluation

Morawski, D. M., Pitbladdo, K., Biancki, E. M., Lieberman, S. L., Novic, J. P., & Bobrove, H. (1996). Hip fractures and total hip replacement. In L. W. Pedretti (Ed.), *Occupational therapy: Practice skills for physical dysfunction* (4th Ed., p. 740). St. Louis, MO: CV Mosby Year Book.

Motor dexterity (upper extremity):

✧ *The Box and Block Test*

Mathiowetz, V., Volland, G., Kashman, N., & Weber, K. (1985). Adult norms for the Box and Block Test of manual dexterity. *Am J Occup Ther, 39,* 386-391.

✧ *Nine Hole Peg Test of Finger Dexterity*

Mathiowetz, V., Weber, K., Kashman, N., & Volland, G. (1985). Adult norms for the Nine Hole Peg Test of finger dexterity. *Occupational Therapy Journal of Research, 5,* 24-38.

Joint range measurement form for the upper extremity:

✧ *Joint Range Measurements* (with permission from the Rehabilitation Institute of Chicago)

Neistadt, M. E. & Crepeau, E. B. (Eds.). (1998). *Willard and Spackman's occupational therapy* (9th Ed., p. 234). Philadelphia: Lippincott & Raven.

Muscle strength grades:

✧ *Muscle Testing Grades*

Pedretti, L. W. (Ed.). (1996). *Occupational therapy: Practice skills for physical dysfunction* (4th Ed., p. 113). New York: CV Mosby Year Book.

✧ Grip and pinch strength (using dynamometers and pinch meters with adult normative data)

Mathiowetz, V., Kashman, N., Volland, G., Weber, K., Dowe, M., & Rogers, S. (1985). Grip and pinch strength: Normative data for adults. *Arch Phys Med Rehabil, 66,* 69-74.

Muscle evaluation:

❖ *Muscle Examination* (Adapted with the express permission and authority of the March of Dimes Birth Defects Foundation)

> Pedretti, L. W. (Ed.). (1996). *Occupational therapy: Practice skills for physical dysfunction* (4th Ed., pp. 114-115). New York, CV Mosby Year Book.

Assessment of motor and process skills:

❖ *Assessment of Motor and Process Skills* (observational measure of real life tasks—the motor exploration and the degree of physical effort that a client experiences during an ADL task. The process aspect reflects the overall level and use of time, space organization and safety as well as the ability to compensate for these problems).

> Fisher, A. C. (1999). *Assessment of motor and process skills* (3rd Ed.). Fort Collins, CO: Three Star.

Suggested reading:

> Bray, K., Fisher, A., & Puron, L. (2001, July/August). The validity of adding new tasks to the assessment of motor and process skills. *Am J Occup Ther, 55*(4), 409-415.

NEUROLOGICAL AND PHYSICAL IMPAIRMENT

Test to determine the level of motor recovery presence of synergistic movements, and any associated reaction of the degree of hypertonicity in the CVA client:

❖ *Brunnstrom Test* (The Hemiplegia Classification and Progress Record)

> Pedretti, L. W. (1996). Movement therapy: The Brunnstrom approach to the treatment of hemiplegia. In L. W. Pedretti (Ed.), *Occupational therapy: Practice skills for physical dysfunction* (4th Ed., pp. 406-408). St. Louis, MO: CV Mosby Year Book.

Test determining abnormal movement patterns, abnormal motor patterns, presence of primitive reflexes, righting reactions, abnormal coordination, protective reactions, equilibrium and postural mechanism (Neurodevelopmental: Bobath):

❖ This type of evaluation's emphasis is upon the quality of movement. The therapist observes changes of tone, postural reactions, and coordination rather than looking at specific joints and muscles.

> Bobath, B. (1978). *Adult hemiplegia: Evaluation and treatment.* London: William Heinemann Medical Books.

Also found in:

> Davis, J. Z. (1996). Neurodevelopmental treatment of adult hemiplegia: The Bobath approach. In L. W. Pedretti (Ed.), *Occupational therapy: Practice skills for physical dysfunction* (4th Ed.). St. Louis, MO: CV Mosby Year Books.

Proprioceptive neuromuscular facilitation evaluation (PNF) techniques (useful when working with Parkinson's disease, arthritis, and CVA):

❖ PNF Evaluation—Follows a sequence from proximal to distal (i.e., vital functions such as breathing, swallowing, voice production, oral and facial musculature, ocular-visual control). Next the head and neck would be considered. Tone, alignment (midline or shift to one side?) and stability are observed throughout the evaluation. Each segment is evaluated individually (in specific movement patterns) as well as in developmental activities in which there is interaction of body segments).

> Davis, J. Z. (1996). Neurodevelopmental treatment of adult hemiplegia: The Bobath approach. In L. W. Pedretti (Ed.), *Occupational therapy: Practice skills for physical dysfunction* (4th Ed., pp. 420-421). St. Louis, MO: CV Mosby Year Books.

Also available:

> Voss, D. E., Ionta, M. K., & Myers, B. J. (1985). *Proprioceptive neuromuscular facilitation* (3rd Ed.). Philadelphia: Harper and Row.

Evaluation using the Rood approach (neuromuscular dysfunction)

✧ The client is evaluated developmentally and treated sequentially. The client does not proceed to the next developmental sensorimotor level until some measure of supraspinal (voluntary) control is achieved. The cephalocaudal rule is followed (intervention begins with the head and proceeds from proximal until the sacral area is reached).

> McCormack, G. I. (1996). The Rood approach to treatment of neuromuscular dysfunction. In L. W. Pedretti (Ed.), *Occupational therapy: Practice skills for physical dysfunction* (4th Ed., pp. 377-399). St. Louis, MO: CV Mosby Year Book.

> Farber, S. (1974). *Sensorimotor evaluation and treatment procedures for allied health personnel.* Indianapolis: Indiana University and Purdue University at the Indianapolis Medical Center.

> Farber, S. (1982). *Neurorehabilitation: A multisensory approach.* Philadelphia: WB Saunders.

OCCUPATIONAL PERFORMANCE/ROLES

Individualized measure of a client's self-perception in occupational performance (with emphasis upon productivity, self-care and leisure):

✧ *Canadian Occupational Performance Measure* (COPM)

> The Canadian Association of Occupational Therapists. (1994). Toronto, Ontario, Canada: ACE Publications.

Also available from:

> The American Occupational Therapy Association

✧ Complete COPM starter kit

✧ COPM training video

✧ COPM video companion workbook

✧ 100 COPM Measure Forms

> 1-877-404-AOTA
>
> www.aota.org

✧ *Occupational Performance History Interview II* (OPHI-II)

> The American Occupational Therapy Association
>
> 1-877-404-AOTA
>
> www.aota.org

✧   *Assessment of Communication and Interaction Skills* (ACIS)
     The American Occupational Therapy Association
     1-877-404-AOTA
     www.aota.org

The use of the occupational role history:

✧   The occupational role history is useful in determining a balance of activities.
     Watanabe, S. (1968). *Activities configuration: Regional institute on the evalua-tion Process*. Final Rep. RSA-123-T-68, New York, American Occupational Therapy Association, Inc.

Clients' perceived roles throughout the life span:

✧   *The Role Checklist*
     Oakley, F., Kielhofner, G., Barris, R., & Reichler, R. K. (1986). The Role Checklist: Development and empirical assessment of reliability. *Occupational Therapy Journal of Research, 6,* 157-170.

PARKINSON'S DISEASE

Parkinson's disease evaluation components:

✧   The Parkinson's disease evaluation process
     Hooks, M. L. (1996). Parkinson's disease. In L. W. Pedretti (Ed.), *Occupational therapy: Practice skills for physical dysfunction.* (4th Ed., pp. 845-851). St. Louis, MO: CV Mosby Year Book.

✧   *ADL Oriented Assessment-of-Mobility Scale* (For those with Parkinson's disease and dementia)
     Pomerov, V. (1990). Development of an ADL Oriented Assessment-of-Mobility Scale suited for use with elderly people with dementia. *Physiotherapy, 76(8),* 446-448.

✧   *The Fatigue Severity Scale*
     Friedman, J. & Friedman, H. (1993). Fatigue in Parkinson's disease. *Neurology, 43,* 2016.

SAFETY IN THE HOME

✧   *The Functional Assessment and Safety Tool* (FAST)—helpful with discharge planning
     Darzins, P., Edwards, M., Lowe, S., McEvoy, E., Rudman, D., & Taipalek, et al. (1994). *Functional assessment and safety tool user's manual.* Hamilton, MC Master University/Hamilton Civic Hospitals

Home safety evaluation:

✧   *Home Safety Evaluation and Home Safety Tips to Prevent Falls—Appendix 3: Module Handouts*
     Mandel, D. R., Jacobson, J. M., Zemke, R., Nelson, L., & Clark, F. (1999). Home and safety evaluation and home safety tips to prevent falls—Appendix 3: Module handouts. *Lifestyle redesign: Implementing the well elderly pro-gram.* Bethesda, MD: American Occupational Therapy Association, Inc.

✧ *The Safety Assessment of Function and the Environment for Rehabilitation (SAFER) Tool*—evaluates the older adult's ability to manage in the home and provides recommendations.

> Oliver, R., Blathwayt, J., Bruckley, C., & Tamaki, T. (1993). Development of the safety assessment of function and the environment (SAFER) tool. *Canadian Journal of Occupational Therapy, 60,* 78-82.

> Letts, L. & Marshall, L. (1995). Evaluating the validity and consistency of the SAFER tool. *Physical and Occupational Therapy in Geriatrics, 13,* 4, 49-66.

✧ *The Home Occupation-Environment Assessment* (HOEA) (useful with clients with dementia)

> Baum, C., Edwards, D., Bradford, T., & Lane, R. (1995). *Home occupation environment assessment (HOEA).* St. Louis: Occupational Therapy Program, Washington University.

> Fax: 314-286-1601

> logsdonb@msnotes.wustl.edu

SENSORY

Evaluation of touch and pressure sensibility in the hand:

✧ *Semmes-Weinstein Monofilament Test* (Recommend the "mini-kit" which is useful in determining the absence or presence of protective sensation)

> Weinstein, S. (1993). Fifty years of somatosensory testing: From the Semmes-Weinstein Monofilaments to the Weinstein Enhanced Sensory Test. *J Hand Ther, 6,* 11-22.

SENSORY STIMULI RESPONSE—MENTAL HEALTH

Self-report assessment that measures the client's behavioral response to sensory stimuli:

✧ *The Adult Sensory Profile*

> Brown, C. & Dunn, W. (1999). *The Adult Sensory Profile: Describing sensory processing in schizophrenia.* Paper presented at the meeting of the American Occupational Therapy Association. Indianapolis, IN.

STEREOGNOSIS

Testing stereognosis

✧ *Recording the Test of Stereognosis*

> Pedretti, L. W., Zoltan, B., & Wheatley, C. J. (1996). Evaluation and treatment of perceptual and perceptual-motor deficits. In L. W. Pedretti (Ed.), *Occupational therapy: Practice skills for physical dysfunction* (4th Ed., p. 234). St. Louis, MO: CV Mosby Year Book.

SEATING/POSITIONING

Evaluation, assessments, and measurement in seating (wheeled mobility seating):
✧　Measurement (e.g., head height, hip width, chest width, etc.) and general evaluation

Perr, A. (1998, October). Elements of seating and wheeled mobility intervention. *OT Practice, 3*(6), 16-24.

✧　Stinnett involves functional activities, neurological status, sitting on side of mat, supine positioning on mat, as well as measurements involving areas such as head height, hip width, chest width, etc.

Stinnett, K. (1999, June). Geriatric seating intervention in the skilled nursing facility. *OT Practice, 4*(6), 40-43.

✧　*A Wheelchair Positioning Assessment Form*

Mayall, J. K. & Desharnais, G. (1995). *Positioning in a wheelchair: A guide for professional care givers of the disabled adult.* Thorofare, NJ: SLACK Incorporated.

✧　Linear seating, cushions, contour seating and molded seating (assessments)

Lange, M. L. (2000, November 6). Seating systems. *OT Practice, 5*(22), 23-24.

✧　Measurements and adaptations (assessment and measurements):

Swedberg, L. M. (1998). Low-tech adaptations for seating and positioning. *OT Practice, 3*(9), 26-31.

VISUAL/PERCEPTUAL FUNCTION

Hemi-inattention (visual focus):
✧　*A Simple Test of Visual Neglect*

Albert, M. L. (1973). A simple test of visual neglect. *Neurology, 23,* 658-664.

Hemi-inattention (functional tasks with visual focus):
✧　*Behavioral Inattention Test* (BIT)

Wilson, B., Cockburn, J., & Halligan, P. *Behavioral Inattention Test* (BIT)

National Rehabilitation Services

117 North Elm St., P.O. Box 1247

Gaylord, MI 49735

517-732-3866

Tests scanning strategy to a broad space (visual focus):
✧　*The Scanboard Test* (Warren)

Warren, M. (1990). Identification of visual scanning deficits in adults after cerebrovascular accident. *Am J Occup Ther, 44,* 391-399.

Attention to visual detail:
✧　*Match* (Match computerized test)

Life Science Associates

1 Fenimore Rd.

Bayport, NY 11705

516-472-2111

Object identification (visual focus):

✧   *Dynamic Assessment of Object Identification*

>   Toglia, J. P. (1989). Visual perception of objects: An approach to assessment and intervention. *Am J Occup Ther, 43,* 587-595.

Tests for constructional praxis:

✧   *The Test of Visual Motor Skills* (TVMS)

>   Gardner, M. F. (1992). *The test of visual—Motor skills* (TVMS). Burlingame, CA: Psychological and Educational Publication.

✧   *The Benton Visual Retention Test*

>   Sivan, A. B. (1992). *The Benton Visual Retention Test.* San Antonio, TX: The Psychological Corporation.

✧   *The Rey Complex Figure*

>   Lezak, M. D. (1983). *Neuropsychological assessment* (2nd Ed.). New York, Oxford University.

✧   *The Three-Dimensional Block Construction Test*

>   Benton, A. L. & Fogel, M. L. (1962). Three-dimensional constructional praxis: A clinical test. *Arch Neurol, 7,* 347.

Screening evaluation for praxial motor planning:

✧   *Perceptual motor evaluation for head injured and other neurologically impaired adults* (Zoltan, B. and Associates). Praxis motor planning.

>   Pedretti, L. W., Zoltan, B., & Wheatley, C. J. (1996). Evaluation and treatment of perceptual and perceptual-motor deficits. In L. W. Pedretti (Ed.), *Occupational therapy: Practice skills for physical dysfunction* (4th Ed., p. 237). St. Louis, MO: CV Mosby Year Book.

Associations and Organizations Relating to Gerontology

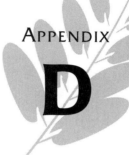

Appendix

D

✧ Aging Design Research Program
AIA/ACSA Council on
Architectural Research
1735 New York Ave. N.W.
Washington, DC 20006

✧ American Association of Retired
Persons (AARP)
601 E. Street N.W.
Washington, DC 20049

✧ American Federation of Home
Health Agencies (AFHHA)
1320 Fenwick Lane, Suite 100
Silver Springs, MD 20910

✧ American Health Care Association
(AHCA)
1201 L St. N.W.
Washington, DC 20005-4101

✧ American Hospital Association
(AHA)
One N. Franklin
Chicago, IL 60606

✧ American Occupational Therapy
Association (AOTA)
4720 Montgomery Lane
P.O. Box 31220
Bethesda, MD 20824

✧ American Psychiatric Association
(APA)
1400 K St. N.W.
Washington, DC 20005

✧ American Society of Hand
Therapists (ASHT)
401 N. Michigan Ave.
Chicago, IL 60611

✧ American Society on Aging (ASA)
833 Market St., Suite 511
San Francisco, CA 94103

✧ Association for Gerontology in
Higher Education (AGHE)
1001 Connecticut Ave. N.W.
Suite 410
Washington, DC 20036-5504

✧ Atlantic Information Services, Inc.
1100 17th St. N.W.
Suite 300
Washington, DC 20036

✧ Canadian Association of
Occupational Therapists (CAOT)
3400-1125 Colonel By Dr. (TTC
Bldg.)
Ottawa, ON K1S 5R1
Canada

✧ Center for Biomedical Ethics
University of Minnesota
UMHC Box 33, Harvard St.
At East River Rd.
Minneapolis, MN 55455

✧ Center for Medical Advocacy
P.O. Box 350
Willimantic, CT 06266

✧ Center for Universal Design
School of Design
North Carolina State University
Campus Box 8613
219 Oberlin Rd.
Raleigh, NC 27695

✧ Congressional Information
Service, Inc. (CIS)
4520 East-West Hwy
Bethesda, MD 20814

✧ Congressional Quarterly (CQ)
Customer Services
1414 22nd St. N.W.
Washington, DC 20037

✧ Families U.S.A
1334 G St. N.W.
Washington, DC 20005

✧ Gerontological Society of America
(GSA)
1275 K St. N.W. Suite 350
Washington, DC 20005

✧ Human Factors and Ergonomics
Society
P.O. Box 1369
Santa Monica, CA 90406

✧ Interdisciplinary Society for the
Advancement of Rehabilitation
and Assistive Technology (RESNA)
1700 N. Moore St., Suite 1540
Arlington, VA 22209

✧ Joint Commission Accreditation of
Healthcare Organizations
(JCAHO)
One Renaissance Blvd.
Oakbrook Terrace, IL 60181

✧ Kennedy Institute of Ethics
National Reference Center for
Bioethics Literature
Georgetown University
Washington, DC 20057

✧ League of Women Voters of the
United States
1730 M. St. N.W.
Washington, DC 20036

✧ National Archive of Computerized Data on Aging (NACDA)
Inter-University Consortium for Political and Social Research
P.O. Box 1248
Ann Arbor, MI 48106

✧ National Association for Home Care (NAHC)
519 C. St. N.E.
Washington, DC 20002

✧ National Center for Health Statistics Centers for Disease Control and Prevention—Public Health Service
U.S. Department of Health and Human Services
6525 Belcrest Rd.
Hyattsville, MD 20782

✧ National Citizens' Coalition for Nursing Home Reform (NCCNHR)
1224 M. St. N.W., Suite 301
Washington, DC 20005

✧ National Council on Disability
1331 F. St. N.W., Suite 1050
Washington, DC 20004

✧ National Council on the Aged, Inc. (NCOA)
600 Maryland Ave. S.W.
West Wing 100
Washington, DC 20024

✧ National Health Council, Inc.
350 5th Ave., Suite 1118
New York, NY 10118

✧ Office of the Federal Register, National Archives and Records Service
General Services Administration
Washington, DC 20002
(Please see U.S. Government Printing Office for access of printed documents)

✧ President's Committee on Employment of People with Disabilities
1331 F. St. N.W., Room 636
Washington, DC 20004

✧ U.S. Architectural and Transportation Barriers Compliance Board
Office of General Counsel (Access Board)
1331 F. St. N.W., Suite 1000
Washington, DC 20004-1111

✧ U.S. Department of Justice
Civil Rights Division
Office on the Americans with Disabilities Act
P.O. Box 66118
Washington, DC 20035-6118

✧ U.S. Government Printing Office
P.O. Box 371954
Pittsburgh, PA 15250
(All government printing including agencies such as the Federal Register and documents from the National Institutes of Health and National Institutes on Aging)

✧ Visiting Nurse Associations of America
3801 E. Florida Ave., Suite 206
Denver, CO 80210

HEALTHY PEOPLE 2010
(UNITED STATES)

Healthy People (HP) 2010 is a nationwide, comprehensive approach to improving the public health for all Americans. HP 2010 is the contribution of the United States to the World Health Organization's (WHO's) "Health for All" strategy.[1]

HP 2010 is under the auspices of the U.S. Department of Health and Human Services (office of the Surgeon General). Its predecessor was HP 2000 in which specific health goals were identified under the guidance of federal, state, and community government efforts. The emphasis was upon developing a comprehensive health care system for all Americans. HP 2010 is a continuation of the HP 2000 initiative. The two major goals of HP 2010 are (1) to increase the quality and years of healthy life and (2) to eliminate health disparities.[1]

Kyler and Merryman recommend that occupational therapists pay particular consideration to the five major central concepts of HP 2010. These are as follows:[1]

1. An individual's health cannot be separated from the health of the community.
2. We can, as a nation, make a difference in the health status of the nation and the individual within a relatively short time period.
3. There still is much, as a nation, that needs to be done.
4. Vital to the success of the HP 2010 is the factor of community partnerships.
5. Professional organizations, religious organizations, and businesses can work together to improve the health of the community (e.g., recycling, participating in health fairs, and assessing school health education).

Kyler and Merryman suggest a number of ways that occupational therapists and certified occupational therapy assistants can contribute (whether it be as an individual, as a department, or as an organization). These consist of:[1]

1. Attending and participating in meetings and special events related to HP 2010
2. Integrating HP 2010 into current clinical intervention and programs

3. Utilizing HP 2010 objectives as part of strategic and operational plans for one's occupational therapy department

4. Incorporating HP 2010 into occupational therapy educational curricula (as well as seminars, workshops, etc.)

5. Volunteering to be part of community and professional organization committees

A major objective of HP 2010 is to monitor the health status of all Americans (using such factors as access to health care professionals, improving the quality of life, the financing of health care and indicators of birth and death rates). Some of the leading health care factors are weight gain and obesity, physical activity, tobacco and substance abuse, mental health, injury and violence, sexual behavior, immunization, environmental life quality, and health care access.[1]

"Health promotion, disease prevention, and curing and rehabilitating persons with illnesses are brought together in one network of integrated services that reaches to the community level. This is the philosophical underpinning of HP 2010."[1, p. CE-2]

When participating in HP 2010, occupational therapy practitioners need to be aware of the International Classification of Functioning and Disability (ICIDH-2) which belongs to the "family" of classifications that was developed by WHO. This language code provides a wide range of information concerning health (e.g., functioning, diagnoses, disability, and reasons for encounter and intervention). It uses a standardized common language which permits communication about health care across the world's sciences and disciplines. An example of this language classification system can be seen in the classification of "functioning" (at the levels of the body or body part, the whole person and the whole person in a social context). It promotes three levels for the concept of disablement (e.g., abnormalities or losses of structure and functioning are termed as impairment, limitations of activities are termed as disabilities and restrictions in participation [which was formerly termed handicaps]). The environment has also been introduced as an additional aspect in classification.[2]

It is of utmost importance for occupational therapists to become familiar with the ICIDH-2 terminology, as this language is understood by all sectors such as finance, direct service, and policy. In relationship to HP 2010, ICIDH-2 is a tool that will help to characterize mental, physical, economic, social, and environmental interventions that will aid in improving people's lives and levels of functioning.[1,3] ICIDH-2 provides a common language for administrators, health care providers, and policy makers that integrates the social and medical models.[1] Therefore it is wise for therapists to learn these terms and make use of them in our day-to-day lives when providing services.

"The focus on managing chronic health conditions, reducing disease, and improving the well-being and self-sufficiency of all of us is a primary goal of HP 2010. Designing a health promotion initiative is the work of many persons."[1, p. CE-3]

There are many opportunities and roles for occupational therapy practitioners in HP 2010. Case-based or programmatic consultation are examples of such roles.[1] The American Occupational Therapy Association is one of 250 national membership organizations that were asked to formally contribute and comment on this initiative. The federal government has been involved in encouraging people to integrate HP 2010 into current educational efforts, programs, communities, and businesses. Nearly all states have work groups. Most of the work groups are at the local health department level (therefore responsive to the communities that they represent). Occupational therapy can play a major role in moving this initiative forward.[1] It is our ethical obligation to participate in this process.

REFERENCES

1. Kyler, P. & Merryman, M. B. (2000, November 6). Healthy People 2010. *OT Practice, 5*(22), CE-1-CE-7.

2. Lollar, D. J. (2000). *Toward consistency in disability: The International Classification of Functioning and Disability—ICIDH-2.* Paper presented at the 2000 American Occupational Therapy Association Annual Conference and Exposition, Seattle, WA.

3. Anonymous. (2000). *Introduction to ICIDH.* New York: World Health Organization.

A simulation game in which players encounter conditions associated with aging. This can promote meaningful discussion and encourage participants to employ a new set of values when experiencing everyday practice.

✧ *What's Your Aging I.Q.?*
   National Institute on Aging
   U.S. Department of Health and Human Services
   National Institutes of Health
   U.S. Government Printing Office, 1991, 281-837/40019
   This resource uses a question/answer format to provide readers with current information concerning aging (see below).

✧ *Consciousness-Raising Programs to Promote Positive Attitudes in Caregivers* (Courtesy S. Lewis, OTR/L, MFA, 1980).
   This resource utilizes discussion techniques and cartoons to stimulate thinking concerning the problems that elderly persons encounter in the community and in institutional living.

✧ Menks, F. (1983, December). Practice concepts: The use of a board game to simulate the experiences of old age. *Gerontologist 23*(6), 565-568.
   This article describes how an occupational therapy educator created, developed, and used a board game to increase an understanding and awareness of some of the common physical and psychosocial experiences of older adults by simulating the gains and losses that are found in old age.

NATIONAL INSTITUTE ON AGING
WHAT'S YOUR AGING I.Q.?

1. Baby boomers are the fastest growing segment of the population.	T	F
2. Families don't bother with their older relatives.	T	F
3. Everyone becomes confused or forgetful if they live long enough.	T	F
4. You can be too old to exercise.	T	F
5. Heart disease is a much bigger problem for older men than for older women.	T	F
6. The older you get, the less you sleep.	T	F
7. People should watch their weight as they age.	T	F
8. Most older people are depressed. Why shouldn't they be?	T	F
9. There's no point in screening older people for cancer because they can't be treated.	T	F
10. Older people take more medications than younger people.	T	F
11. People begin to lose interest in sex around age 55.	T	F
12. If your parents had Alzheimer's disease, you will inevitably get it.	T	F

13. Diet and exercise reduce the risk for osteoporosis.   T   F
14. As your body changes with age, so does your personality.   T   F
15. Older people might as well accept urinary accidents as a fact of life.   T   F
16. Suicide is mainly a problem for teenagers.   T   F
17. Falls and injuries "just happen" to older people.   T   F
18. Everybody get cataracts.   T   F
19. Extremes of heat and cold can be especially dangerous for older people.   T   F
20. "You can't teach an old dog new tricks."   T   F

ANSWERS

1. False.

There are more than 3 million Americans over the age of 85. That number is expected to quadruple by the year 2040, when there will be more than 12 million people in that age group. The population age 85 and older is the fastest growing age group in the United States.

2. False.

Most older people live close to their children and see them often. Many live with their spouses. An estimated 80 % of men and 60 % of women live in family settings. Only 5 % of the older population live in nursing homes.

3. False

Alzheimer's disease or other conditions that result in irreversible damage to the brain can cause confusion and serious forgetfulness in old age. But at least 100 other problems can bring on the same symptoms. A minor head injury, high fever, poor nutrition, adverse drug reactions, and depression also can lead to confusion. These conditions are treatable, however, and the confusion they cause can be eliminated.

4. False.

Exercise at any age can help strengthen the heart and lungs and lower blood pressure. It also can improve muscle strength and, if carefully chosen, lessen bone loss with age. See a physician before beginning a new exercise program.

5. False.

The risk of heart disease increases dramatically for women after menopause. By age 65, both men and women have a one in three chance of showing symptoms. But risks can be significantly reduced by following a healthy diet and exercising.

6. False.

In later life, it's the quality of sleep that declines, not total sleep time. Researchers have found that sleep tends to become more fragmented as people age. A number of reports suggest that older people are less likely than younger people to stay awake throughout the day and that older people tend to take more naps than younger people.

7. True.

Most people gain weight as they age. Because of changes in the body and decreasing physical activity, older people usually need fewer calories. Still, a balanced diet is important. Older people require essential nutrients just like younger adults. You should be concerned about your weight if there has been an involuntary gain or loss of 10 pounds in the past 6 months.

8.   False.

Most older people are not depressed. When it does occur, depression is treatable throughout the life cycle using a variety of approaches, such as family support, psychotherapy, or antidepressant medications. A physician can determine whether the depression is caused by medication an older person might be taking, by physical illness, stress, or other factors.

9.   False.

Many older people can beat cancer, especially if it's found early. Over half of all cancers occur in people 65 and older, which means that screening for cancer in this age group is especially important.

10.   True.

Older people often have a combination of conditions that require drugs. They consume 25 % of all medications and can have many more problems with adverse reactions. Check with your doctor to make sure all drugs and dosages are appropriate.

11.   False.

Most older people can lead an active, satisfying sex life.

12.   False.

The overwhelming number of people with Alzheimer's disease have not inherited the disorder. In a few families, scientists have seen an extremely high incidence of the disease and have identified genes in these families which they think may be responsible.

13.   True.

Women are at particular risk for osteoporosis. They can help prevent bone loss by eating foods rich in calcium and exercising regularly throughout life. Foods such as milk and other dairy products, dark green leafy vegetables, salmon, sardines, and tofu promote new bone growth. Activities such as walking, biking, and simple exercises to strengthen the upper body also can be effective.

14.   False.

Research has found that, except for the changes that can result from Alzheimer's disease and other forms of dementia, personality is one of the few constants of life. That is, you are likely to age much as you've lived.

15.   False.

Urinary incontinence is a symptom, not a disease. Usually, it is caused by specific changes in body function that can result from infection, diseases, pregnancy, or the use of certain medications. A variety of intervention options are available for people who seek medical attention.

16.   False.

Suicide is most prevalent among people age 65 and older. An older person's concern with suicide should be taken very seriously and professional help should be sought quickly.

17.   False.

Falls are the most common cause of injuries among people over age 65. But many of these injuries, which result in broken bones, can be avoided. Regular vision and hearing tests and good safety habits can help prevent accidents. Knowing whether your medications affect balance and coordination also is a good idea.

18.   False.

Not everyone gets cataracts, although a great many older people do. Eighteen percent of people between the ages of 65 and 74 have cataracts, while more than 40 %

of those between 75 and 85 have the problem. Cataracts can be treated very success-fully with surgery; more than 90 % of people say they can see better after the proce-dure.

19. True.

The body's thermostat tends to function less efficiently with age, making the older person's body less able to adapt to heat or cold.

20. False.

People at any age can learn new information and skills. Research indicates that older people can obtain new skills and improve old ones, including how to use a com-puter.

A CONSCIOUSNESS-RAISING TRAINING PROGRAM CONCERNING AGING

Specific objectives are to:

✧ Become aware of advocacy in rendering service to the older person

✧ Identify a number of social concerns that affect the older person

✧ Compare society's views on aging with personal views

✧ Identify and discuss the effect of institutionalization upon the older person

Exploring Attitudes Through Discussion

✧ Time: 20 minutes

✧ Equipment needed: A blackboard, chalk, eraser, paper, and pencils

✧ Group size: Recommended range four to 40 participants

The trainer states the following: "Within the next 2 minutes, write down all the char-acteristics or thoughts that come to your mind when you hear the worlds 'old person.' Begin writing."

At the end of the 2 minutes the trainer says, "Stop writing. I am now going to ask each one of you what you have written." The trainer proceeds to ask each participant what he or she has written, and records this on the blackboard. However, a specific characteristic needs to only be written once. The characteristics are then compared and discussed in terms of what is commonly considered by today's society as having posi-tive or negative attributes.

This exercise explores attitudes toward the older person that most people hold. It offers a time for reflection, expression, and understanding of long-held beliefs of soci-ety's values. For instance, a discussion concerning comparison of a young face (smooth skin and full hair color) to an old face (wrinkled skin and gray hair) reveals that our society, based upon youth orientation, often regards the aging process as undesirable. The cosmetic industry has developed a number of options (i.e., hair dye, lotions to smooth the skin) for those people who wish to camouflage the signs of aging.

EXPLORING ATTITUDES THROUGH CARTOONS AND DISCUSSION

✧   Time: Approximately 100 minutes (7 minutes per cartoon)

✧   Materials needed: A copy of the set of 14 cartoons for each participant.

The trainer states the following: "The use of the cartoon, or the caricature, has been helpful in stimulating people to think about political and social conditions. The lithographs of the great French artist Honoré Daumier are constant reminders of the use of professional power over the lay person. Although they are over 100 years old, many of these works, depicting injustice, are as fresh and vital today as the day they were first created.

"American culture has utilized the cartoon as a way of poking fun at current lifestyles and attitudes. Today, we are going to view 14 cartoons that were especially created to help us think about some of the problems that older people encounter in the community and in institutional living. These cartoons in no way reflect upon a single institution, agency, center, or profession. Rather, their purpose is to shock us into an in-depth examination of current attitudes and practices that relate to the older adult. Caregivers, in particular, have a vital role to play, and need to think of themselves not only in terms of rendering services, but also in terms of assuming an advocate role.

"Each cartoon will be viewed separately, and a brief discussion will follow."

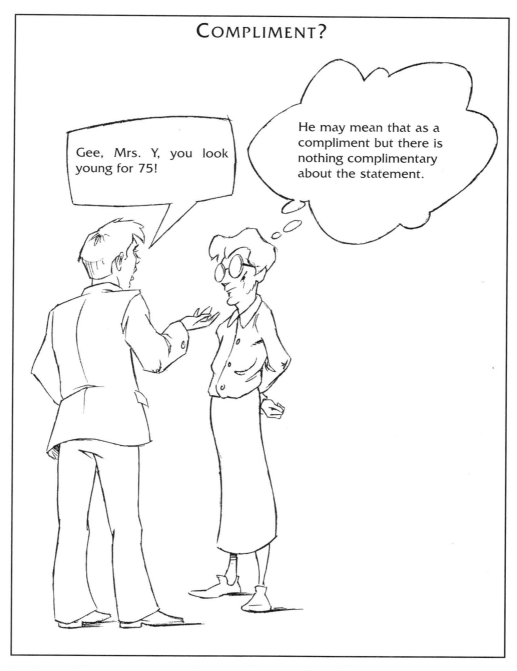

COMPLIMENT?

Gee, Mrs. Y, you look young for 75!

He may mean that as a compliment but there is nothing complimentary about the statement.

Read as participants view cartoon: In our culture, youth and beauty are considered to be synonymous. If someone wants to pay a compliment to an older adult, he or she will often say how young that person looks. If one could learn to say, "Gee, Mrs. Y, you look great," and eliminate any references to young or old, then perhaps ageism would wane.

Discussion:

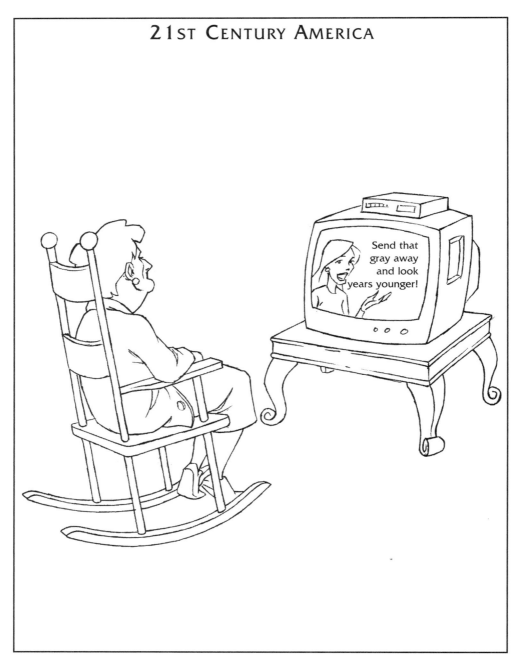

Here again, we see the effects of a culture that worships the youthful body. Constant advertisements on television and in other communication media remind us that gray is ugly—something that needs to be camouflaged. Is it a crime to be old? Why does our society make people feel ashamed of wrinkled bodies and graying hair?

Discussion:

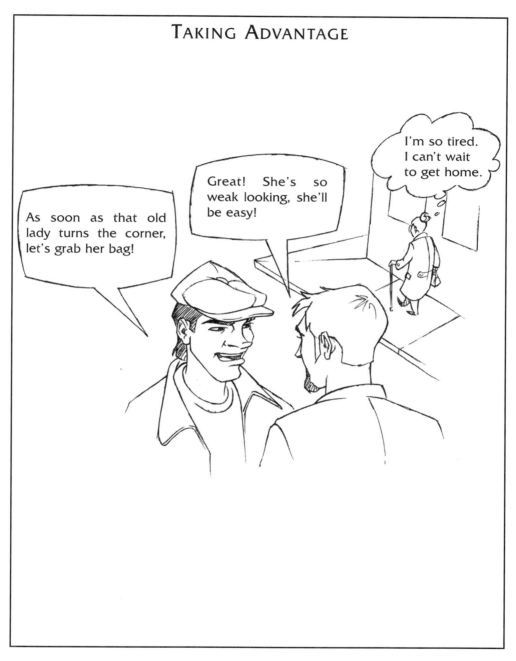

Street crime has become a constant fear of many elderly. The slow gait and bent frame that is often associated with aging makes many older adults easy targets for purse or wallet snatching. Because of this fear, a growing number of older people have become afraid to venture out at night or to use public parks.

Discussion:

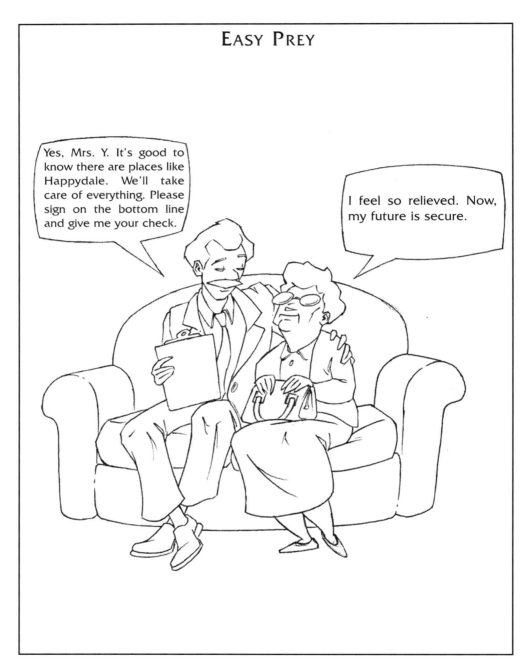

Swindling old people out of their savings by promising them great returns on their investments, "full" retirement programs, and full health coverage through a multitude of health insurance policies has become the practice of many people who believe that the elderly are vulnerable to such action.

Discussion:

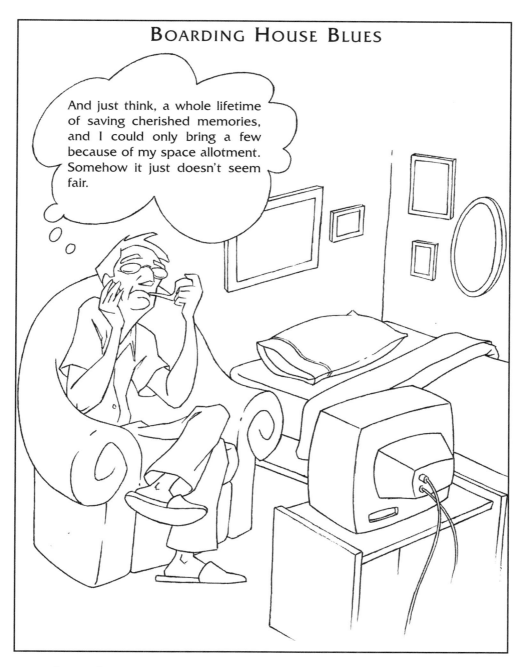

For financial reasons many older adults end their days in retirement hotels or boarding homes. Often they are limited as to what they can bring with them, and cherished mementos of a lifetime may have to be discarded.

Discussion:

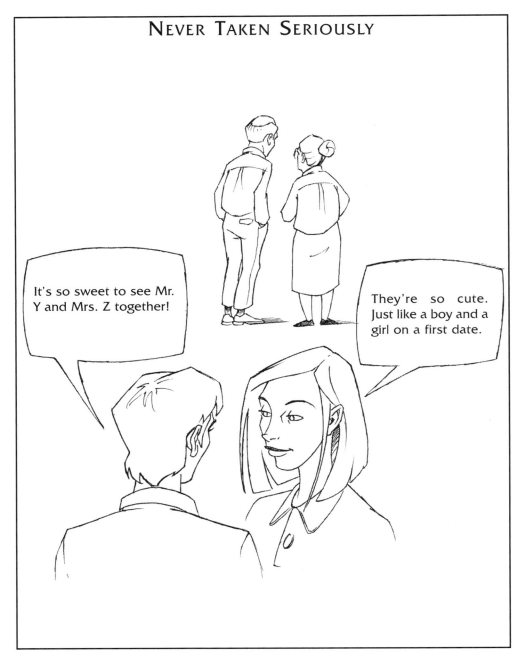

For many younger people, sex and the elderly seems to be an unrealistic concern. Instead, older adult relationships are often thought of in terms of a young boy and girl—sort of sexless and "cute."

Discussion:

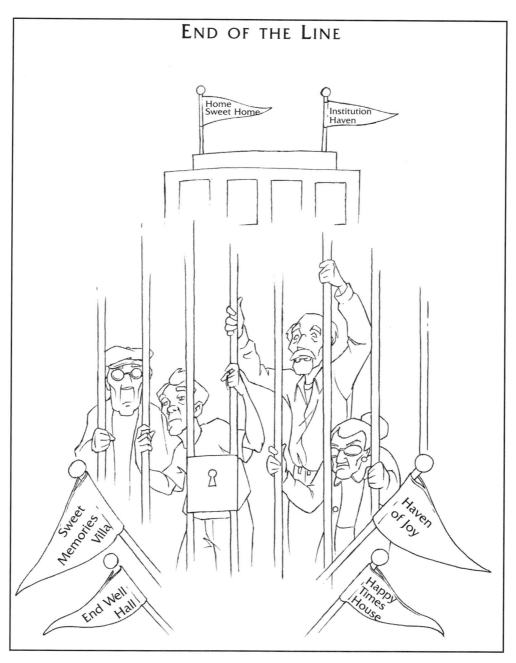

With the decline of the extended family and the rise of the nuclear family, increasing numbers of at-risk older adults are being cared for in institutions. A large number of these facilities use names that evoke thoughts of a paradise-like lifestyle. Many older people who need the services of a medical facility feel that they are being abandoned by their family, friends, and society, and fear the very thought of institutional living.

Discussion:

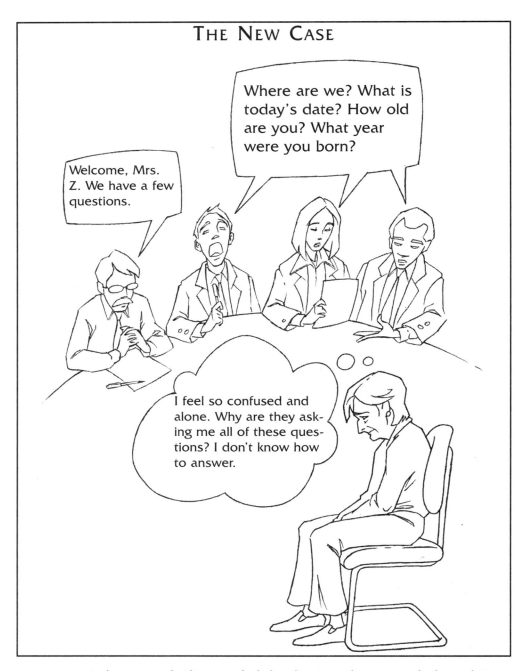

A new arrival to a care facility may feel shy, disoriented, angry, or frightened. Even when well-intended questions to discover the extent of a disability are asked, the new resident may not be able to respond appropriately.

Discussion:

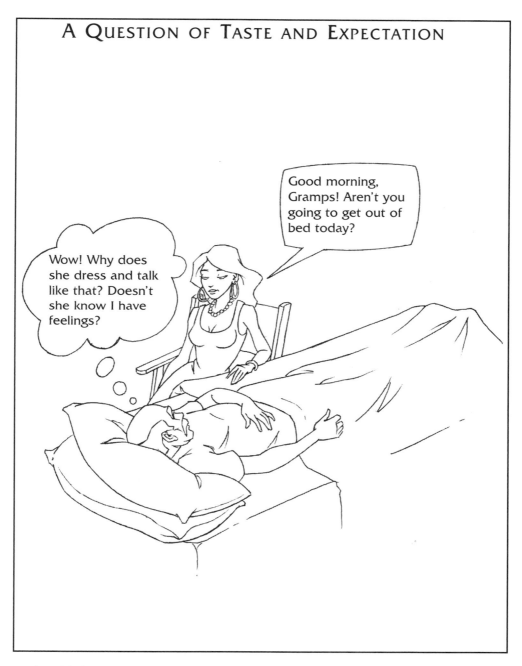

The elderly resident is not often thought of in terms of being able to react sexually. Therefore, many staff members may not be aware that their manners or clothing style might sexually arouse their clients.

Discussion:

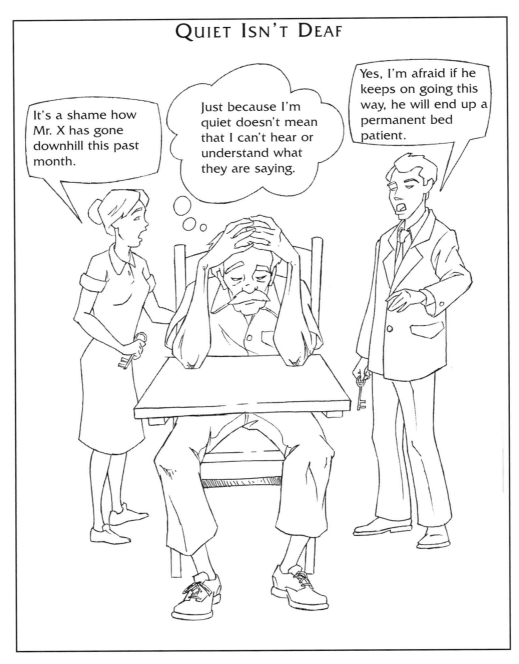

There are times when well-meaning staff may talk about a resident who appears to be unresponsive in his or her presence. Often, staff personnel may not realize that although this person does not act responsively, he or she may be perfectly capable of understanding all that is being said.

Discussion:

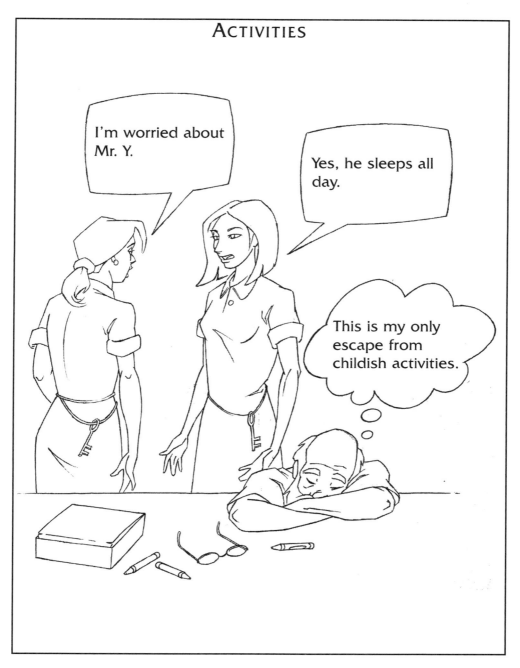

Activities for older adults should not be an echo of childhood. Instead, they should be thought of in terms of stimulation and challenge. Staff should ask the question, "Would I like this for myself?" Activities should concur with acknowledgment of the resident's ability and ethnic background, and should have some prestigious value to the client.

Discussion:

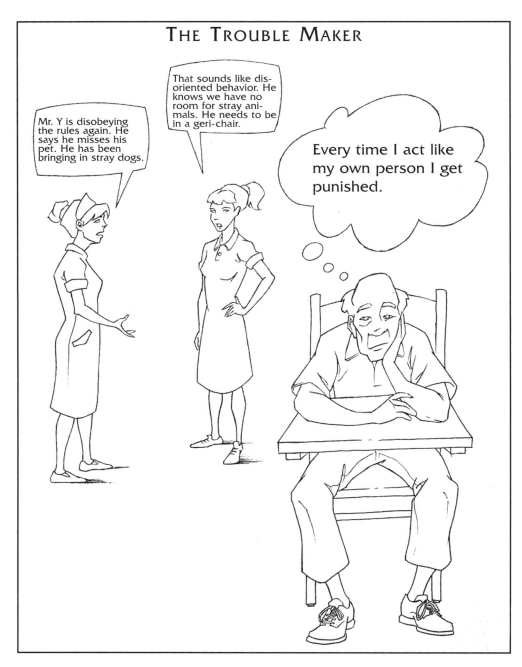

Living in institutions usually means following the rules of the facility. Sometimes it is difficult to individualize and respond to each resident's request. Behavior that is interpreted as disoriented may be a reflection upon the resident's inability to cope with the restrictions of institutional living. The geri-chair is often used to help restrain confused, disoriented, wandering residents, particularly those who have a history of falls.

Discussion:

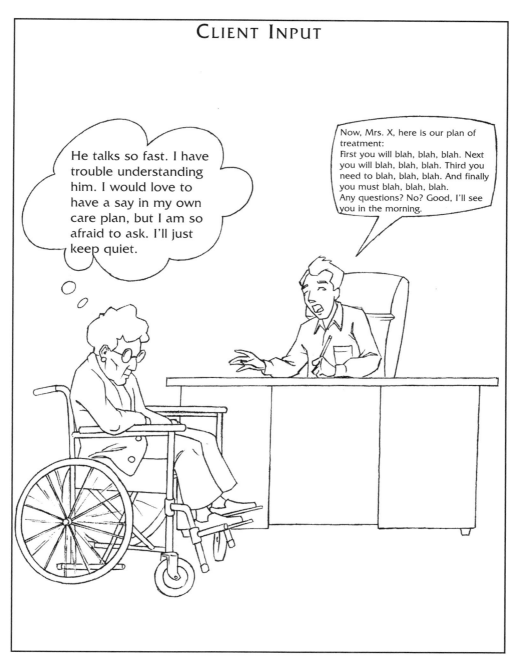

When talking to older people with multiple problems, staff members need to speak slowly and clearly and wait for the older person's response so that he or she may have a true opportunity to participate in he or she own intervention plan.

Discussion:

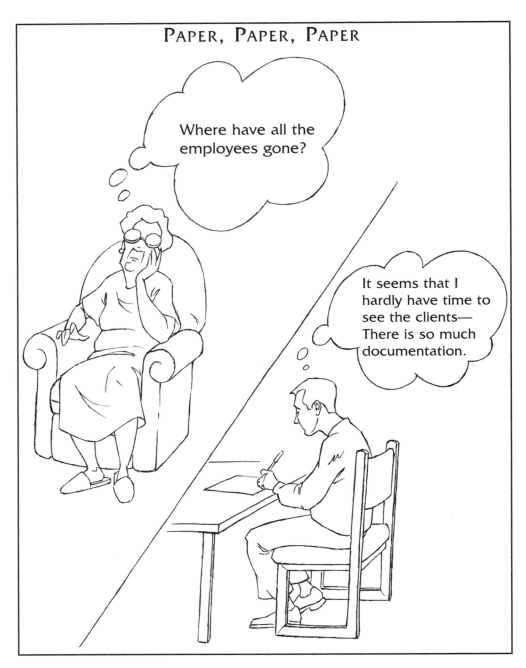

Paperwork involving both documentation of progress notes and the completion of private and public health forms has increasingly cut in on staff/client time.

Discussion:

EXERCISE COMPONENTS FOR WELL-BEING AND FITNESS

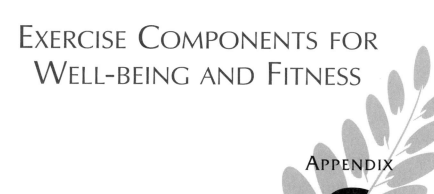

APPENDIX

G

DEVELOPING A HEALTHY LIFESTYLE

Make certain that the client has received medical clearance before participating in all activities.

Category	How to Develop
Cardiovascular endurance	Aerobic exercise is utilized to increase oxygen usage by the body. Activities of large muscles are performed repetitively so that the heart rate is increased at a targeted appropriate range for 20 to 30 minutes (a minimum of three times weekly). This involves the use of large muscle groups that are at low tension with sufficient oxygen to sustain the activities over a specific time period. Aerobic exercise includes activities such as aerobic walking, tennis, skiing, bicycling and swimming.[1,2]
Muscular endurance	Aerobic activities (swimming, bicycling, aerobic walking) are to be utilized.[1,2]
Muscular strength (strength training)	An appropriate level of stimulus is provided to a muscle, as well as a time period for recovery, to permit muscle growth. Muscular strength is developed through isometrics, isokinetics, and weight training (e.g., free weights, dynabands, pilates, tubing, circuit machines, and sculpting classes).[1,2]
Flexibility	Flexibility involves range of motion in a series of joints or in a single joint. This includes the change of ratio of length to tension in muscle groups or within a single muscle. Yoga, tai chi, physioball classes, water aerobics, swimming, and proprioceptive neuromuscular functioning are examples of flexibility training.[1,2]

Category	*How to Develop*
Balance and coordination	Balance and coordination are believed to be related to central, peripheral, sensory, and motor input—with strength being linked as a strong component. Activities such as dancing, racquet sports, yoga, tai chi, chi gong, golf, swimming, balance boards, walking on a painted line, and physioballs promote balance and coordination.[1,2]

The benefits from appropriate exercise are:[1,2]

✧ Improvement of psychological well-being (reduces stress, provides appropriate release of one's emotions, and improves one's ability to increase periods of alertness)

✧ Increased bone density

✧ Decreased body fat

✧ Decreased constipation

✧ Reduced edema

✧ Improved flexibility

✧ Decreased blood pressure

✧ Increased cardiac output

✧ Increased aerobic capacity and reduction in the tendency to form blood clots

✧ Decreased resting heart rate (the number of times the heart beats per minute)

✧ Increased metabolism

✧ Increased oxygen to body and brain tissues to promote healing and alertness

✧ Increased speed of movement, reaction time, and range of motion

✧ Increased muscular endurance and strength

✧ If carried out in a group setting, exercise can promote socialization.[1,2]

REFERENCES

1. Lewis, S. (1989). *Elder care in occupational therapy,* (pp. 105-108). Thorofare, NJ: SLACK Incorporated.
2. Toto, P.E. (2000, May/June). *To the point . . . Healthy life style redesign begins with you* (pp. 1-3). Penn Point: Pennsylvania Occupational Therapy Association.

SUPPLIES

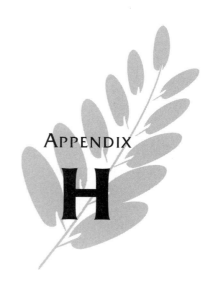

APPENDIX

H

ARTS AND CRAFTS

- Arts for All
  10 S. 5th St.
  P.O. Box 767
  Bayfield, WI 54814
  715-779-9526
  fax: 715-799-9527
  www.zotartz.com
- Dick Blick Art Materials
  P.O. Box 1267
  Galesburg, IL 61402
  1-800-447-8192
  fax: 1-800-621-8293
  www.dickblick.com
- Imaginart
  307 Arizona St.
  Bisbee, AZ 85603
  1-800-828-1376
  fax: 1-800-737-1376
  www.imaginartonline.com

- NARSAD Artwork/NARSAD
  (Mental Health)
  761 West Lambert Rd.
  Brega, CA 92821
  714-529-5571
  fax: 714-990-0791
  www.mhsource.com/narsadart.html
- Perler Beads/Dimensions
  1801 N. 12th St.
  Reading, PA 19604
  1-800-523-8452
  www.perlerbeads.com
- S and S Worldwide, Inc.
  75 Mill St.
  Colchester, CT 06415
  860-537-3451
  fax: 860-537-2563
  www.ssww.com

Computer Technology/ Computer Generated Information

✧ Abledata
8630 Fento St., Suite 930
Silver Spring, MD 20910
1-800-277-0216
fax: 301-608-8958
www.abledata.com
A complete and comprehensive database on assistive devices in North America (more than 27,000 products are available)

✧ Applied Learning Corp
1376 Glen Hardie Rd.
Wayne, PA 19087
Tel: & fax: 610-688-6866
The Malton family of adaptive keyboards

✧ Brain Train
727 Twin Ridge Lane.
Richmond, VA 23235
804-320-0105
fax: 804-320-0242
www.braintrain.com
Computerized mental exercise (Captain's log, Sound Smart, and Smart Driver)

✧ Chart Links
74 Forbes Ave.
New Haven, CT 06512
203-469-0707
fax: 203-469-2921
www.chartlinks.com
Software for a variety of needs, such as case management, team conference, rehabilitation scheduling, and occupational therapy (Products are compliant with JCAHO, CARF, and PPS)

✧ Justay Computer Solutions, Inc.
P.O. Box 1155
Burlington, MA 01803
718-750-8454
www.justay.com
Evalwriter—computer software to reduce time required to generate an evaluation

✧ Advanced Therapy Product
P.O. Box 3420
Glen Allen, VA
804-747-8574
www.atpwork.com
Driving Simulators feature the STISIMD Drive Interactive Driving System by Systems Technology, Inc., that are capable of measuring and assessing many components used in driving (e.g., reaction time, maintained lane position, divided attention, etc.)

✧ Doron Precision System
P.O. Box 400
174 Court St.
Binghamton, NY 13902-0400
607-772-1610
fax: 607-772-6758
www.doronprecision.com

✧ Forward Motions, Inc.
214 Valley St.
Dayton, OH 45404
1-877-FMI-VANS
www.forwardmotion.com
Handicapped accessible vehicles

DRESSING, BATHING, GROOMING, SELF-FEEDING, AND TOILETING

❖ Alimed, Inc.
297 High St.
Dedham, MA 02026
781-329-2900
fax: 1-800-437-2966
Jbretz@alimed.com
Including Ableware by MADDAK

❖ Bed-Check Corp.
307 E. Brady
Tulsa, OK 74120
1-800-523-7956
fax: 918-582-9828
cheryl@bedcheck.com

❖ Borin-Halbich, Inc. (medication containers)
2617 North Pioneer Lane
Spokane, WA 99216
509-922-1114
fax: 509-922-4846

❖ Desi's Secret (adaptive needs clothing)
119 Vermeer Dr.
Langhorne, PA 19047
215-752-5232
fax: 215-752-9812
www.desisecret.com

❖ Duralife, Inc.
195 Phillips Park Dr.
S. Williamsport, PA 17702
570-323-9743
fax: 570-323-9762
www.duralife-usa.com
Wheeled shower/commode chairs, bath chairs, transfer benches, and shower gurneys

❖ Dycem (non-slip materials)
83 Gilbane St.
Warwick, RI 02886
401-738-4420
fax: 401-739-9634
www.dycem.com

❖ Fashion Ease (adaptive clothing)
Division of M and M Health Care Apparel Company
1541 60th St.
Brooklyn, NY 11219
718-853-6376
fax: 718-436-2067
www.fashionease.com

❖ Functional Solutions (North Coast)
Adaptive Equipment
NCM Consumer Products Division
P.O. Box 6070
San Jose, CA 95150
1-800-235-7054
fax: 408-938-9923
www.ncmedical.com

❖ iCan, Inc.
870 Bowers
Birmington, MI 48009
248-594-4226 x128
fax: 248-594-2034
www.iCan.com
Internet company provides a comprehensive collection of products.

❖ Imaginart (daily living, feeding, swallowing)
307 Arizona St.
Bisbee, AZ 85603
1-800-826-1376
fax: 1-800-737-1376
www.imaginartonline.com

❖ Inglis Drink-Aide
2600 Belmont Ave.
Philadelphia, PA 19131
1-800-336-7022
fax: 215-878-6231
www.drink-aide.com

✧ Lighthouse (visionary solutions)
111 E. 59th St., 12th Floor
New York, NY 10022
1-888-770-7660
www.lighthouse.org

✧ Jordan's Mobility Solutions, Inc. (feeding)
P.O. Box 132772
Tyler, TX 75713
903-526-2100
fax: 903-526-2103
www.disabilityaccessories.com

✧ MADDAK, Inc.
6 Industrial Rd.
Pequannock, NJ 07440
973-628-7600
fax: 973-305-0841
www.maddak.com
Manufacturer of Ableware assistive devices, home health care, and rehabilitation products.

✧ PETA U.K Ltd./Mechanaids Co., Inc.
21-1 Hampden Dr.
South Easton, MA 02375
1-800-227-0877
fax: 508-238-1752
www.peta-uk.com
Full range special needs scissors, kitchen utensils, and garden tools

✧ Providence Spillproof
P.O. Box 40672
Providence, RI 40672
1-888-843-5287
fax: 401-521-0522
www.kcup.com
Spillproof Kennedy, Nosey Cups, Independence Mugs/Lids, and Specialty Urinals

✧ Reliant Medical Products, Inc.
500 Beacon Parkway W.
Birmingham, AL 35209
205-943-5126
www.reliantmedicalproducts.com
Swallowing disorders (e.g., Limited Flow Drinking Cup)

✧ Sammons Preston— "Enrichments" (ADL Equipment)
4 Sammons Court
P.O. Box 5071
Bolingbrook, IL 60440
1-800-323-5547
fax: 1-800-547-4333
www.sammonspreston.com
Sammons Preston has recently been acquired by the Ability One Corporation. Its name will remain the same.

GROUND TRANSPORTATION

✧ Accessible Transportation
P.O. Box 292
Zionsville, PA 18092
215-679-0467
fax: 215- 619-0467
www.accessibletransport.com

A resource that lists all of the private and public transit companies, charter, bus tour, and water raft operators across the United States that have accessible lift equipment vehicles.

Home Modification/Home Adaptation to improve function

✧ Barrier Free Lifts, Inc.
9230 Prince William St.
Manassas, VA 20110
1-800-582-8732
fax: 703-367-7861
www.bflift.com
lift and transfer products

✧ Dolomite Home Care Products
4081 Calle Tesoro, Unit N
Camarillo, CA 93012
805-388-0612
fax: 805-388-4614
www.dolomitehcp.com
Bath lifts (aquatic),shower commodes, and walkers

✧ Extended Home Living Services
5230 Capital Dr.
Wheeling, IL 60090
847-215-9490
fax: 847-215-9632
www.ehls.com
Accessibility contractor-specializing in home modification solutions. CASPAR, innovative home assessment protocol is available.

✧ Contact: Margaret A. Christenson, MFH, OTR, FAOTA, President
Lifease, Inc.
St. Paul, MI
1-800-961-3273

Software home assessment (EASE 3.0). This program has the ability to select and produce reports of appropriate idea and product solutions that are based upon a client's functional capacity and home setting.

✧ Liko, Inc.
842 Upper Union St., Suite 4
Franklin, MA 02038
1-888-545-6671
fax: 508-528-6642
www.liko.com
Liko, Inc., offers a full line of lifts such as portable, ceiling mounted, sit-to-stand and multipurpose.

✧ MedTek, LLC
3003 Northway Dr.
Baltimore, MD 21234
410-426-7834
Stair lifts, ramps vehicle lifts

✧ Total Access
319 West Gay St.
West Chester, PA 19380
1-800-651-5666
fax: 610-738-3329
www.totalaccess.baweb.com
Specializing in creating accessible environments for those with disabilities

Physical Rehabilitation (Equipment/Supplies)

✧ Alimed, Inc.
297 High St.
Dedham, MA 02026
781-329-2900
fax: 1-800-437-2966
Jbretz@alimed.com

✧ American Orthopedic Appliance Group, Inc.
234 Main St.
Cornwall, NY 12518
845-534-9087
fax: 845-534-4800
www.thera-glove.com
Thera-Glove Hand and Wrist Supports

❖ Ball Dynamics International
14215 Mead St.
Longmont, CO 80504
1-800-752-2255
fax: 1-877-223-2962
www.balldynamics.com
Therapeutic Balls

❖ Baltimore Therapeutic Equipment
Co.
7455-L New Ridge Rd.
Hanover, MD 21076
410-850-0333
fax: 410-850-5244
www.bteco.com
BTE Equipment

❖ BWA Technologies, Inc.
3935 New Bear Ave., Suite 255
Raleigh, NC 27610
919-250-0944
fax: 919-255-9806
www.bwa.technologies.com
(weighted glove)

❖ Cube Integrations
114 Bank St.
Batavia, NY 14020
716-345-1487
fax: 716-344-1400
Cubeintegrations@usa.net
Integrative therapy tool used to
enhance fine/visual/gross motor
skills, language, and cognition.

❖ Fluidotherapy
The Chattanooga Group, Inc.
4717 Adams Rd.
Hixson, TN 37343
1-800-592-7329
fax: 1-800-242-8329
www.chattgroup.com
Dry heat therapy

❖ Gottfried Medical, Inc.
P.O. Box 8966
4105 West Alexis Rd.

Toledo, OH 43623
1-800-537-1968
fax: 419-474-8822
www.gottfriedmedical.com
Surgical elastic supports, pressure
garments

❖ Hansmann Industries, Inc.
130 Union St.
North Vale, NJ 07647
201-767-0255 x47
fax: 201-767-1369
www.hansmann.com
Manufacturer of rehab equipment

❖ Hipsaver
1-800-358-4477
www.hipsaver.com
hipsaver@msn.com
Pads over each trochanter dissipate falls

❖ Interactive Metronome, Inc.
2300 Weston Rd.
Weston, FL 33311
954-385-4660
fax: 954-385-4674
www.interactivemetronome.com
Useful with motor planning, timing technology, and sequencing

❖ Invacare Corporation (Corporate
Office)
One Invacare Way
Elyria, OH 44035
1-800-333-6900
fax: 440-329-6568
www.invacare.com

❖ JACE Systems
55 Carnegie Plaza
Cherry Hill, NJ 08003-1020
1-800-800-4276
www.jacesystems.com
Specialists in upper-extremities
therapies (Design manufacturer
and distribution of CPM equipment)

✧ Joint Active Systems, Inc.
2600 S. Raney St.
Effingham, IL 62401
1-800-879-0117
fax: 217-347-3384
Mwhotz@bonuttiresearch.com
Devices designed to improve ROM by utilizing principles of SPS and stress relaxation (at the same time reducing joint compression and providing soft tissue lengthening)

✧ Jump-In
10315 Moon Lake Court
Pinckney, MI 48169
734-878-0166
fax: 734-878-0169
Jumpin@htonline.com
www.jump-in-products.com
Products for physical and sensory restoration

✧ Kinesio USA Corp. Ltd.
11005 Spain, N.E., Suite 2
Albuquerque, NM 87111
505-856-2029
fax: 505-856-2983
www.kinesiotaping.com
Production of kinesio taping that is used for pain management, muscular rehabilitation, and edema

✧ Maddak, Inc.
6 Industrial Rd.
Pequannock, NJ 07440
973-628-7600
fax: 973-305-0841
www.maddak.com
Manufacturer of rehabilitation products; home health care and Ableware assistive devices

✧ McKie Splints
P.O. Box 16046
Duluth, M.N. 55816

1-888-477-5468
fax: 1-888-477-5468
Manufactures neoprene thumb splints and supinalor straps

✧ MedDev Corporation
730 N. Pastoria Ave.
Sunnyvale, CA 94088
1-800-543-2789
fax: 408-730-9732
www.meddev-corp.com
Offers a variety of hand therapy exercises

✧ North Coast Medical, Inc.
18305 Sutter Blvd.
Morgan Hill, CA 95032
1-800-821-9319
fax: 1-877-213-9300
www.ncmedical.com
Promotes a wide variety of therapeutic equipment and supplies for the physically disabled client. Orthotic rehabilitation products.

✧ OCUTECH VES
109 Conner Dr., Suite 2105
Chapel Hill, NC 27514
1-800-326-6460
www.ocutech.com
Provides visual improvement in conditions such as macular degeneration, diabetic retinopathy, and high myopia

✧ Orthotic Rehabilitation Products, Inc.
7002 E. Broadway
Tampa, FL 33619
1-800-597-2547
fax: 1-800-841-1295
www.orthoticrehab.com
Manufactures a full line of orthotic devices (a.k.a. Orthotic Rehab)

✧ Otto Bock
3000 Xenium Lane N.

Minneapolis, MN 55441
612-519-6175
fax: 612-519-6152
Provides orthotic equipment (including wheelchair armrests)

✧ Pencil Grip
P.O. Box 67096
Los Angeles, CA 90067
310-315-3545
fax: 310-315-0607
asherp@thepencilgrip.com
Evokes full hand and arm action while reducing cramping and stress

✧ Restorative Care of America
11236 47th St. N.
Clearwater, FL 33762
1-800-627-1595
fax: 727-573-1886
www.rcai.com
Manufacturers prefabricated orthotic devices

✧ Sammons Preston
4 Sammons Court
Bolingbrook, IL 60440
1-800-323-5547
fax: 630-226-1389
www.sammonspreston.com
Promotes a wide variety of therapeutic equipment and supplies for the physically disabled client. Sammons Preston has recently been acquired by the Ability One Corporation. Its name will remain the same.

✧ Sprint/Rothhammer
P.O. Box 3840
San Luis Obispo, CA 93403
1-800-235-2156
fax: 805-541-5330
www.sprintaquatics.com
Aquatherapy rehabilitation

✧ Stretchwell, Inc.

P.O. Box 104
Newton, PA 18940
1-888-396-2430
fax: 215-675-8042
www.stretchwell.com
Manufactures therapy bands, fitness balls, "Fit-Lastic" therapy products

✧ Smith and Nephew Rehabilitation
N104 W13400 Donges Bay Rd.
Germantown, WI 53022
1-800-558-8633
fax: 1-800-545-7758
www.smith-nephew.com/us/rehab
Promotes a wide variety of therapeutic equipment and supplies for the physically disabled client. Smith and Nephew has recently been acquired by the Ability One Corporation and will be called by its original name, Rolyan.

✧ Thera-Band Products/
Hygenic Corp.
1245 Home Ave.
Akron, OH 44310
330-633-8460
fax: 330-633-9359
www.thera-band.com
Manufactures all Thera-Band products (including swim and land equipment)

✧ Therapeutic Dimensions
P.O. Box 365
Spokane, WA 99210
509-323-9275
fax: 509-323-9277
Promotes upper body exercisers (e.g., Range Master, Pull-ez shoulder pulleys and Thera-loop door anchor for banding and tubing exercise)

✧ Therapro, Inc.
225 Arlington St.
Framingham, MA 01702

508-872-9494

fax: 508-875-2062

www.theraproducts.com

Provides adaptive equipment and activities to promote sensation and perception

✧ Wenzelite Rehab Supplies

3815 15th Ave.

Brooklyn, NY 11232

718-768-8002

fax: 718-768-8020

www.wenzelite.com

Adult (bariatric 700-lb capacity) safety rollers

RECREATION/LEISURE/SPORTS

✧ Flaghouse
601 Flaghouse Dr.
Hasbrouck Heights, NJ 07604
201-329-7529
fax: 201-288-3897
www.flaghouse.com
TheraGym Balls, Snoezelen, Recreational, and Leisure supplies

✧ S and S Worldwide
75 Mill St.
Colchester, CT 06415
860-537-3451
fax: 860-537-2563
www.ssww.com
Sensory recreation items. Claudia Allen Diagnostic Module products, sports and hobby equipment.

SEATING, POSITIONING, MOBILITY

✧ Broda Seating
385 Phillip St.
Waterloo, ON N2L 5R8
Canada
1-800-668-0637
fax: 519-746-8616
www.brodaseating.com
Manufactures seating systems and health care chairs to meet the needs of long-term care clients.

✧ Danmer Products, Inc.
221 Jackson Industrial Dr.
Ann Arbor, MI 48103
734-761-1990
fax: 734-761-8977
Manufactures seating/positioning equipment, floatation devices.

✧ Electric Mobility Corporation
One Mobility Corporation
591 Mantua Blvd.
Sewell, NJ 08080
1-800-662-4548
fax: 856-468-2075

www.fascalscooters.com
Provides electric mobility products.

✧ Homecrest Industries
P.O. Box 350
140 Madison Ave.
Wadena, MN 56482
1-800-346-4852
fax: 1-800-346-4858
www.homecrest.com
Rock 'n Lo wheelchair (three chairs in one—tilt-in-space, rocking chair, and transport)

✧ Invacare Corporation (Corporate Office)
One Invacare Way
Elyria, OH 44035
1-800-333-6900
fax: 440-329-6568
www.invacare.com
Provides wheelchairs for various needs as well as molded seating (such as Pin Dot Contor U).

❖ The Jay Cushion /The Jay Back
Jay Sunrise Medical
7477A East Dry Creek Pkwy
Longmont, CO 80503
1-800-456-8165
fax: 1-800-200-4114
www.sunrisemedical.com
Provides contoured cushions for seating.

❖ Matrix
Matrix, Peach Medical
1-800-253-6217
www.concentric.Me/ ˜Matrix
Provides carved foam seating.

❖ McCarty's SacroEase LLC
3929 Industrial Ave.
Coeur d'Aleve, ID 83815
1-800-635-3557
fax: 208-664-6891
www.mccartys.com
Provides SacroEase Posture
Correction Seats and Comfort Ease Splints.

❖ Medco (Division of KKC Inc.)
12051 Forestgate Dr.
Dallas, TX 75243
972-235-1033
fax: 972-235-9644
Manufactures polystyrene bead-filled, patented products to position clients.

❖ Mulholland Positioning Systems
P.O. Box 391
215 N. 12th St.
Santa Paula, CA 93061
1-800-543-4769
fax: 805-933-1082
www.mulhollandinc.com

❖ Posey Company
5635 Peck Rd.
Arcadia, CA 91006
626-443-3143

fax: 626-443-5064
www.posey.com
Manufactures items such as non-slip matting, posture supports, positioning aids, and wheelchair accessories.

❖ Position Dynamics
2636 289th Place
Adel, IA 50003
515-993-5001
fax: 515-993-4172
www.PositionDynamics.com
Manufactures a power tilt, tilt and recline, and recline seating system that can be mounted on power wheelchairs.

❖ Rubbermaid Healthcare Products
3124 Valley Ave.
Winchester , VA 22601
540-542-8322
fax: 540-542-8838
www.healthcareproducts.com
Provides a wide variety of home health care products and mobility aids.

❖ Skil-Care Corp.
29 Wells Ave.
Yonkers, NY 10701
914-963-2040
fax: 914-963-2567
Develops wheelchair cushions and positioning devices.

❖ Supracor, Inc.
2050 Corporate Court
San Jose, CA 95131-1753
408-432-1616,   1-800-787-7266
fax: 408-432-1975
www.supracor.com
Provides Stimulate honeycomb pressure relief and positioning cushions and other items such as "breathable" sheet for customized seating and positioning.

✧ Symmetrix Back/Roho Group
The Roho Group
100 Florida St.
Belleville, IL 62221
1-800-851-3449
www.therohogroup.com
Provides pod seating (placed at various angles and locations to support the trunk as well as a variety of other types of seating).

✧ Wheelchairs of Kansas
204 W. 2nd St.
P.O. Box 320
Elles, KS 67637
1-800-537-6454

fax: 1-800-337-2447
www.wheelchairsofkansas.com
Manufactures large wheelchairs as well as standard.

✧ Varilite
4000 First Ave. S.
Seattle, WA 98134
1-800-827-4548
fax: 206-343-5795
www.varilite.com
Manufactures vibration and impact reduction cushions (e.g., seat cushions, back supports, belts, drop seats, solid inserts, ankle-positioning devices).

SERVICE DOGS

✧ Canine Companions for Independence
P.O. Box 205
Farmingdale, NY 11735
631-694-6938
fax: 631-694-0308
www.caninecompanions.org
Breeds, trains, and places highly skilled assistance dogs with disabled individuals.

✧ Delta Society
289 Perimeter Rd. E.
Renton, WA 98055
425-687-2344
fax: 425-235-1076
www.deltasociety.org
Provides information concerning animal activities, therapy and how to use Pet Partners team in therapy protocols.

TELEPHONE COMMUNICATIONS

✧ Ameriphone, Inc.
12082 Western Ave.
Garden Grove, CA 92841
714-230-1506
fax: 714-897-4703
Products include ADA compliance kits, amplified telephone, remote control phones, notification sys-

tems, and emergency response telephones.

✧ Lifeline Systems MS/22
111 Lawrence St.
Framingham, MA 01702
1-877-419-5565
Provides personal response and support services.

TIME MANAGEMENT

✧ Time Timer
7707 Camargo Road
Cincinnati, OH 45243
Tel.: 513-561-2599

fax: 513-561-4699
www.timetimer.com
Provides visual deception of elapsed time.

TOILET LEVATORS

✧ LCM Distribution Ltd.
14102 8th St., N.E.
Calgary, Alberta T2A 7W6, Canada
1-888-726-4646
www.medichair.com

✧ Medway Corporation
103 Grayback Lane.
Amherst, OH 44001
1-800-817-3118
www.medwaycorp.com

URINARY INCONTINENCE

✧ Neotonus, Inc.
835 B Franklin Court
Merietta, GA 30067
770-428-7356
fax: 770-425-5264
www.neotonus.com
NeoHealth (Wellness for Seniors, a Division of Neotonus, Inc.) provides onsite urinary incontinence programs through NeoControl.

✧ NeuroControl Corporation
8333 Rockside Rd., 1st Floor
Cleveland, OH 44125
216-912-0101
fax: 216-912-0129
www.neurocontrol.com
Markets implantable devices to restore function to paralyzed muscles (NeuroControl VOLARE Bladder System).

VARIOUS MODULAR RAMP SYSTEMS

✧ Van Duerr Industries
820 West 7th St.
Chicago, CA 95928

530-893-1596
fax: 530-893-1560
www.vanduerr.com

VISUAL DYSFUNCTION

✧ Elia Life Technology
354 E. 66th St., Suite 4A
New York, NY 10021
212-327-2550
fax: 212-861-0426
www.elialife.com
Provides materials such as a tactile alphabet which can be learned much quicker than the Braille alphabet.

✧ Eschenbach
904 Ethan Allen Hwy.
Ridgefield, CT 06877
203-438-7471
fax: 203-438-1670
Manufactures and distributes magnifiers, filters, telescopes, video magnifiers for the visually impaired, and diagnostic kits for eye care and rehabilitation professionals.

✧ Lighthouse International
111 E. 59th St., 12th Floor
New York, NY 10022
1-888-770-7660
www.lighthouse.org
Provides materials for the visually impaired through stores and catalogs.

✧ National Library Service for the Blind and Physically Handicapped (Free Talking Books)
1-800-424-8567
www.loc.gov/nls

✧ Optelec U.S., Inc.
6 Liberty Way
Westford, MA 01886
1-800-828-1056
fax: 978-692-6073
www.optelec.com
Provides magnification for the visually impaired (including "Clear View" products that feature easy-to-use controls which are helpful to individuals with macular degeneration and other low-vision conditions) to enhance independence in reading and writing.

✧ Recording for the Blind and Dyslexic
20 Roszel Rd.
Princeton, NJ 08540
609-520-8079
fax: 609-243-7056
www.rfbd.org
Serves persons who cannot read standard print effectively due to visual perceptual or other physical disability. The educational and professional library makes available taped texts to individuals with membership.

✧ Stereo Optical Co.
3539 N. Kenton Ave.
Chicago, IL 60641
773-777-2869
fax: 773-777-4985
www.stereooptical.com
Provides portable vision testers (Optic Vision Testers—tests acuities, phorias, depth and color perception as well as contrast sensitivity).

✧ Video Eye Corporation
Dept. USN
10211 W. Emerald
Boise, ID 83704
1-800-416-0758
fax: 208-377-1528
Provides the Video Eye power magnification system.

LIVING ARRANGEMENTS AND THE ELDERLY

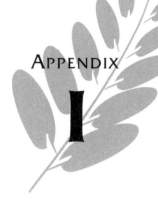

APPENDIX

I

LIVING ARRANGEMENTS

Type (Name)	Definition	Features
Personal resident unit	Owner occupied units	Single home/condominium
Single room occupancy	Retirement hotel (renter)	Usually older hotel. Single room (with/without bath)
Retirement communities	Commercial retirement villages	May be owner/renter occupied. Social center (pool, golf, tennis, community center)
Life care contract and founder's fee communities	Private sector, full services with medical center on grounds. Apartment/cottage type living arrangement (may be religiously affiliated or totally commercial)	Usually large lump sum required upon entry. Monthly maintenance fee. Social, cleaning, and dining services. Medical center/nursing care center on grounds (may require extra fee)

Living Arrangements and the Elderly
(continued)

Type (Name)	Definition	Features
Social programs	Federal, state, or religiously affiliated to provide care	Foster homes, adopt-a-grandparent programs, sheltered housing, domiciliary care
Emergency shelters	Safe environment for victims of elder abuse	Immediate care for abused elders
Family arrangements	Family setting	Usually living with adult child and his or her family
Congregate housing	Group living—residents do the same thing at the same time (meals served communally)	Common dining room and central kitchen. May be federally, locally, or religiously supported
Purchase retirement housing	Commercially private self-contained communities	Basic shopping amenities, activity programs, on-site medical care
Rent-subsidy programs	Rent is subsidized by the federal government	1965 Housing Act and 1974 Housing Act (includes Section 8—which encourages the use of existing housing stock)
Intermediate housing	Remodeled apartments clustered in an area conveniently located near geriatric services	Provides a more protected and structured environment than a boarding home
Personal care home	Home for individuals with chronic disabilities or conditions that require assistance with activities of daily living	A nurse is available for medication needs and a physician may be on call. All meals are provided, and assistance is given for daily activities as needed
Alternative housing	Broad range of living arrangements—common to most is a small environment, decent physical facilities, and utilization of existing housing stock	House sharing (owner renting space to another), commune (residential cooperative)
Boarding home	Privately operated homes	Renter is supplied with a room, board, and usually shared bath. The number of boarders may vary
Halfway house	Room and shared bath. Renter may be supported by an agency	More structure and support than a boarding home. May have a program coordinator on site

LIVING ARRANGEMENTS AND THE ELDERLY (CONTINUED)

Type (Name)	Definition	Features
Assisted care facility (sometimes referred to as personal care)	Private or religiously affiliated living arrangement for those needing assistance with medication, activities of daily living, or cognitive problems	A nurse is available for medication needs, and a physician may be on call. All meals are provided, and assistance is given for activities of daily living and cognitive management
Nursing home	May be for profit, nonprofit, county, state, federal, private, religiously affiliated. May provide skilled care and chronic care	Nursing staff around the clock. Physicians available on a regular basis and for emergencies. Therapies, dietician, social workers, activities workers available as needed within specific guidelines. Nursing aides or CNAs available for ADLs as needed.

REFERENCE

Lewis, S. (1989). *Elder care in occupational therapy* (pp. 28-29). Thorofare, NJ: SLACK Incorporated.

MODIFYING AND DESIGNING LIVING ARRANGEMENTS

APPENDIX

J

To prevent slipping and tripping:

✧   Mark bright-colored tape at edge of steps, at thresholds, and on appliance controls.

✧   Provide light switches at the top and the bottom of stairs as well as handrails on both sides.

✧   Paint outside steps with paint that has a bright contrasting color and a rough texture or use abrasive tape. Whenever possible paint and tape should have reflective qualities for night use.

✧   Install wall-to-wall indoor-outdoor carpeting in the bathroom to prevent slipping or spillage that cannot be seen.

✧   Place grab bars (of contrasting colors) around shower/tub.

✧   Use a contrasting bath mat over the tub edge to increase and improve visibility.

✧   Utilize a nonskid mat of contrasting color so that foot placement is appropriate and accurate.

✧   Mark the top and bottom of landings of stairs with a different surface or color.

✧   Provide uniform stair height that has uniform tread widths.

✧   Provide rises on stairs that are a maximum of 7 inches high and 11 inches deep.

✧   Provide a lighted pathway from the bedroom to the bathroom (night light).

✧   Install a hand-held flexible shower hose with on/off switch that can be controlled at the showerhead.

✧   Fasten all carpets firmly and utilize carpeting that has tight, short loops/pile.

✧   Apply nonskid backing/tape on rugs.

✧   Mark or eliminate all uneven surfaces.

✧ Mark the edges of steps and thresholds with bright colored tape.

✧ Increase lighting so that all areas are visible and avoid glare.

✧ Provide a toilet seat of contrasting color.

✧ Utilize nonskid shower/tub surfaces.

✧ Keep major paths of movement in the home open (do not clutter or place fur-niture in the way of needed walk-through space), eliminate low-profile furniture or move it out of access routes.

✧ Provide decals on glass doors to indicate that the space is not open.

✧ Utilize exterior ramps, when needed, that are at least of a scale of 1:20 (one inch of height for every 20 inches of length).

✧ Indoor ramps require a maximum grade ratio that is 1:12. A level platform top would allow an adequate ratio for wheelchair maneuverability.

✧ Utilize no threshold shower stalls that use shower curtains instead of sliding glass or plexiglas doors.

To promote balance and safety:

✧ Ensure that door widths permit wheelchair passage.

✧ Provide walkways and hallways with a smooth, even, continuous route that is at least 48 inches wide.

✧ Utilize flush doorjambs.

✧ Provide grab bars as needed (especially in the shower/tub and toilet seat area).

✧ Ensure that the toilet seat is a comfortable height.

✧ Secure all furniture.

✧ Ensure that ramps are appropriately aligned.

✧ Ensure proper seat height for all furniture and wheelchairs.

✧ Provide chairs that have a firm support and armrests (useful when arising from chair).

✧ Provide slow-closing elevator doors with sensitive reopening mechanisms that do not swing forcefully shut.

To prevent accidents or personal attack:

✧ Utilize emergency electronic devices and telephones in bedroom, kitchen, and bathroom areas.

✧ Have emergency numbers available in large print at telephone area.

To prevent gas leakage, water overflow, fires, burns, and scalding:

✧ Provide controlled temperature in showers, tubs, and sinks.

✧ Use safety shut-off for gas burners.

✧ Mark hot water faucets in red.

✧ Provide stove burner controls in front of the stove.

✧ Install a tap water overflow alarm.

✧ Utilize bright colored tape to mark the on/off positions of appliance controls (stove, electric fry pan, microwave).

To prevent back, hip, knee joint, and hand strain and to promote energy conservation:

✧　When there is a client need, provide a floor-to-ceiling pole that can be used to assist with dressing and transfers.

✧　Provide convenient clothing and small article storage in a manner so as to avoid bending.

✧　Use doorknobs that are levered.

✧　Purchase refrigerators that do not have low drawers; side-by-side styles are helpful.

✧　Use raised toilet seats with grab bars at toilet area.

✧　Place mirrors at eye level.

✧　Install a mirror with an extension arm on wall (bedroom and/or bathroom areas).

✧　Mount a hair dryer on the wall so it does not have to be held.

✧　Provide countertops at an appropriate level for the client (consider wheelchair if that is applicable).

✧　Make space for a chair/stool near counters.

To separate the foreground from the background:

✧　Increase utilization of color contrast (e.g., dark knobs on light cabinets, surfaces of edges or steps, at thresholds; on light switches and on appliance controls).

✧　Utilize contrasting textures when needed.

✧　Provide large dials on stoves, ovens, and microwaves for easy reading.

To provide good illumination, prevent glare, and ensure safety:

✧　Install automatic or pull chain lights in closets.

✧　Avoid exposed bulbs (use horizontally lowered window shades, frosted bulbs, shaded lamps, valance lighting, and cone lighting to prevent glare).

✧　Provide task lighting where extra illumination is required.

✧　Increase lighting (multiple bulbs or higher wattage) as needed.

✧　Utilize switches that provide adjustable intensity for light with different tasks.

✧　Install window treatments and awnings on outside windows with direct sunlight that permit light filtering.

✧　Provide illuminated switches (lights and appliances and any other electrical equipment). Make certain that all electrical wires are out of access routes, uncluttered, and clearly visible.

✧　Make certain there are nightlights at the corners of the bedroom, leading to the bathroom, and inside the bathroom.

✧　Avoid high-glossed floors/utilize nonreflective floor tiles.

✧　Maximize the use of natural light.

✧　Avoid placing objects that provide glare (television, clocks, glass-covered pictures and mirrors) near light sources.

✧　Avoid fluorescent lights when possible.

✧　Put placemats on shiny Formica work surfaces and tabletops.

In addition to the previous table dealing with modifying living areas, the following information is recommended:

In *Occupational Therapy Treatment Goals for the Physically and Cognitively Disabled* there is an exceedingly useful resource titled "Environmental Compensations: Architectural Barriers/Safety" that promotes the application of architectural adaptations for individuals with physical disabilities and varying cognitive levels.[1]

REFERENCE

1. Blue, T. (1992). Teaching the physically disabled. In C. K. Allen, C. A. Earhart, & T. Blue (Eds.), *Occupational therapy treatment goals for the physically and cognitively disabled* (pp. 263-267). Bethesda, MD: The American Occupational Therapy Association, Inc.

SUGGESTED READING

Holm, M. B., Rogers, J. C., & James, A. B. (1998) Treatment of occupational performance areas. In M. E. Neistadt & E. B. Crepeau (Eds.), *Willard and Spackman's occupational therapy* (9th Ed., pp. 323-375). Philadelphia: Lippincott.

Lewis, S. (1989). *Elder care in occupational therapy* (p. 31). Thorofare, NJ: SLACK Incorporated.

Sevigny, J. (2000, March 1). The value of OT in home safety: More than just an assessment. *OT Practice* 5(6), 10-13.

Shamberg, S. L. & Shamberg, A. (1996, June). Blueprints for independence: Carefully planned environmental modification can improve functional performance. *OT Practice, 1*(6), 22-29.

Universal Design

In 1993, *universal design* was defined by architect Ronald Mace as "an approach that incorporates products as well as building features and elements which, to the greatest extent possible, can be used by everyone."[1, p. 12] In a similar fashion, the Center for Universal Design in Raleigh, NC, defines universal design as "the design of products and environments to be usable by all people to the greatest extent possible without the need for adaptation or specialized design."[2, p. 1]

In the 1970s, Ronald Mace established a company called Barrier Free Environments. In the 1980s, Mr. Mace proposed the concept of a center for accessible housing. This later became the Center for Universal Design. In 1995, a group of designer architects, environmental design researchers and engineers initiated work on developing a set of seven universal design principles. These principles, published in 1997, are summarized as follows:[2-5]

1. *Equitable usage*: Ensures equitable use and is marketable to persons with diverse abilities. An example of this would be power doors with sensors at entrances.

2. *Flexible usage*: Accommodates a wide range of abilities and individual preferences (e.g., is the product adaptable for both left-handed and right-handed persons? Is the product able to accommodate to the user's pace and accuracy?).

3. *Intuitive and simple use*: The design is readily understood (regardless of the user's knowledge, experience, current concentration level, or language skills). The intent of the space or product is immediately obvious (e.g., an appliance with a switch or dial that is in plain view, well labeled, and easily used).

4. *Perceptible information*: The design needs to communicate necessary information, in an effective manner, to the user (regardless of the user's sensory abilities or ambient conditions). An example of this would include the product being able to provide appropriate tactile, written, and verbal cues for usage directions (such as visual, tactile, and audible controls on a thermostat).

5. *Tolerance for error*: The design needs to minimize hazards and adverse visible consequences of unintentional or accidental use. Elements should be arranged to minimize errors and hazards. The most used elements, the most accessible elements, and the most hazardous elements need to be eliminated, shielded, or isolated. Warnings of errors and hazards need to be provided, fail-safe features need to be utilized, and unconscious action in tasks that require vigilance should be discouraged. A double-cut car key which can be easily inserted into a recessed keyhole (either way will work) serves as a specific example of this principle.

6. *Low physical efforts*: The product or shape should have the capacity to be used in an efficient and comfortable manner with a minimal amount of fatigue. These designs should allow the user to maintain a neutral body position, use reasonable operating forces, minimize sustained physical effort, and minimize repetitive actions. Some examples of this principle are touch lamps that operate without a switch or loop and lever handles on faucets and doors.

7. *Size and space for approach and use*: There needs to be adequate space for maneuverability (approach, reach, and manipulation) without regard to the user's body size, posture, or mobility (whether an individual ambulates unaided or uses a wheelchair or assistive device). Four guidelines are appropriate when using this principle—a clear sight line to important elements for any standing or seated user should be provided, accommodate variations in grip and hand size, all reach components should be comfortable for any standing or seated user, and there should be adequate space for personal assistance or the use of assistive devices. Examples of this principle include installing wide gates at train or subway stations, placing controls on the front, and clearing floor space near and around dumpsters and mailboxes.

Since the inception of the Americans with Disabilities Act of 1990 (Public Law 101-336, July 26, 1990, in which a national mandate to end discrimination against persons with disabilities [including civil rights protection in public accommodations, employment, services provided by local and state governments, private and public transportation, and telecommunication relay services]) was established, occupational therapy practitioners have been increasingly involved in consultancy with industry, business, and in the home (as such occupational therapy practitioners are becoming ever more involved in the area of universal design).[3,4]

In her article, "Embracing Universal Design," Christenson illustrates the fact that previously there had been other approaches to describe specialized design. These included transgenerational design (focus on accommodating older individuals—with this approach environments and products are designed to be compatible with the sensory and physical impairments that limit major life activities that are usually associated with the aging process) and barrier-free or adaptable housing (consciously designed to eliminate barriers by adjusting or adding certain elements).[3]

Historically, the field of occupational therapy has focused upon assistive technology. *Assistive technology*, a person-specific approach that includes an array of products that compensate and/or help an individual function with a disability, can include such items as a jar opener for persons with arthritis or a long-handled shoehorn for individuals who experience difficulty reaching their feet while trying to put on their shoes.[3]

The definition for assistive technology that is used by the American Occupational Association was established by the Technology-Related Assistance for Individuals with

Disabilities Act of 1988. This definition is as follows: "Assistive technology is an item, piece of equipment, or product system, whether acquired commercially off the shelf, modified, or customized, that is used to increase, maintain, or improve functional capabilities of individuals with disabilities."[3, p. 14, 6]

Christenson provides an excellent description of the differences and overlaps among barrier-free housing, assistive technology, and universal design. A barrier-free shower base that is flush with the floor was installed in an apartment that was designed for a broad base of users. It was constructed of reinforced white fiberglass with a center drain. The manufacturer had advertised this shower as barrier-free, as it was designed for wheelchair users. However, it had a smooth but slippery surface when wet. While this shower base was suitable for wheelchair users, it was unsafe for ambulatory persons. It was necessary for the ambulatory individual to place decals on the shower floor or use a shower mat on the floor to prevent slipping. In this instance, the shower mat and the decal were assistive technology, as they were products that had to be added to compensate for the problem of falling or slipping. However, if the manufacturer had textured the shower surface, it would have been a universally designed item.[3]

The role of occupational therapy with universal design is one that offers great promise, for we therapists "are uniquely suited to provide services involving universal design due to our background in task analysis, assessment of person-environment fit, and knowledge of human anatomy and physiology and the disease process."[4, p. 3] Also, we are knowledgeable of the strategies for adapting environments to increase independence in older persons who experience the changes that are associated with aging.[4]

Occupational therapists have the opportunity to work in many venues. The workplace is an area in which older workers will most likely need universal design assistance: to prevent injury, to reduce health care related expenses, and to promote cost savings due to less retrofitting. Examples of universal design in the workplace can include automatic elevators, automatic doors, adjustable work station, and furniture, storage units that are easily movable; a proper lighting level with a minimum amount of glare, telephone and electrical outlets that are within easy reach from a seated and standing position, and emergency systems that are easily perceived by all persons through the use of tactile, visual, and auditory cues.[4]

Universal design usage in the home environment is another avenue where occupational therapists can utilize their expertise. Universal design in the home follows the same basic principles as that of the workplace. Some examples include raising the dishwasher to prevent bending; installing raised outlets throughout the home; adding color-coordinated grab bars and level-controlled faucets in the bathroom; providing an environmental control unit near the bed to allow the user to control the television, lights, and fan when lying down; providing wider hallways and wider doorways throughout the home; and installing no-threshold showers.[3,4] Aesthetics and function are the keys to providing a universally designed home. Most people want to feel that their home is home-like. No one wants to feel that his or her home looks stigmatized or institutionalized.[4]

Universal design and ergonomics go hand-in-hand at the workplace, at home, and in community areas. In these settings universal design and ergonomics promote an environment that "becomes more user-friendly and adapts to the person rather than the person adapting to the environment. Universal design also ensures that environments are usable by the majority of persons with less need for specialized solutions."[4, p. 4]

A team approach involving universal design concepts (consisting of occupational therapists, gerontologists, designers, architects, and building professionals) and using an assessment of clients' homes as well as the identification of specific modifications has been addressed in the newly developed Assessment Survey Process for Aging Residents (CASPAR).[7] This assessment process is concerned with the basic universal design concepts in improving living arrangements for older adults. Traci Rosenfelt, OTR/L, MOT, has been involved in coordinating the National Institute on Aging funded project that developed CASPAR.[8] This useful assessment provides ample information regarding: activities of daily living; consumer priorities; the ability to participate in home-specific occupations; and the layout, space, and design of the residence (in order to specify home modification).[7] "CASPAR makes it possible for occupational therapists to conduct accurate functional and environmental assessments that enable home modifications specialists to provide individualized, cost-effective, detailed solutions without traveling to the client's home. As a result CASPAR can be used anywhere in the country to assess homes and specify modifications."[8, p. 18]

This assessment is especially useful in areas that might not have trained home modification providers but where local builders are available to install or construct the modifications that are recommended by extended home living services (EHLS) or other specialists in home modification. CASPAR can be used by occupational therapists to collect information regarding a client's problems and abilities and the home environment.

The questions included in this assessment act as a guide, and comment sections are available for therapist use. Information collected revolves around mobility issues (that represent the types of modifications that are usually made by modification specialists), and sensory and cognitive abilities (as these can affect the appropriateness of mobility-related modifications). Together, the client, the family, and the occupational therapist categorize and identify high priority areas of the home that need changes. This assessment also involves the therapist taking simple photographs and select measurements of problem areas. The CASPAR video and a training guide are available to assist the therapist in this process.

At the completion of the CASPAR assessment the therapist or client forwards this information to a home modification specialist.[8] A staff that consists of occupational therapists, architects, allied health professionals, and remodeling experts review the material and consult with the occupational therapist and the client in order to develop proposed solutions (e.g., the analysis of the home, rationale, and recommendations for the best solutions; alternative solutions; product specifications; comparative costs; architectural drawings—if necessary; vendor information; drawings; and installation specifications). The proposed solutions are sent back to the client or the occupational therapist. This type of detailed information enables a local contractor, handyman, or remodeler to make appropriate, attractive, and cost-effective home modifications. Once the recommendations are completed, it is the client who is responsible for selecting an on-site contractor to construct the modifications. Support from the EHLS staff is available, as needed, to the contractor and the client, as the project is completed.[8] CASPAR is a vehicle that is useful to occupational therapists who are serving clients in need of home modifications.

The opportunities for occupational therapists to participate in environments that utilize universal design concepts are enormous. This is a unique area in which occupational therapy practitioners can use their skills in consulting with architects, developers, and builders in planned communities (e.g., assisted living facilities, retirement housing).[4] "Occupational therapist are well-suited to provide consultation to older adults and to assist them with remodeling an existing home, or building a new one that incorporates safety and comfort features that will support them throughout their later years.[14, p. 4]

REFERENCES

1. Mace, R. (1998). *Universal design: Housing for the lifespan of all people.* Washington, DC: U.S. Department of Housing and Urban Affairs.
2. Connel, B., Jones, M., Mace, R., Mueller, J., Mullick, A., Ostroff, E., et al. (1997, April 1).*The principles of universal design.* Raleigh, NC: The Center for Universal Design.
3. Christenson, M. A. (1999, November 9). Embracing universal design. *OT Practice 4*(9), 12-15, 25.
4. Swartz, T. (2001, March). Universal design and the aging worker. *Gerontology Special Interest Section Quarterly, 24*(1), 3-4.
5. Miller, D. M. (2001, October 1). Safety the American way. *Advance for Occupational Therapy Practitioners 17*(20), 7-8.
6. Technology-Related Assistance for Individuals with Disabilities Act of 1988. Pub. L. 100-407;29 U.S.C. 2002
7. Anonymous. (2002). *Comprehensive Assessment and Solution Process for Aging Residents (CASPAR).* Wheeling, IL: Extended Home Living Services.
8. Pynoos, J., Sanford, J., & Rosenfelt, T. (2002, April 8). A team approach for home modifications. *OT Practice 7*(7), 15-19.

RESOURCES

✧ The Center for Universal Design
North Carolina State University
College of Design
P.O. Box 8613
Raleigh, NC 27695
1-800-647-6777
www.design.ncsu.edu/cud

✧ The National Resource Center for Supportive Housing and Home Modification
The Andrus Gerontology Center
University of Southern California
3715 McClintock Ave.
Los Angeles, CA 90089
213-740-1364
fax: 213-740-7069
www.homemods.org

✧ Long distance learning (including an online certificate program in home modifications) is currently available at: 213-740-1364
mhenke@usc.edu

✧ Another excellent resource is to attend courses, workshops, and conferences at local institutions of higher learning that offer content in universal design concepts, supportive housing, and home modification. One may find excellent resources right in his or her own "backyard."

For example, this author recently attended one such two-day workshop at Philadelphia University, titled, "Beyond Ramps: Designing Spaces to Enhance Competency." This university also offers a certificate in "Environmental Adaptation Through Design" to occupational therapy practitioners (OTR and COTA).

Philadelphia University (Continuing Professional Education)

School House Lane and Henry Ave.

Philadelphia, PA 19144

1-215-951-6853

www.PhilaU.edu/ot

Assisted Living Facilities and Occupational Therapy

Appendix

L

Assisted living facilities (ALFs), a relatively new option for older adults in the United States, have been common in northern European countries such as Sweden and Denmark for decades. In Denmark, occupational and physical therapy are a part of the daily routine within this setting.[1]

The Assisted Living Federation of America (ALFA) considers an ALF to be a combination of housing that provides personalized support services and health care designed to meet both scheduled and unscheduled needs of those who require help with daily living activities.[2]

The growing industry of ALFs in the United States is related to a number of factors such as:[2]

✧ The increasing number of persons that are 85 years and older
✧ The changing roles of women (who have long been the caregivers for aging relatives)
✧ Elders living alone due to being divorced or widowed or having never married

The following principles of care are espoused by the ALFA:[2]

✧ Foster independence for each resident
✧ Offer cost-effective quality care that is custom designed to meet each individual's needs
✧ Promote the individuality of each resident, and at the same time treat each resident with respect and dignity
✧ Protect the privacy of each resident
✧ Allow each resident the right to choose his or her lifestyle
✧ Provide a safe, residential environment

✧   Involve friends and family (as appropriate) in care planning and the implementation of care

✧   Ensure that the assisted living residence is a valuable asset to the community

More than 1 million Americans live in an estimated 20,000 ALFs.[2] An average resident's profile is that of an 84.2-year-old woman who had moved from her own home and who now needs assistance with 1.3 to 2.6 activities of daily living. It is expected that this individual will live in the ALF for approximately 2.6 years. Preceding admission to an ALF, the average resident has demonstrated decline in meal preparation, medication management, and bathing.[2,3]

Assisted living is an industry where individuals receive "assistance" with daily activities such as medication management, dressing, bathing, nutritious meals, and housework. There also needs to be careful attendance to strategies for residents to remain socially, physically, and mentally active.[4,5]

A major mission of assisted living is to provide a safe environment that has a residential tone (non-institutional), to foster independence, and to provide for family involvement.[4]

Fagan suggests a number of factors for occupational therapy practitioners to be aware of when considering a particular ALF as a potential workplace. First, one needs to ascertain the quality of services that are already offered by the ALF. Next, the capabilities of the staff to carry out any recommendations that the practitioner may make is of extreme importance. Third, it needs to be discerned if the compensation for occupational therapy services is appropriate.[6] Fagan suggests a number of questions that are useful to ask when determining the suitability of the ALF as a worksite.

1. Does the ALF have licensed practical or registered nurses available on a regularly scheduled basis to oversee the wellness and health needs of the residents? These regulations vary from state to state, as some states may require only that a nurse is available (this could include the use of the telephone), while other states have no such requirements. Some states permit the use of visiting nurses on an as-needed basis (from a home health agency).

2. If there is no regularly scheduled nurse in the facility, is there an individual who is responsible for assigning home health aides or nursing assistants to help the residents? Are there enough personnel to carry out the programs that the occupational therapy consultant would recommend?[6]

3. Is the ALF owned by an individual, a nonprofit organization, a small organization, or a for-profit chain? Individual facilities may have the ability to enter into agreements and arrangements with providers, but most need to obtain approval from corporate management. An ALF that is owned by an individual or a small organization will, most likely, have more autonomy in decision making regarding the delivery of services.[6]

4. Will the on-site management team of the ALF be supportive of programs that the occupational therapy practitioner may recommend? Will the team be helpful in finding solutions to any areas of improvement that are suggested by the practitioner? Is the management team willing to listen and implement the practitioner's suggestions?[6]

5. Financial arrangements for services need to be specifically detailed when discussing any type of arrangement. Questions to be asked include the following:

Will the facility pay the practitioner for all of his or her time? Will the practitioner be billing individual residents as an occupational therapist in private practice? Is the therapist able to bill all of the insurance plans that enroll the residents? If a resident is enrolled in a health maintenance organization (HMO), will the therapist be able to treat that resident or will the HMO refer the resident to a participating provider?[6]

DIRECT INTERVENTION SERVICES

When considering working in an ALF setting, there are many avenues of service from which therapists may choose. These involve: direct intervention, consultative services, health promotion (wellness and prevention services), environmental adaptation/design (this includes providing direct recommendations and guidance to the facility, as well as assisting clients in identifying environmental and physical design features that will support their independence), and providing services of a collaborative nature with the activities staff. Each one of these facets will be individually discussed in the following paragraphs.[6,7]

Fagan details a variety of direct intervention options in ALF. These occupational therapy services can be provided to those residents who are experiencing a decline in occupational performance by an occupational therapy practitioner from a rehabilitation or home health agency (either employed by these agencies or as a private contractor for these agencies) or a therapist in private practice. This type of intervention is usually reimbursed by Medicare, Medicare HMOs, and some private health insurance plans when criteria are met and when developed in conjunction with a physician's care plan.[6] Areas of direct intervention intervention usually focus upon familiar activities of daily living skills (bathing, grooming, dressing, toileting, and functional mobility involved in performing activities of daily living) and instrumental activities of daily living (laundry, community reintegration, and money management).[5] Enhancing a resident's ability to adapt to favored leisure skills (e.g., embroidery, knitting, painting, writing, card playing) in the wake of declining vision, fine motor skills, and endurance is another venue for remediation.[6]

Besides referrals for physical decline, referrals in direct intervention may also include: functional continence retraining, powered or scooter mobility training, low-vision remediation, and psychosocial needs (especially needs of depression).[6] Within the realm of intervention in the ALF is the area of environmental adaptation to promote competency in activities of daily living for those residents experiencing a decrease in strength, range of motion, or fine motor skills. The most frequently used adaptations include lever-style doorknobs and faucets, adapted key holders, bigger light switches, illuminated light switches, focused lighting, raised toilet seats or levators, bed assist bars, grab bars in strategic locations, and bath benches. In addition a therapist may also be asked to customize specific adaptations for special client needs.[6]

CONSULTIVE SERVICES

Consultation services to ALFs is another important role for occupational therapists. In this type of work setting, a consultant therapist may be hired for a set number of hours per month (or week) or for a special project. Often the AFL administrator may have predetermined objectives for specific needs (e.g., development of a falls prevention program, instructing staff in methods to encourage resident independence with dressing and bathing, involvement in the admissions/resident assessment process, involvement and development of a dementia care program, and developing an aquatics program [if the AFL has its own pool or buses residents to a community pool suitably heated for older adults]). At other times a therapist may be asked to help solve problems regarding a specific resident's needs. In situations such as this, it is wise to thoroughly review state licensure laws and professional liability insurance regulations regarding the need for obtaining physician's orders when providing services to residents on a consultation basis.[6]

Consultation opportunities relating to health promotion and wellness are other kinds of services that therapists can provide. Lifestyle redesign (as exemplified by the University of Southern California program and detailed in Unit I of this text) and health education management (e.g., medication management, stress management, the empowerment of the residents to maintain and enhance their quality of life and independence, the prevention of potential health problems, and the empowerment of the residents to make informed choices concerning matters that are important to them) provide a skilled and powerful approach for therapists to promote wellness.[6,8]

Consultation services involving collaboration with the activities staff of ALFs offer another way in which therapists can utilize their professional expertise. Many ALFs do not have a recreational therapist on staff. Instead there is a reliance on activities personnel who may have minimal formal training. While some of these staff members may possess excellent skills, others may need and benefit from assistance and planning appropriate activities for residents with physical problems or for those diagnosed with dementia or other types of cognitive impairments. Of special note are those with Alzheimer's disease. In many instances the occupational therapist may need to assess the skills of each resident (e.g., the Allen Cognitive Level Test[9]) to determine appropriate group selection and to assist the activities staff member with the adaptation of activities as needed by each resident.[6]

Environmental design and environmental adaptation are two of the most exciting and promising areas of expansion for therapists. Although occupational therapy has been concerned with and involved in barrier-free design and the promotion of adaptive environments to address impairment for a long time, this area of concern has also seen great advancement in promoting wellness.[6,10] Fagan explores the fact that occupational therapy practitioners have been trained to understand the functional impact of impairment (e.g., low or impaired vision resulting from disease or conditions such as cataracts, macular degeneration, glaucoma, retinopathy, and other impairments such as disability due to hemiplegia, Parkinson's disease, and degenerative joint disease). These conditions may result in the restriction of a resident's ability to open heavy doors, use the bathroom safely, or find one's way through darkened hallways.

Solving problems, such as a resident not being able to distinguish where a chair stops and the floor begins, or not being able to rise from a chair or sofa that is too soft and too low readily falls into the practitioner's domain. Therapists who work with architects, interior designers, and construction companies during new construction have the opportunity to recommend features that are able to improve the functional use of a building. This may also be cost saving in that it may prevent the need for further widespread adaptations throughout the facility.[6]

Chialastri and Kolodner posited yet another dimension for occupational therapy's involvement of universal design and adaptation. They sought "to discover a comprehensive tool that could be used to survey ALFs to compare design features that have an impact on a person's occupational performance and independence."[7, p. 2] This tool can be used in a number of ways, such as a tool to help an older adult and family members determine which ALF is best suited for the needs of the prospective resident, and to provide therapists and ALF administrators with much needed information as to the appropriateness of building spaces (both inside and outside).[7]

This pilot tool consisted of a 72-item physical environment assessment checklist with further coding within each category to give functional meaning to the design feature. The seven categories, derived from constructed concepts found in the literature and clinical experience are: the dwelling unit, the bathroom, the gardens, the corridors, the cultural environment, the public space, and the social environment. The functional meaning codes encompassed the following concepts: safety and security, self-maintenance role, accessibility, leisure-pursuer role, and socializer role.[7] Many items on the checklist could be coded in more than one category. Three ALFs were selected for utilization of the pilot tool. Some general considerations resulted from the use of this survey. Despite the fact that bathrooms are the most common location for self-maintenance activities (e.g., bathing, showering, toilet hygiene, oral hygiene, and grooming), the bathrooms in all three facilities were generally small. No facility had adequate counter space to store frequently used items (e.g., lotion, cosmetics, cologne, toothpaste). This lack of storage space reduces consumer choice and hinders independence. Also, elevated toilet seats were not available as a standard feature (limiting the ease of sit-to-stand transfers). The color contrast between the walls and grab bars was minimal (making it difficult for those residents with decreased visual acuity to distinguish the difference between the wall and the grab bar). No facility used the option of placing shower water controls low and toward the outside of the shower stall so that a resident would be able to adjust the water pressure and temperature before entering the shower.[7]

Another area that did not score well in the three facilities was the resident personal laundry room. No facility had sufficient and accessible counter space to permit the folding of laundry from a seated position. Nor did these facilities have front-load washers.[7] While Chialastri and Kolodner believe that this pilot tool needs to be refined and a more extensive survey is needed to validate the findings, it is my opinion that this is an excellent example of how occupational therapy can intervene in providing a way to determine environmental deficits that can affect independence and ease in performing everyday living activities. With this type of information facilities can better understand the needs of older, physically challenged residents in performing valued functional activities. Adaptations can then be rendered that can improve the occupational performance of late life residents.

In summary, ALFs offer a work setting with a wide opportunity for therapists to expand on in an ever-growing and much-needed service area.

REFERENCES

1. Regnier, V. A. (1994). *Assisted living housing for the elderly: Design innovations from the United States and Europe*. New York: Wiley.
2. Anonymous. (2000). *What is assisted living?* Fairfax, VA: Assisted Living Federation of America.
3. Anonymous. (1998). *National survey of assisted living residents. Who is the customer?* Annapolis, MD: National Investment Conference for the Seniors Housing and Care Industry.

4. Cassidy, J., Kolodner, E. (1999). Assisted living 101: Profile of a growth industry. *Gerontology Special Interest Section Quarterly, 22*(2),1-4.

5. Fagan, L. (1999). Assisted living 102: Experiences of an occupational therapist. Gerontology *Special Interest Section Quarterly, 22*(3), 1-3.

6. Fagan, L. A. (2001, February 19). OT's role in assisted living facilities. *OT Practice* 6(4), 33-38.

7. Chialastri, P. D. & Kolodner, E. L. (2002, September). Assisted living facilities: Function or fiction? *Gerontology Special Interest Section Quarterly, 24*(3), 1-4.

8. Butin, D. & Montgomery, A. (1997, September) Health promotion programs for older adults: The Oxford Health Plan's Model for innovative programming. *Gerontology Special Interest Section Quarterly, 3*, 1-3.

9. Allen, C. K. (1982). Independence through activity: The practice of occupational therapy (psychiatry). *Am J Occup Ther, 36*, 731-739.

10. Cooper, B. A., Cohen, U., & Hasselkus, B. R. (1991). Barrier free design: A review and critique of the occupational therapy perspective. *Am J Occup Ther, 45*, 344-350.

RESOURCES

✧　American Association of Homes and Services for the Aging
　　202-783-2242
　　www.aahsa.org

✧　American Health Care Association
　　202-842-4444
　　www.ahca.org

✧　Assisted Living Federation of America
　　703-691-8100
　　www.alfa.org

Ways in Which Color Contrast Can Be Achieved

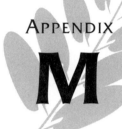

Appendix M

Characteristic Name	Description
Hue	The actual color
Light/dark	Lightness or darkness of a color
Warm/cool	Warm—colors closest to the red end of the spectrum (yellow, orange, red). Cool—colors farthest from the warm end (green, violet, blue)
Complementary	Colors that appear opposite each other on the color wheel (e.g., yellow and violet, red and green, orange and blue)
Simultaneous	Colors placed next to each other that can generate the complement of each (e.g., red and green can interplay so that each appears more red or green)
Saturation	The degree or purity of a color (e.g., pale colors are more noticeable when placed next to colors that contain greater amounts of pigment)
Extension	Refers to the size of areas being contrasted (e.g., light colors on a dark ground are more visible than equal-sized dark areas placed on a light ground)[1-4]

References

1. Lewis, S. (1989). *Elder care in occupational therapy* (p. 93). Thorofare, NJ: SLACK Incorporated.
2. Itten, J. (1970). The art of color (a translation). In F. F. Biren (Ed.), *The elements of color*. New York: Van Nostrand Reinhold.
3. Cooper, B. A. (1985, April). A model for implementing color contrast in the environment of the elderly. *Am J Occup Ther, 39*(4), pp. 33-63.
4. www.lighthouse.org/colorcontrast.htm

Rethinking Preretirement Planning and the Role of Occupational Therapy

Appendix N

In her article, "Preretirement Planning: How to Create a New Role for OT," Carol A. Leslie, OTR/L discusses her involvement in presenting a preretirement planning program for the employees of a major corporation.[1]

Because occupational therapists "focus on the total of life decisions relating to motivators, self-care, home maintenance, chores, career, finances, hobbies, social ability, friendships, faith, problem solving, future plans, health, illness management, and all of the other roles that create the canvas of one's existence," our contributions to preretirement planning can be significant, practical, and all-encompassing.[1, p. 16]

If a company agrees on a collective fee up front, there may not be a need for employee co-pay or third party payer issues.[1]

When initiating a program Leslie suggests the following:

1. Create a list of potential occupational therapy services useful for preretirement employees (e.g., wellness, occupation-based functions and coping).
2. Send a letter of inquiry to the targeted companies' director of human resources, chief of operations officer, occupational health nurse, or director of benefits to request a meeting so that the list can be reviewed and explore the concept of a presentation to the employees.

If the proposal is declined, accept it gracefully and ask for feedback on how occupational therapy services could be more beneficial to the employees and the company. On the other hand, if the proposal is accepted, it is important to prepare. Even if one does not have all of the answers, it is important to present potential solutions to common problems. Likewise, it is essential that one demonstrates that he or she understands the company's decision-making process (even if one does not have all of the answers).

"During negotiations, you must underpromise and overdeliver."[1, p. 18] Whenever one is asked something that he or she may be unsure of, it is wise to suggest that this situation needs to be "checked on" and that there will be an answer within 48 hours. This provides the potential presenter with time to think the situation through.[1]

Understanding the business or industry culture is essential. The corporate world has its own language, and disregarding this may lead to failure. Therefore, each company's product and language should be a part of one's presentations. Leslie emphasizes that we refrain from clinical terms, as these connote to lay individuals: problems, weakness, and illness (i.e., use terms like cognitive reframing to emphasize coaching a successful person. This should be used versus improving or "fixing" an impaired or dysfunctional individual). "Rigidly holding onto the clinical model will limit you to the once-a-year medical seminar, only to be booked if a particular condition (e.g., stroke rehabilitation, chronic pain management) is of interest to employees."[1, p. 17] It is important to focus upon basic human adaptation to retirement versus a psychological or psychosocial adaptation. Leslie suggests camouflaging a clinical basis with everyday language so that employees can be helped to rediscover and find roles that are meaningful to them.[1]

In terms of the financial aspects, it is essential to make one's proposal easy to apply, nonthreatening, practical, and financially viable. Some fiscal years run from July through June while others may run from January through December. It is imperative to become aware of targeted companies' fiscal year, as this cycle will affect their billing and spending.[1]

Throughout most of the Western industrialized world, individuals have viewed jobs as a measure of success and one's ability to be a provider. Therefore, much of one's worth may hinge on what one does (not on core values and character). These beliefs influence how one thinks about him- or herself; one is a human doer not a human being.[1] If one removes the ability of what one does through retirement, one can become at a loss for ways to feel worthy. This loss can lead to hopelessness and depression. "Retirement can be unexpectedly daunting and lonely. Anticipated days of nothing to do quickly lose their appeal without purposeful activities and roles."[1, p. 17]

The retirement experience is heavily affected by role performance, personal motivation, and physical demands. Leslie highlights a number of areas to consider for preretirement sessions:[1]

- Quality of life parameters
- Typical aging and atypical aging (such as simple forgetfulness versus Alzheimer's disease, needing a new lens prescription versus macular degeneration, achy joints versus osteoporosis)
- Societal expectations of performance during each of life's decades
- How each prospective retiree defines his or her own mastery (efficacy)
- Motor abilities (e.g., dancing, swimming, sports, crafts, home maintenance, baking, gardening, cooking, water aerobics)
- Cognitive abilities (reading, money management, chess, bridge)
- Faith in healing and healthy aging, the role of human connectedness, coping with change
- Gender differences in coping
- Risks due to long-term problems such as smoking, obesity, or alcohol dependency
- The benefits of a healthy diet
- Financial stressors and/or advantages (such as increased prescription costs, half-

price movie tickets, half-price travel fares, early bird restaurant specials, relocation to warmer climates [snow birds])

✧ Relationship issues (e.g., widows, widowers, divorcees may have needs for dat-
ing skills enhancement, assertiveness training, social mores discussions,
addressing adult children's reactions to new partners, HIV protection, changes
in spouses' roles, as a homemaker spouse [who never retires] may bear some
resentment toward a retiree's anxiety over having "not much to do")

Some of these topics may need to be discussed with the company so as to ensure
that they are considered appropriate for presentation. If any are considered undesirable
for discussion by the company, then one could provide handouts of available community resources.[1]

"Focusing on wellness, instead of illness, is essential during preretirement planning.
Volunteerism or part-time employment can be a wonderful alternative to the pressures
of the previous job while enhancing feelings of fulfillment, connectedness, worth, and
experiences."[1, p. 18] Preretirement employees should be encouraged to consider these
possibilities before they retire. Engaging in life roles that foster one's sense of personal
impact on his or her environment is a paramount need of all of us.[1]

Susan Cantor Bachner had developed an inventive preretirement intervention program that continues to be important and useful, entitled the Tactical Activity Planning
Program (TAP). Bachner divides this program into four sequential areas—fact find,
assessment, option search, and strategies. Its basic concept is to help each participant
legitimize new activity patterning for retirement. This program deals with personal
adjustment issues involving the meaningful use of time and role adjustment. Activity
analysis is used as a tool for assessment and planning.[2]

Fact find, the first stage, involves the logging of 1 week's activities so that a current
activity configuration can be assessed. Information includes all types of activities—
work, play or recreation, chores, talking on the telephone, television viewing, and even
daydreaming. A five-part day (divided into morning, early afternoon, late afternoon,
early evening, and late evening) examination expresses a wide variation of tasks,
demands, habits, and energy levels. Because the client who is involved in this process
has no predetermined time slots, a more accurate picture of attention span, pace, and
involvements can be gleaned.[2]

In stage two, the assessment is composed of four separate parts. These are:

✧ Source of motivation (this involves the categorizing of each activity into the following statements—"I want to," "I must," "Someone else wants me to," and
"Someone else says I must")

✧ Self-rating (there is a corresponding self-rating of the outcome of each activity
in terms of how the participant perceives the quality of the results or the feelings generated/associated with the activity. This ranges from poor, fair, good,
very good, to excellent)

✧ Profile (this involves an in-depth look at the characteristics and possibilities of
the activities. Some examples of possible profile items might include creative
versus routine activity, low versus high energy level, an opportunity to earn
money, an activity one prefers to perform by him- or herself versus one that is
done with others)

✧ Synthesis of the preceding information (this section requires the participants to
indicate if the activity listed [with its corresponding motivations, ratings, and

profiles] is something that should be kept or maintained, or undesirable and needing change

The third stage, labeled option search, reexamines items that have been listed as needing change. The following types of questions serve as catalysts to stimulate new ideas:[2]

- ✧   Can this activity be adapted? If so, how?
- ✧   Are there new ways to use this activity as it is or are there new uses for it?
- ✧   What would happen if parts were subtracted, slowed down, or eliminated?
- ✧   Can different activities, different people, and different locations be substituted?
- ✧   Is it possible to turn the activity backward?

To summarize, there are at least six ways to change activities (alternate uses, adaptations, subtractions, substitutions, combinations, and rearrangements).[2]

The fourth and final stage, strategies, evolves from option search in that the participant makes a selection of one or two of the most useful options. Underneath each statement that reflects the desired change, the participant should list a minimum of five sequential steps that will be needed in order to reach the desired goal. Participants should be encouraged to think in sequentially and concrete related steps, as this enhances the change process.[2]

In summation, TAP is a nonthreatening teaching tool for well and healthy individuals planning to retire. Because the input is from the perspective of the individual participant, there are no threatening or intrusive value judgments. This preretirement process requires that realistic goals be developed and that the participant be expected to supply the concrete steps that will lead to goal realization.[2, p. 187] TAP has great value in that it assists the prospective retiree in understanding the relationship in life between leisure time activities and work. This type of intervention is helpful in preventing feelings of despondency, worthlessness, and the development of identity problems because the participant has been made aware, through this process, of how to effectively use his or her time in a healthful and purposeful manner.

Bachner reminds us that "Individuals invest for many years in a preparatory process for an occupation on which their identity will be based."[2, p. 187] Before retirement from work concludes, these individuals must "with similar preparation explore and then legitimize a new activity patterning for retirement."[2] Although this description of TAP was written in 1986, this preretirement program still shines through the years. It is an inventive and pragmatic approach (with an emphasis on client-centered control and development) that can help participants to explore and plan for life after work.

As Leslie states, "Preretirement planning embodies all that is occupational therapy. No other profession is so closely aligned with life roles, purposeful activity, and maximizing function, which are essential elements for successful retirement."[1, p. 18]

The education of preretirement employees on issues that may arise when work has ceased is helpful in enhancing these individuals' abilities to not only solve problems but also thrive at this transitional time.[2] This is a service area for our profession that is needed and in which we have much expertise. Indeed, it is a specialty area unto itself.

REFERENCES

1. Leslie, C. A. (2002, February 25). Preretirement planning: How to create a new role for OT. *OT Practice 7*(4), 16-18.

2. Bachner, S. C. (1986). Retirement activity planning. In L. J. Davis & M. Kirkland (Eds.), *The role of occupational therapy with the elderly* (pp. 182-185). Rockville, MD: The American Occupational Therapy Association, Inc.

SUGGESTED READING

American Occupational Therapy Association. (1997). Fundamental concepts of occupational therapy: Occupation, purposeful activity and function (statement). *Am J Occup Ther, 51,* 864-866.

American Occupational Therapy Association. (1989). Occupational therapy in the promotion of health and the prevention of disease and disability (position paper). *Am J Occup Ther, 49,* 1011-1013.

Jonsson, H., Josephsson, S., & Kielhofner. (2002). Narrative and experience in an occupational transition: A longitudinal study of the retirement process. *Am J Occup Ther, 55,* 424-432.

LOOKING BEYOND TRADITIONAL INTERVENTION IN CARDIOVASCULAR ACCIDENTS

NEW WAYS OF LOOKING AT INTERVENTION

Clinicians need to always look for new and/or adapted methods and techniques of therapy (especially when considering improving upper extremity functioning with older adults whose diagnosis is hemiplegia). There are a number of effective approaches that can be used when treating older individuals with this condition.

TYING MOVEMENT TO FUNCTION

In a recent article, "Improving Upper Extremity Function in Adult Hemiplegia," Jan Davis focuses upon bridging the gap between movement and function from the onset of intervention and through the recovery process.[1]

Initiating Intervention

First, it is necessary to identify the major problem areas. Because individuals who are recovering from a stroke may have many common problem areas beyond dysfunction of motor control (e.g., cognition, biomechanical limitations, motor planning, or premorbid conditions), detecting the key problem areas is a major concern. These can be discerned through accurate and specific observations, as well as moving and handling the client. "It is important not only to *look* for limitations, but also to try to *feel* limitations in range of motion, resistance to movement, or changes in muscle tone."[1, p. 8] It is essential to be able to analyze normal movement and the components that are a part of normal movement (within a functional context). It is this ability that leads to a good evaluation and effective intervention strategies. When one looks at the movement patterns that deviate from normal patterns, it is important to ask the right questions. Some of these are: Why does this pattern deviate from normal patterns? Is there an orthopedic problem? Is the problem due to environmental restrictions? Was the problem premorbid?[1]

The next step involves prioritizing the key problem areas and determining which has the greatest effect on limiting functional gains (e.g., fear, cognitive impairment, neglect, or sensory loss). After the problems have been prioritized, it is important to make a determination as to which problems can most realistically be remediated within the time constraints that have been allotted.[1]

Promoting functional recovery of the involved upper extremity before there is a return of movement plays a vital role in the rehabilitation process.[1] "The more opportunities we take to incorporate the weak side into everyday real-life functional tasks, the more possibilities for laying a foundation to promote the highest level of recovery."[1, p. 9] The focus of intervention in the early stage of recovery (and thereafter) includes the following strategies:

1. Increase the awareness of the affected side.
2. Learn to incorporate or integrate the involved side into activities along with the stronger side.
3. Prepare for function by beginning with improving trunk control, weight-shifting, and proximal stability.[1]

Modifying the environment can be an essential first step in encouraging an awareness of the affected side. Positioning the bed so that the client's affected side is toward the door, nightstand, and television encourages family members and staff to approach from the affected side. This, in turn, helps to improve the client's awareness of the involved side. In addition, the client must turn toward the affected side when reaching for the telephone or water. This action facilitates trunk rotation and weight bearing. Using this type of positioning enhances the client's ability to decrease neglect and learn to compensate if a visual field cut should be present.[1]

Davis recommends three ways in which the nonfunctional upper extremity can be incorporated into everyday functional tasks/activities.[1] It is always important to include the involved upper extremity during these tasks. *Weight bearing/stabilizing* is one method that can be used to facilitate weight bearing over the affected side, as it encourages the use of the involved side and also improves the client's awareness of the affected side. An example of this occurs when the clinician positions the client with the involved arm supported and used as a stabilizer by placing that arm on a table (or other surface) that is within the client's visual field. Clients who are positioned in this manner are very likely to continue to spontaneously include the involved arm in tasks. Another method, *guided movement*, promotes normal sensory information while at the same time it facilitates normal movement patterns. Also, it encourages compensation for visual field cut(s) and is useful in improving function and awareness of the affected side. Guiding occurs when the clinician places his or her hand over the client's hand so that objects may be manipulated correctly during a task. This method is very effective with individuals who experience difficulty with motor planning, apraxia, and visual field cuts. Besides encouraging more normal movement patterns, guiding can be extremely helpful with clients who experience aphasia (as it eliminates a need for verbal prompts).[1]

Davis recommends that the following six steps be employed by clinicians when using the guiding method:[1]

1. The clinician should place his or her hand completely over the client's involved hand (down to the fingertips if this is possible).

2. The client should be moved by the clinician in as normal a movement as possible.

3. Talking should be kept at a minimum. Feedback should be allowed to come from the task/activity.

4. The practitioner should sit or stand where his/her movements are most similar to the client's.

5. The clinician should be sensitive to the client's movements. The practitioner should move together with the client in a normal sequence and movement.

6. The clinician should guide both the involved and uninvolved hand whenever possible.

The third method, *bilateral use of the upper extremities*, promotes symmetry while at the same time allowing the client to incorporate the affected side without the clinician's assistance. This method is useful in facilitating dynamic trunk control. It also promotes awareness of the involved side and serves to better integrate both sides of the body. Upper extremity bilateral activities such as wiping the table, shaving, or washing windows are useful when incorporating this method.[1]

IMPROVING FUNCTION AFTER THE INITIAL STAGES OF INTERVENTION ARE CONCLUDED

Improving function once movement has begun is a major objective in the recovery of the client with a cerebrovascular accident (CVA). After identifying the major problem areas, the clinician and the client collaborate to determine the movements or motion that they want to facilitate. Davis recommends using the intervention principles of neurodevelopmental treatment (NDT) that was developed by Berta and Karel Bobath (as it is based on normal movement and development).[2] Davis summarizes this approach (please refer to Unit 3, where the Bobath method has been discussed in greater detail) as the promotion of "the highest level of functional recovery for a client by helping him or her to relearn normal patterns of movement and avoiding the abnormal compensatory movement patterns commonly seen after stroke."[1, p. 10] NDT provides the foundation for considering the whole individual and understanding that proximal control and development help to improve distal function.

Once the specific upper extremity movement for facilitation has been selected, it is important to choose a starting position that will most efficiently and effectively reach the objective (this position may be sidelying, supine, sitting, or standing). The practitioner can then ask the client to attempt a selective movement such as wrist extension, elbow flexion, supination, or pronation. The clinician would then take the client through the movement so that he or she can begin to experience how that movement "feels." As the client attempts to move, the therapist moves, facilitates, guides, and inhibits the upper extremity as needed in order to achieve controlled movement.[1]

When working with upper extremity movement, it is necessary to identify the components necessary for proximal control. The therapist needs to determine where to place his or her hands so that the client's movement can be effectively facilitated.[1] Davis states that the best way to learn specific facilitation techniques is through video-tape demonstrations and hands-on practice in workshops.[1]

Movement can readily be incorporated into functional activity (e.g., if working on selective elbow flexion, the client might practice bringing the phone up to his or her ear). Davis prefers functional activities (which she calls tools) taken from everyday life situations to improve upper extremity function and movement. Davis recommends the following suggestions to facilitate functional activity:[1]

- ✧ The client should be in a good starting position (be exact).
- ✧ One should not proceed too quickly (slightly slower than normal generally makes a good pace).
- ✧ Variations should not be assumed to be wrong (there are a great number of variations of normal movement).
- ✧ The clinician should facilitate, inhibit, and guide the client through the functional activity.
- ✧ The practitioner should modify the position of the client to elicit more appropriate movements, and modify the activity to elicit better movements. The client's movements should not just be the only movements that are modified.
- ✧ Activities that require the same movements that the clinician is trying to elicit are the most helpful.
- ✧ Activities that are appropriate to the client's skill level are the most beneficial as more complex activities require greater skill.
- ✧ The difficulty of the activity may be increased as the client improves.
- ✧ The practitioner should anticipate the next step in the activity (i.e., the movement that is needed) and be ready to facilitate it.
- ✧ Last, but certainly not least, the activity must have meaning to the client. The client must understand the purpose of the activity and be motivated to participate in it.

Davis has given us much pause for thought as she incorporates meaningful and functional activities to promote recovery in the client with CVA. Her concluding remarks are very telling: "To be the most effective and elicit the best results, a problem-solving approach must be used that includes taking in information, interpreting the information, and designing and implementing an intervention program that not only facilitates upper extremity movement, but also ties that movement to function."[1, p. 12]

Constraint-Induced Movement Therapy and Occupational Therapy

In Unit 3 the work of Edward Taub, PhD concerning the rehabilitation of upper extremity function after a CVA was discussed. Currently occupational therapists are beginning to consider and utilize this type of therapy.[3]

Constraint-induced movement therapy (CIMT) is an intervention approach that constrains the unaffected arm (either by mitt or sling). At this writing it is a highly controversial concept because it is still in the research phase.[3] However, Joyce Sabari, PhD, OTR, BCN, and Leslie A. Kane, MA, OTR, witnessed the dramatic results of a case of natural CIMT that occurred in a 79-year-old woman who had a pontine stroke while standing on a city street. During this episode the client fell and fractured her right shoulder. Orthopedic intervention called for her arm to be immobilized, which is basically the same protocol as that used by CIMT.[4] Immediately after the CVA the woman was completely unable to care for herself and her frustration level was exceedingly high. However, by the time she left the hospital, the individual (whose arm was still in a sling) was able to feed herself, dress herself, and use a computer and mouse. This was all due to the return of strength and control of the affected arm.[4]

Taub coined the term *learned nonuse* to connote the concept that learned nonuse occurs during the first few weeks following a CVA because compensation begins almost immediately after the incident.[5-8]

Most studies involving CIMT techniques have been done with a small group of participants (who have upper extremity dysfunction in one arm due to a stroke). In Dr. Taub's study there are very strict requirements such as:

1. Participants must have no cognitive deficits.
2. The protocol consisted of 2-week intervention periods where the non-affected arm was constrained for 90% of waking hours.
3. Participants had therapy for at least 6 hours a day—5 days a week.

In therapy the participants practiced tiny movements that would enhance their ability to reach out, grasp, and move items. These individuals regained three-quarters of their normal use of their paralyzed arms in just 2 weeks. The participants also showed growth changes in their brains (as demonstrated by pre- and post-therapy brain mapping techniques). Six months post therapy these achievements were still retained.[5-8]

Taub's intervention is two-pronged. One prong focuses upon taking away the compensating arm and forcing the participant to use the affected arm. The other prong involves promoting an incentive for the participant to want to move his or her affected arm. This is needed in order for the central nervous system to be able to reorganize. This does not happen spontaneously as there needs to be a response to confronting a challenge or needing a goal.[3] Sabari states that, "The goal of therapy is to structure the challenges so that the demands of the task and environment are going to stimulate the person's brain to begin to figure out a way to get the muscles to move the arm. This is what OT is all about."[3, p. 8]

Michele Hahn, MSOT, OTR/L is currently involved in CIMT research at Washington University in St. Louis (funded by the National Institutes of Health). This study is complex and involves three levels of therapy and a higher level of CIMT. Hahn cautions that it is too early to make gross generalizations about this form of intervention, "because it's not for everybody, and it is too soon to tell."[3, p. 8]

Hahn goes on to relate that a major aspect of CIMT involves *shaping*. The clinician looks at a particular movement the client is working on and pinpoints where it becomes difficult. The clinician then isolates this point of difficulty and asks the client to rehearse or repeat the movement. The client then practices the movement that was difficult in blocks of time (perhaps 40 to 45 minutes) and at random. Hahn states that "this is where some people are going to get back the normalcy of their movements… shaping is a key piece."[3, p. 9] Therapy also progresses to encouraging the client to perform functional tasks. Hahn clearly manifests, "If you have someone do shaping all day and nothing functional, it's just exercise. What OTs bring to this is their knowledge in purposeful activity and motor learning. It's about understanding activity, what it does to people, and how it motivates them."[3, p. 9]

At present CIMT is typically not covered by insurance companies. However, there still is a demand for CIMT. Hahn runs a private program out of Washington University for which participants pay out of pocket. Dr. Taub also runs the Taub Training Clinic at the University of Alabama as a direct pay service.[8] While work in CIMT is still in a nascent state, its prospects look promising, and it represents a new area of remediation that should prove helpful to impaired elders.

Conclusion

In summary, the two approaches discussed in this appendix offer interesting, effective, and promising methods for approaching intervention with those older adults who experience upper extremity dysfunction due to CVA.

References

1. Davis, J. (2001, December 17). Improving upper-extremity function in adult hemiplegia. *OT Practice, 6*(22), 8-12.

2. Bobath, K. (1980). *A neurological basis for the treatment of cerebral palsy*. London: Heinemann.

3. Gourley, M. (2002, February 11). Regaining upper-extremity function through constraint-induced movement therapy. *OT Practice 7*(3), 7-9.

4. Sabari, J., Kane, L., Flanagan, S. R., & Steinberg, A. (2001). Constraint-induced motor relearning after stroke: A naturalistic case report. *Arch Phys Med Rehabil, 82*, 524-528.

5. Kunkel, A., Kopp, B., Muller, G., Villringer, K., Villringer, K., Taub, E., et al. (1999). Constraint-induced movement therapy for motor recovery in chronic stroke patients. *Arch Phys Med Rehabil, 80*, 624-628.

6. Dromerick, A. W., Edwards, D. F., & Hahn, M. (2000). Does the application of constraint-induced movement therapy during acute rehabilitation reduce arm impairment after ischemic stroke? *Stroke, 31*, 2984-2988.

7. Blakeslee, S. (2000, June 2). Study offers hope for use of limbs disabled by stroke: Therapy is found to work in 2 to 3 weeks. *The New York Times (The National Report)*, A12.

8. Anonymous. (1998). Taub training clinic. *UAB Health System*. Retrieved November 20, 2001 from: http://www.health.uab.edu/show.asp?durki=43761.

An Emerging Opportunity: Life Care Management and Occupational Therapy

Life care management, a more hands-on approach to client care than traditional case management, includes a variety of services to the frail elderly, such as:[1]

1. A comprehensive evaluation of the client and family
2. An ongoing relationship with the client and family
3. Knowledge of community resources
4. Increased communication with other health care professionals
5. The ability to target specific types of care when needed
6. The enhancement of the primary care physician's role while at the same time providing care across the health care continuum

Life care managers "work with patients and their families to help plan their future so that the patients aren't simply reacting to unanticipated predicaments."[1, p. 28]

In the past decade, health care provider organizations have come to realize that clients need to be kept as healthy as possible. Necessary services need to be provided as cost effectively as possible.[2]

As a result of this trend the concept of health promotion and wellness came to the forefront in the health care community. To combat the reality that chronic health conditions require ongoing health care services and that clients who fall into this category are at high risk for catastrophic health care events, health care providers began looking for more effective means in managing diseases that would affect this population through regular health maintenance and prevention procedures. Disease management programs that targeted clients with conditions such as asthma, diabetes, and congestive heart failure have resulted in reduced health care expenditures and positive clinical outcomes.[3,4]

Sue Parker, OTR/L (a life care manager for the Frail Older Adult Management program [FOAM] at the Crozer Keystone Health System in southeastern Pennsylvania) and

Heisner, OTR/L (the Operations Manager of Rehabilitation Services at Delaware County Memorial Hospital—one of five hospitals in the Crozer Keystone Health System) have detailed the development of the FOAM in which the sickest of the sick frail elderly would be followed. "The program goal was to create a standardized, cost-effective, continuum-based program that provides comprehensive, continuous care management to a high-risk population of frail older adults."[1, p. 28] Heisner was an instrumental member of the FOAM resource team (composed of a geriatrician, a social worker, a geriatric nurse practitioner, a dietician, rehabilitation therapists, and a home care representative). Through Heisner's contributions (which included helping other professional team members understand the unique role that occupational therapy had to offer), it was decided that an occupational therapist could fill the role of one of two life care managers. Heisner suggested that a nurse practitioner, an occupational therapist, or a social worker would be good candidates. Sue Parker, an occupational therapist, was chosen after intense interviewing by three physicians and the current care manager.

The life care manager is responsible for:[1]

1. An initial evaluation (that explores psychosocial, medical, pharmacological, functional, nutritional, literacy, pain, caregiver, family, environmental, and quality of life issues)

2. The development of an individualized care plan (the focus of which rests upon each client's individual goals and needs)

3. Consideration of any elements that may interfere with the stipulated goals while managing the chronic disease state

The care plan is sent to the client's primary care physician. Within this care plan the physician is provided with a comprehensive "picture" of the client such as: the client's story; medications found in the home; current medical, psychosocial, and functional status; and some assessment results such as found in the Geriatric Depression Score, the Mini Mental State Exam, and any other relevant information.[1]

In the article "Life Care Management and OT: A Perfect Match," Parker cites a case review that provides an example of occupational therapy "on the job" as a life care manager. Ms. X, a client enrolled in the FOAM program, was terribly lonely. She had recently been moved (by her family) from her "unsafe" home in the city where she had lived most of her life but where crime had begun to become a major issue. In her new "safer environment" she was unfamiliar with the surroundings, as she did not drive nor did she know how to get around. Her rent had increased to 80% of her income, and she was looking for a way to earn some money to pay some of her bills. Parker connected Ms. X with a "granny program." This provided her with a stipend to be a "helper" in a school for children that had special needs for 5 days a week. The client, once again connected to a meaningful and purposeful life, was earning an income. "Because occupational therapists look at meaningful and purposeful activities as an essential component to health and well-being, this was a perfect match and a perfect solution."[1, p. 31]

Since its inception the FOAM program has saved the system money. There also has been an increase in the clients' mental health status as measured by the quality of life indicators of the SF-12.[5] The program has generated more business than can be handled. At present two life care managers follow 130 clients.[1]

"Occupational therapists are a perfect match for providing needed intervention—we know how to break down activities to match the functional abilities of our clients."[1, p. 31] Life care management represents a new and growing avenue for occupational therapy involvement.

REFERENCES

1. Parker, S. & Heisner, C. (2002, April 29). Life care management and OT. *OT Practice 7*(8), 28-32.

2. Berwick, D. M. (1996). Quality of health care. Part 5: Payment by capitation and the quality of care. *N Engl J Med, 335*, 1227-1231.

3. Edelman, C. L. & Gaven, C. S. (1994). Health policy and the delivery system. In C. Edelman & C. Mandle (Eds.), *Health promotion throughout the life span* (pp. 47-70). St. Louis, MO: Mosby.

4. Zitter, M. (1997). A new paradigm in health care delivery: Disease management. In W. Todd & D. Nash (Eds.), *Disease management: A systems approach to improving patient outcomes* (pp. 82-90). San Francisco: Jossey-Bass.

5. Ware, J. E. (1993). *SF-12 health survey*. Lincoln, RI: Quality Metric.

.

CLIENT-CENTERED PRACTICE

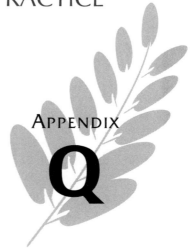

APPENDIX

Q

Client-centered therapy was first developed and introduced by Dr. Carl R. Rogers as a psychotherapeutic interaction method. It has also been termed nondirective counseling. It focuses on providing an understanding relationship within which the client may clarify his or her feelings. "The method is called 'client-centered' because it focuses on the client as a present person, and 'nondirective' because it believes in a minimum of intervention or direction on the part of the therapist."[1, p. 517] The psychotherapist should bring certain attitudes toward the client. Among these are interest, attentiveness, understanding, nonevaluativeness (does not express approval or disapproval); and the lack of talking about his or her own affairs or interests. "The interview belongs to the client."[1, p. 505] The psychotherapist must master the art of listening (such as becoming aware of the client's sensitivities and feelings). The clinician's job in this type of psychotherapy is to show an understanding of the client's expressions by clarifying the feelings behind them.[1] Rogers has led the way in understanding that it is the client's self-perceptions and feelings that are of the utmost importance in achieving appropriate and meaningful remediation.

In occupational therapy occupation-based practice focuses upon the concept of client-centeredness. Client-centered occupational therapy practice has been defined as "an approach to service which embraces a philosophy of respect for and partnership with people receiving services."[2, p. 253] The following recommendations (as affirmed by Law and Mills) represent ways in which occupational therapy personnel can promote a client-centered philosophy:[3]

1. Clients and their caregivers have the ultimate responsibility for decisions concerning services and daily occupations.

2. Clients and their caregivers must be shown the utmost respect (including the choices they make).

3.   Participation by the caregiver and client is to be facilitated and enhanced in all aspects of service delivery.

4.   Information, emotional support, and physical comfort should be provided.

5.   The focus upon intervention rests upon the person-environment-occupation relationship.

6.   The delivery of service needs to be individualized and flexible.

7.   Caregivers and their clients need to be empowered to solve occupational performance issues.

In regard to recommendation number 5, which emphasizes the importance of the person-environment-occupation fit, it is important to consider how the client views the variables that occur in each therapeutic activity (such as motivation, activity tolerance, novelty, importance, and quality). These will directly affect a client's participation in his or her remediation program. The person-activity-environment fit is also important as it refers to the match among the abilities and skills of the individual, the various demands of the activity, and the characteristics of the social, physical, and cultural environments.[4]

Chisholm, Dolhi, and Schreiber say that a therapist's ability to provide occupation-based (which they consider to definitely be integral with a client-centered approach) intervention is enhanced significantly when an assessment/evaluation tool is used that measures, identifies, and prioritizes what the client needs to do, wants to do, and is expected to do.[5] One such tool is the Canadian Occupational Performance Measure (COPM). This tool is an individualized client-centered outcome measure that is designed to detect a change in a client's self-perception over time.[5] Specifics as to where to purchase this item can be found in Appendix C.

Michelle L. Lange describes how she uses a client-centered evaluation approach when performing an evaluation involving assistive technology and switch access. "A switch evaluation begins with the client. To determine the best switch type and location, it is important to know what assistive technology the client wants to access and how he or she will use it."[6, p. CE-5] Whenever possible ask the family and the client to discuss or indicate what has previously worked, what has not worked, and why. The client should then be asked to demonstrate to the therapist a movement that he or she believes may work.[6] It is easy to see how relevant this approach is in incorporating client and caregiver input and preference into the process of evaluating appropriate and meaningful client needs and functioning level. With this type of exploration and interview an assistive device (in this case a switch) can be chosen that will be useful to the client.

I was fortunate to personally hear Rogers speak about the client-centered process as a therapeutic modality. In relation to this, the importance of client input and discussion as part of the therapeutic process became a dominant feature in the geriatric intervention program that I developed at a large state mental hospital in Pennsylvania. My first publication, "A Patient-Determined Approach to Geriatric Activity Programming Within a State Hospital" (published in the *Gerontologist*), described the importance of providing an avenue in which elderly institutionalized clients were involved in the decision-making process of their own therapeutic program. It was the belief that elderly chronic clients were "capable, with support, of making decisions that affect their life situations," that was the focal point of the program. These elder inpatients/clients became involved in occupations that were meaningful to them. Further, "It is a self-determined atmosphere that aids in defeating institutionalized dependency and patron-ization."[7, p. 146]

The program was designed to offer services to a maximum of 35 female clients who functioned on multiple levels. Diagnoses included schizophrenia, organic brain syndrome (due to circulatory disturbances or epilepsy), mental retardation, and depression. Impaired vision and hearing, low fatigue tolerance, and loss of range of motion in the upper and lower extremities were some of the physical limitations these clients experienced. The mean age of the 35 clients initially admitted into the program was 72 years. The age range was from 61 to 88. The length of the most recent continuous hospitalization ranged from less than 1 year to 45 years. The mean stay was 24 years.

Interrelated group settings, united by one basic group (known as the Basic Socialization Club) form the elements upon which the program was structured. The Basic Socialization Club was heterogeneously composed of all program members (35). It acted as a funnel for the remainder of the activities. It was within this group that the members determined (with therapist support and assistance as needed) what other therapeutic activity settings would be appropriate. The Basic Socialization Club's activities consisted of communal singing, exercise, reality reinforcement in the recognition of personal identification, discussion of current events, and the daily participation of one of the members as a host or hostess in serving snacks to other group members.[7]

Group direction, names, and purposes of each activity (which the clients called clubs) were discussed and decided upon by all group members and the therapist. Unlike the Basic Socialization Club, the rest of the therapeutic activity settings remained small (10 persons at the most in a group, with an average of 7 individuals). Some of the therapeutic groups that developed as a result of the client's specific interests were:

❖ *The variety club*: Individual participants were encouraged to make projects/gifts (using arts and crafts modalities) for themselves, friends, or family members.

❖ *The cooking club*: Members were involved in the weekly planning, preparation, serving, and clean-up of an entire luncheon meal. Trips to the local supermarket added a realistic dimension that aided in making the cooking club a total experience. As one member remarked, "It's nice to know that I can make some decisions concerning my own meals."[7, p. 147]

❖ *The ecology and garden club*: Group participants were responsible for plant care, flower arranging, the outdoor raising of vegetables (which were used in the cooking group), and nature study (this included discussion of findings from nature walks).

❖ *The friendship club*: Members were concerned with the physical and emotional well-being of the residents in the building. Projects included the beautification of the building (such as posters or hanging baskets), writing to recently discharged members, and sending get well wishes to clients who were in the local community hospital.

❖ *The grooming club*: Clients were provided with opportunities for developing a sense of responsibility and concern for their appearance. Hairstyling, make-up application, nail care, perfume utilization, washing and dental care, dressing techniques, and appropriate clothes choice were some of the specific activities of this group.[7]

In general, many of these therapeutic activity groups became a platform for achieving a number of therapy goals. Some of these included improving a comprehension of cause and effect relationships (e.g., if one burns food in a cooking group, he or she will soon realize that it is necessary to "watch the pot" in order to prevent this from happening again); the improvement of eye-hand coordination skills; socialization skill improvement, increasing of attention span, and improvement of muscle tone (e.g., by promoting a structured involvement in meaningful occupations a client has the opportunity to develop and reinforce appropriate physical and social skills).

Some group members were involved in transfer placement to other less restrictive community residential care settings (e.g., nursing homes and boarding homes). One-to-one discussions (between the therapist and the client) concerning the transfer process were important aspects of this process. As one member told me, "The clubs and community trips have helped me feel more interested in the things around me and have helped me feel more confident about myself."[7, p. 149] The Friendship Club's members were involved in writing to participants who had been discharged from the hospital to other settings. This helped to serve as a supporting link to a former member who was in the process of adapting to new living situations.

In conclusion, the client-centered program of elderly chronic mentally ill clients empowered these individuals to "take hold of their own intervention as much as possible." Motivation to do "for oneself" (instead of depending on others) was a primary factor in helping many of these late life adults to achieve higher functioning levels. This also led to the promotion of an improved sense of self. While this program was initiated at a time when state hospitals had very large geriatric populations, programs that use a client-centered approach will continue to encourage older adults to improve their self-esteem, self-confidence, and functioning levels.

Whether the setting is home based, in an acute care hospital, or in any other type of environment, it is through the client-centered approach that the client actively participates in "taking charge" of his or her own intervention issues. Remediation efforts are more readily and more meaningfully achieved when the client's input is the driving force behind the intervention process.

REFERENCES

1. Shaffer, L. F. & Shoben, E. J. (1956). *The psychology of adjustment: A dynamic and experimental approach to personality and mental hygiene* (2nd Ed., pp. 505-506, 517-519). Boston: Houghton-Mifflin Company.

2. Law, M., Baptise, S., & Mills, J. (1995). Client-centered practice: What does it mean and does it make a difference? *Canadian Journal of Occupational Therapy, 62*, 250-257.

3. Law, M. & Mills, J. (1998). Client-centered occupational therapy. In M. Law (Ed.), *Client-centered occupational therapy* (pp. 1-18). Thorofare, NJ: SLACK Incorporated.

4. Dunn, W., Foto, M., Hinojosa, J., Schell, B., Kohlman-Thomson, L., Hertfelder, M. (1994). Uniform Terminology for Occupational Therapy (3rd Ed.). *Am J Occup Ther, 48*, 1047-1054.

5. Chisholm, D., Dolhi, C., & Schreiber, J. (2000, January). Creating occupation-based opportunities in a medical model clinical practice setting. *OT Practice 5*(1), CE-1-CE-7.

6. Lange, M. L. (2002, February). Assistive technology and switch access. Occupational therapy evaluation. *OT Practice, 7*(3), CE-1-CE-8.

7. Lewis, S. (1975, April). A patient-determined approach to geriatric activity programming within a state hospital. *The Gerontologist, 15*, 146-149.

SUGGESTED READING

Rogers, C. R. (1951). *Client-centered therapy*. Boston: Houghton Mifflin.

Wood, W. (Ed.). (1998). Occupation-centered practice and education (special issue). *Am J Occup Ther, 52*(5).

Wood, W. (Ed.). (1998). Occupation-centered research (special issue). *Am J Occup Ther, 52*(6).

OT/OTA ROLES AND RELATIONSHIPS

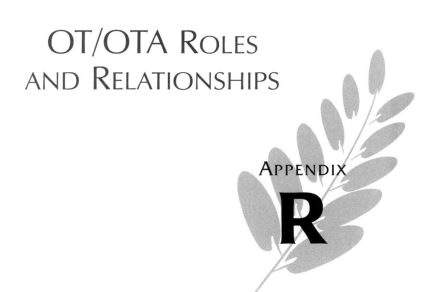

APPENDIX

R

(As Developed by the Commission on Practice, January 2002, and adopted by the Representative Assembly, 2002, M8, and hereby synthesized and summarized by this author.)

GENERAL STATEMENT

The delivery of occupational therapy services is a collaborative process between the occupational therapist (OT) and the occupational therapy assistant (OTA). It is understood that variations in role delineation of the OT and the OTA may change from setting to setting within the boundaries of the following parameters.[1,2]

PARAMETERS FOR SUPERVISION: A SUMMARY

1. Supervision, a cooperative process between two or more persons, is a joint effort to establish, maintain, and or alleviate a level of performance and competence. The supervisor possesses the competence, experience, education, authority, and credentials in excess of those possessed by the supervisee.[1,2]

2. The supervisory process of the OTA is focused upon ensuring the effective and safe delivery of occupational therapy services that fosters development and professional competence.[1,2]

3. The OT is responsible for developing a plan for supervision that includes input from the OTA regarding: the frequency of supervisory contact, the methods and/or types of supervision, and the content areas that need to be addressed.[1,2] The amount of and type of supervision may also be derived from the following

factors: the job setting (e.g., skilled nursing facilities, acute care in a general hospital, a rehabilitation hospital or center), each state's individual practice act, and federal and state regulations regarding the job site.[1,2] Frequency, content, and methods of supervision may also depend upon: the skills of the OT and the OTA, the needs and complexity of the client, and the needs of the practice setting.

4. In order to ensure effective supervision of the OTA a variety of methods and types of supervision should be employed. This can include: observation, co-treatment, dialogue/discussion, and instruction/teaching.[1,2]

5. The supervisory plan needs to be documented and a log of the supervisory contacts needs to be kept. This supervisory log should include the methods and frequency of supervision that is utilized.[1,2]

Roles and Responsibilities of the OT and the OTA

General Considerations

1. It is the OT who is accountable for the safety and effectiveness of the delivery of occupational therapy services, and it is the OT who is responsible for the overall delivery of occupational therapy services.[1]

2. The OT is directly involved in service delivery during the initial evaluation and on a regular basis throughout the entire intervention process.[1]

3. The OTA delivers occupational therapy services while under the supervision of the OT.[1]

4. The OT is responsible for specifically selecting and delegating which occupational therapy services the OTA will engage in. When delegating these services to the OTA, the OT needs to consider the following:

   ⅄ The skill, knowledge, and competence of the OTA

   ⅄ The complexity of the client's needs and condition

   ⅄ The complexity and nature of the intervention[1]

5. Prior to the delegation of service delivery to the OTA, service competency must be documented and demonstrated between the OT and the OTA. The factors that are utilized in assessing service delivery competency are: the judgment and clinical reasoning that is needed during the service delivery process and the performance of specific assessments, techniques, and intervention methods that are contemplated on being used. Service competency must be reassessed and monitored on a regular basis.[1]

6. "The role delineation and responsibilities of the OT and the OTA remain unchanged regardless of the setting in which occupational therapy services are delivered (i.e., traditional, nontraditional, or newly emerging practice settings)."[1, p. 10]

Responsibilities and Roles During the Evaluation Process

1. The OT directs and is ultimately responsible for the evaluation process. It is the OT who makes the client's initial contact during the occupational therapy evaluation. It is at this contact that the following are determined:
   - ⮤ The need for service
   - ⮤ The problems that need to be addressed within the domain of occupational therapy
   - ⮤ With client input, the client's priorities and goals
   - ⮤ The priorities of intervention
   - ⮤ Any other specific assessments that are needed
   - ⮤ Specific assessment tasks that can be delegated to the OTA[1]
2. The OTA can contribute to the evaluation process by implementing specifically delegated assessments (for which service competency had previously been established).[1]
3. The OT is responsible for interpreting the information that is provided by the OTA into the evaluation decision-making process.[1]
4. The OT initiates, completes the evaluation, interprets the data, and develops the intervention plan (regardless of the skill set of the OTA).[1]

RESPONSIBILITIES AND ROLES DURING INTERVENTION PLANNING

1. The OT is responsible for the development of the occupational therapy intervention plan.[1]
2. The OT and the client develop the plan on a collaborative basis.[1]
3. As appropriate, the OTA can provide input into the intervention plan.[1]

RESPONSIBILITIES AND ROLES DURING INTERVENTION IMPLEMENTATION

1. The OT is responsible for implementing occupational therapy intervention.[1]
2. The OT may delegate various aspects of the occupational therapy intervention for the OTA. This delegation is dependent upon the OTA's documented and demonstrated competency in providing service.[1]
3. The OTA may implement delegated aspects of intervention (in which service competency has been established through demonstration and documentation).[1]

RESPONSIBILITIES AND ROLES WHEN REVIEWING INTERVENTION

1. The OT is responsible for determining the need to discontinue or continue services.[1]

2. The OTA contributes to this process by providing information concerning the client's response to intervention. This will further aid the OT in his or her decision making.[1]

RESPONSIBILITIES AND ROLES CONCERNING OUTCOME EVALUATION

1. The OT is responsible for selecting and measuring outcomes that are related to the client's ability to meaningfully engage in occupation.[1]
2. The OTA is responsible for knowing and understanding the client's targeted occupational therapy outcomes. The OTA is also responsible for providing information that is related to outcome achievement.[1]

"OTs carry the responsibility for determining the appropriate use of the OTA. Supervision, however, is viewed as a collaborative process between the OT and the OTA, which fosters growth and development and assures the provision of quality occupational therapy."[2, p. 6] Simply signing off on the OTAs notes is not good supervision. Observing the OTA and providing feedback and guidance (as needed) offers a more constructive course and relationship. I have worked with five OTAs (two in the mental health setting and three in the skilled nursing facility setting). In all situations I found that all of these OTAs were outstanding at providing quality of care to clients. Because it is the OT who is ultimately responsible for all aspects of the provision of services, it is wise to develop an excellent rapport between the OT and the OTA. This includes respect, trust, and an appreciation for the duties and responsibilities between each team member. However, if any type of problem should develop, the weight of bearing this responsibility will rest solely on the shoulders of the OT. Therefore, the OT must be diligent in knowing all aspects involving service delivery and communications with others. It has been my deep gratification to have had the opportunity to work with these dedicated and knowledgeable individuals.

OT/OTA TEAM DEVELOPMENT IN THE SKILLED NURSING FACILITY SETTING

Pam Toto, MS, OTR/L, BCG and Diane M. Hill, COTA/L, AP have written an excellent article that explores the relationship between the OT and the OTA in skilled nursing facilities (SNFs).[3] Not only are these thoughts valuable for the SNF setting, but the application to other job settings is just as valuable. Both Toto and Hill place great importance on communication as a critical variable for facilitating effective OT and OTA relationships. However, as these authors demonstrate, there are (due to time constraints) significantly reduced opportunities for traditional methods of sharing information. Toto and Hill suggest a number of ways that can be developed to share information:

1. Store information in a communication book or a central area.
2. Communication boards and checklist notes provide easily accessible visual information concerning the direct and indirect status of a client.
3. Checklist forms can aid in managing documentation, managing billing details, and as a clinical tool to ensure that performance areas, components, and goals are met.

4. Wall-mounted laminated boards can provide valuable information to all team members regarding evaluation and discharge date, intervention minutes for each day, and quick identification of specified caseload assignments.

5. Voice mail, e-mail, and regularly scheduled telephone conferences are helpful in keeping disruptions to a minimum during valuable direct client care times.[3]

Further, the authors suggest that to maintain efficiency one should provide information in only one format.[3] Another method of communication is through hands-on opportunities (regarding client care). If possible, the OT should provide hands-on intervention a minimum of once a week for each client. For example, the OT and OTA could split the client's intervention period (the OT would address the issues that most significantly impact upgrading the intervention plan or impact goal changes). This can reduce the amount of non-billable communication between the OTA and the OT. Following this type of format the OT can actually observe functional changes instead of relying on second-hand information when performing documentation and discharge planning duties.[3]

Flexibility is another area of concern that affects the OT and OTA relationship. "OT/OTA teams must continuously analyze admission patterns and schedule workdays and hours to provide the best intervention time at the best time to meet their client's goals. Weekend and evening services should be rotated at least within the department if not among the interdisciplinary team."[3, p. 2]

Another way to build good rapport is for the OTA and the OT to be aware of the AOTA Code of Ethics and to base their working relationship on the values expressed in this code.[4] "Awareness of these principles decreases the risk of unintentional noncompliance. OT and OTA collaboration can promote a powerful relationship when both parties embrace positive ethical and moral decision making and problem solving."[3, p. 2]

Conflict resolution is another area that Toto and Hill address. When conflict does arise, negotiation and assertive communication can be very helpful. Consensual integration of both parties' ideas is the most effective way of dealing with these types of problems.[3] Hanft and Banks were able to identify expectations of OTAs and OTs that they felt were critical in forming successful teamwork. OTAs expected OTs "to share professional knowledge, help link interventions to meaningful outcomes, support OTA value and dependability, and provide for tangible supervision."[5, pp. 32-33] The OT's expectation involved the OTA asking questions, following the intervention plan, and providing feedback for any types of modifications.[5] Conflict resolution strategies are helpful in building ways to conduct a successful solution to problem areas.[6] Some strategies include:

1. Mutually agreeing at the outset to seek resolution
2. Identifying and avoiding trigger points (words or actions that can cause a negative response)
3. Practicing and respecting active listening
4. Being open minded and relaxed
5. Summarizing and reflecting

Changing strategies that facilitate a more occupation based work environment can often result in increased job satisfaction and improved service delivery between the OTA and the OT. An example of this involves changing the work environment to allow for an easier engagement in meaningful occupation-based interventional strategies (e.g., rearranging physical space for activities and supplies such as extra clothing, golfing equipment, board games, horticultural materials, and grooming kits [these kits can actually reduce "set-up" time]).[3,7]

Collaborative interdisciplinary teamwork is another approach in providing meaningful intervention for both the client and the staff members. Interdisciplinary team members strive to work together on the same goals (which have been prioritized and identified by each client). An example of this could be physical therapy concentrating on ambulation to and from the bathroom with the client in his or her room while occupational therapy would focus upon dynamic balance for lower body dressing and hygiene.[3]

Maintaining even productivity percentages between the OTA and the OT by managing intervention minutes throughout the week is an important aspect in promoting team harmony and balancing services. Thus, consistent productivity with adequate time for non-billable necessities (e.g., screenings, ordering supplies, filing, performing inservices for the facility, attending interdisciplinary meetings, and participating in care conferences with the client and the family) can more readily occur. Balanced caseloads help to promote the concept of "fairness" between the OTA and the OT.[3]

Another addition to an occupational therapy program (which can be employed by either the OT or the OTA) is the use of volunteers. These individuals can help in a multitude of ways (e.g., role of coach, mentor, or motivator for those receiving care; filling, photocopying, client transport, and the organizing of department supplies/materials).[3]

The roles and relationships between the OTA and the OT must be based on mutual respect, cooperation, and an acknowledgment of each individual's special duties and talents. Toto and Hill have provided some very specific strategies for enhancing this relationship.[3] In order to provide the most effective and efficient services to clients, it is essential to develop this relationship to its fullest. We share a rich and meaningful background, and our clients need responsible, caring occupational therapy staff who are unencumbered with negative feelings based on mistrust and not being considered worthy caregivers. "OT/OTA teams remain invaluable for clients in the SNF setting. Stewardship of success lies in your hands."[3, p. 4]

REFERENCES

1. Anonymous. (2002, August 19). New supervision and roles documents (parameters for appropriate supervision of the occupational therapy assistant; Roles and responsibilities of the occupational therapist and the occupational therapy assistant during the delivery of occupational therapy services—Developed by the Commission on Practice, January 2002). *OT Practice, 7*, 9-10.

2. Anonymous. (2001, October 1). Decision tree: To assist in determining appropriate use and supervision of an occupational therapy assistant (OTA). *OT Practice 6*(18), 6.

3. Toto, P. & Hill, D. M. (2001, June). OT/OTA team building in the SNF environment: Meeting the challenge. *Gerontology Special Interest Section Quarterly, 24*,1-4.

4. Anonymous. (2000). *Occupational therapy Code of Ethics—2000* (Revised). Bethesda, MD: The American Occupational Therapy Association, Inc.

5. Hanft, B. & Banks, B. (1999). Competent supervision: A collaborative process. *OT Practice, 4*, 31-34.

6. Crist, P. (1998, February 16). Hearing understanding, resolving. *Advance for Occupational Therapy Practitioners, 5*.

7. Westropp, J. & Lindstrom, P. R. (1999, March). Renewed energy following an epiphany at annual conference. *Gerontology Special Interest Section Quarterly, 22*,1-3.

SUGGESTED READING

American Occupational Therapy Association. (1993). Occupational Therapy roles. *Am J Occup Ther, 47,* 1087-1099.

Gilkeson, G. (1997). *Occupational therapy leadership*. Philadelphia: FA Davis.

Anonymous. (1999). Standards for Continuing Competence. *Am J Occup Ther, 53,* 599-600.

Toto, P. & Hill, D. M. (2001, July 2). Successful OT-OTA partnerships: Staying afloat in a sea of ethical challenges. *OT Practice* 6(12), 9-12.

EVIDENCE-BASED PRACTICE

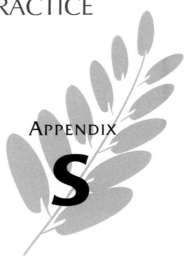

TERMS

Perhaps one of the best definitions in understanding the term evidence-based practice is used by Sackett and associates. They believe evidence-based practice to be a "conscientious, explicit, and judicious use of current best evidence in making decisions about the care of individual clients. The practice of evidence-based [health care] means integrating individual clinical expertise with the best available external clinical evidence from systematic research."[1, p. 2]

In her article, "Evidence-Based Practice: What Can it Mean For Me?" Law aptly discusses that the prime goal of evidence-based practice "is to ensure that external research evidence is critically evaluated, understood, and used in applicable clinical situations. The goal is not to negate clinical reasoning and experience."[2, p. 16]

Law points out that there are a number of reasons or beliefs concerning evidence-based practice that may cause difficulty for occupational therapy practitioners. These are as follows:

1. There may be a perception that evidence-based practice is already part of the clinician's routine and is being carried out to the best of the practitioner's abilities. Many clinicians tend to rely more on the expertise of others in the field than on literature searches.[1,2]

2. Another belief is that evidence-based practice is not possible for front-line clinicians because of the skill and time that is required to search and appraise the research.[2] Sackett and associates state that clinicians who develop selective clients can readily practice evidence-based intervention and care.[1]

The use of evidence-based practice should lead to clients receiving the most appropriate occupational therapy intervention rather than intervention that costs less (use of the best available evidence—not simply information that is gleaned from randomized clinical trials).[1,2] In occupational therapy, when evidence-based occupational therapy is working well, it "is the marriage of external research evidence with clinical reasoning and client participation to ensure that occupational therapy services provided meet the needs of the person receiving them."[2, p. 17]

INTEGRATING EVIDENCE INTO OCCUPATIONAL THERAPY PRACTICE

Taylor describes four steps for incorporating evidence in to the practice of occupational therapy. They are as follows:[2,3]

✧   The clinician should begin by asking a clinical question about a specific client's problem.

✧   Next, the practitioner should search for evidence or information concerning the specific problem.

✧   The clinician should then critically appraise the evidence to determine its usefulness.

✧   Last, the practitioner should apply these findings to his or her practice.

To understand how these recommendations can be put into practice, Law suggests the following scenario. A referral is received for client "X" stating that he or she requires occupational therapy services to increase independence in his or her home and community. The first step involves the clinical question of "What assessment is the best to use for identifying the client's functional abilities?" It is essential to ensure that the assessment provides information concerning the client's occupations (e.g., what the client wants and needs to do and is having difficulty performing).[2,3] Next, the practitioner should search for information concerning the specific problem as related to the assessment procedure. One can begin this search by looking at a minimum of two textbooks that are already at hand. Because it is imperative to learn about the client's perspective regarding his or her occupational performance, the Occupational Performance History Interview and the Canadian Occupational Performance Measure could provide excellent possibilities as starting places.[2,4,5] The National Library of Medicine PubMed system (www.ncbi.nlm.nih.gov/PubMed/) can be quite useful when one is searching for information regarding medical questions. In this case, by using the names of these assessments as key words, one can find an article that illustrates the development of the Occupation Performance History Interview as well as an article that describes narratives with persons who have mental health issues.[2,4,6] For the Canadian Occupational Performance Measure one can locate an article that examines its validity within a community-based practice.[2,7] After the articles and manuals are obtained, one can review both assessments to determine their validity and applicability to the specific situation.

The clinician should then critically appraise the evidence to determine its usefulness. An outcome measuring rating form and guidelines to assist one in completing this review are available from McMaster University and can be downloaded at: www.fhs.mcmaster.ca/canchild/publications/outcome_measures.html

The use of this critical appraisal form can aid one in deciding which assessment is most useful for each particular client (considering the diagnosis, the problem area, and the setting).[2]

After the appropriate assessment has been conducted, the therapist must ask another critical question. This is: What occupational therapy intervention approach will be the most effective (again, considering the diagnoses, setting, and findings from the assessment)?[2] The therapist is then advised to return to the PubMed website to search for articles that contain key words (such as occupational therapy and the specific diagnoses that relate to the individual client, e.g., "occupational therapy and hip fracture"). This search could glean five or six articles based on the topic at question. To critically appraise a research article that includes a specific intervention technique that was used in a study, one can turn to a quantitative review form and guidelines that are available from the Evidence-Based Occupational Therapy Group at McMaster University. This can be downloaded from the following site: www.fhs.mcmaster.ca/rehab/ebp/

After reviewing this article, the therapist can decide if these findings will be applicable and meaningful to the specific clinical situation at hand.[2]

In their article "Getting Started in Evidence-Based Practice," Abreu and Chang explore Law's and Taylor's thoughts on evidence-based practice and its use in clinical practice. They describe five steps to the evidence-based practice process.[8] These consist of:

1. *Formulating the question.* This can be an area or topic relating to: etiology and harm, therapy and prevention, economic analysis, diagnosis, and prognosis. The question should contain four parts: the problem and/or the client, the exposure or intervention, the comparison exposure or intervention (if relevant), and the outcome.[8,9] Law has suggested questions such as: For clients with "X" condition, will "Y" intervention be more effective than "Z" intervention and will this result in leading to outcome or increasing function in outcome?[8,10] "The best outcomes provide the best evidence for practice. The best practice provides occupational therapists and occupational therapist assistants with the opportunity to render better client care."[8, p. CE-2,11] Intervention questions should relate to effectiveness and efficacy.[8]

2. *Searching and sorting evidence.* This step in evidence-based practice involves searching and sorting for the best current evidence that is related to the care of individual clients. In regard to the search aspects, Abreu and Chang suggest the following: make connections with occupational therapy schools for Internet code access as well as for free access to public databases (e.g., PubMed) and specialized services such as the Cochrane Collaboration, which is an international organization made up of health professionals, consumers, and librarians who prepare, ensure, and maintain accessibility of reviews and health care interventions. The Cochrane Library is an online collection of information that can be accessed through university libraries and CD-ROM.[8] Other databases that require access codes that may be of interest to occupational therapy clinicians is the Cumulative Index to Nursing and Allied Health (known as CINAHL) and MEDLINE. Sorting involves ranking the evidence in order to clarify the type of research support that is available and the degree to which it is able to solve the research question. Systematic reviews are also part of the sorting process, as these reviews attempt to summarize unpublished and published materials.[8] Meta-analysis is another method for exploring evidence-based research. This method "refers to a variety of survey methods of research studies on similar topics using statistical techniques designed to synthesize and compare quantitative findings."[8, p. CE-4]

3. *Appraising the evidence critically.* This step involves criticizing and interpreting the evidence. Factors involving this include the power of the study, if the assignment of the subjects was random, and if the study's outcome has clinical significance (95% likelihood that a particular effect has a relationship to a particular intervention). Critical appraisal also involves determining the rigor or quality of the design.[8,10]

4. *Applying scientific research of findings to practice.* This step involves the systematic integration of the evidence with client and institutional factors. "The strength of this methodology is that it can help determine the best practice using the most rigorous quantitative research methodology as the highest index for evidence."[8, p. CE-5]

5. *Re-assessing the EBP process.* The last step is to evaluate the whole process (starting from step 1 through step 4).[8]

Developing a Critical Basis for Clinical Information

Initially searching and reviewing evidence to aid in making a practical decision is time consuming. However, in time this pattern can become part of one's clinical routine. The skill in searching for evidence and then critically appraising the findings, as well as learning to apply this information to one's practice, will increase.[2] If these findings are documented, "You and others can use them in the future without redoing the search and critical appraisal. As the volume of occupational therapy research increases, it is likely that there will be more critical reviews of the literature or meta-analyses that will provide research summaries for clinical use."[2, p. 17]

Both the Canadian Occupational Therapy Foundation and the American Occupational Therapy Association are currently funding critical reviews of occupational therapy literature. It is hoped that the availability of these reviews will greatly expand access of research information summaries that can then be used in the practice of occupational therapy.[2]

Utilizing Evidence-Based Practice Strategies in the United States

In an article entitled "Moving Toward Evidence-Based Practice," Pamela Toto discusses the importance of developing a wider interest in the use of evidence-based practice with older adults. She states that the *Gerontology Special Interest Section Quarterly* (AOTA) "will begin to include brief reviews of diagnoses, clinical problems and environmental issues associated with the geriatric population. These reviews are intended to provide basic information about the tool with regard to function, purpose, value, and reliability and validity in support of evidence-based practice."[11, p. 4]

Within the same article Toto describes the Community Health Promotion Risk Appraisal as developed by Guralnik and associates.[12] This is a 10-minute screening tool that uses test scores for standing balance, walking speed, and one's ability to rise from a chair. It includes a protocol and disability scales that were created by Jack Guralnik, MD, Chief of the Epidemiology and Demographics Office of the National Institute on

Aging. In a study involving 400 older adults over a 4-year period Guralnik and associates provided strong evidence that "measures of lower extremity function can be used to predict the subsequent onset of disability in activities of daily living (i.e., bed-to-chair transfers, using the toilet, bathing, walking across a small room)."[11, p. 4, 12]

Toto then describes how this risk appraisal was helpful when she was involved in a community health promotion program. The goal in this setting was to introduce the importance of fitness as a deterrent to any future disability. At the same time, this tool was used to encourage older adults to join the community wellness program with which she was associated. Toto asserts that occupational therapy practitioners who work in both nontraditional and traditional practice settings can utilize this screening tool to justify preventive interventions as well as to identify clients who are at risk for functional declines.[11]

EVIDENCE-BASED PRACTICE STRATEGIES IN CANADA

A community rehabilitation agency in Toronto, Ontario, Canada, has been involved in developing a method for collecting and applying available evidence of intervention effectiveness in occupational therapy practice.[13] Two informational systems were utilized: the Service Outcome System and the Client Feedback System.[13]

The Community Occupational Therapists and Associates (COTA) Comprehensive Rehabilitation and Mental Health Services had recently expanded to include other disciplines such as physical therapy, speech-language pathology, dietetics, social work, case management, and network therapy.[13] At present there are five specialty teams: mental health, physical medicine, pediatrics, school-based consultation, and psychogeriatrics.[13] Two sources of information (functional changes in clients after intervention and the client's perception of and satisfaction with the service delivery) were identified. Various clinical teams, which included occupational therapists, managers, clients, their family members, and a researcher, were responsible for designing the information systems while the agency was responsible for implementing and evaluating the systems.[13]

The service outcome system utilized a pretest and a posttest to measure the effect, impact, and/or consequences of services on users. All outcome measures were administered by the occupational therapist who visited the client. Measures were conducted at least twice (at admission and at discharge). For those clients who were longer term, re-evaluations are also used to calculate changes that occur over time.[13] Four criteria were used in selecting outcome measures. The criteria are:

1. Can capture anticipated or probable changes
2. Is practical for use in daily practice
3. Is suitable to the client population
4. Has demonstrated psychometric characteristics

Using these criteria, six measures for different clinical areas were selected:[13]

✧ The *Le système de mesure de l'autonomie fonctinnelle* (SMAF) was used to measure physical dysfunction.

> Herbert, R., Currier, R., & Bilodeau, A. (1998). The Functional Autonomy Measurement System [SMAF]: Description and validation of an instrument for the measurement of handicaps. *Age and Aging, 17*, 293-302.

✧   The Canadian Occupational Performance Measure was utilized to detect changes in a client's self-perception of his or her ability to perform functional activities that are meaningful to the individual (occupational performance) over time.

　　Law, M., Baptiste, S., Carswell, A., McColl, M., Polatajko, H., Pollock, N. (1998). *Canadian Occupational Performance Measure.* (3rd Ed.). Ottawa, ON: CAOT Publications ACE.

✧   The Quality of Life Interview

　　Lehman, A. F. (1998). A quality of life interview for the chronically mentally ill. *Evaluation and Program Planning, 11,* 51-62.

✧   The Life Skills Profile was the outcome measure for mental health.

　　Rosen, A., Hadzi-Pavlovic, D., & Parker, G. (1989). The Life Skills Profile: A measure assessing function and disability in schizophrenia. *Schizophrenia Bulletin, 15,* 325-337.

✧   The Burden Scale for Family Caregivers was used for psychogeriatric services.

　　Grasel, E. (1995). Somatic symptoms and caregiving strain among family caregivers of older clients with progressive nursing needs. *Archives of Gerontology and Geriatrics, 21,* 253-266.

✧   Presently the Safety Assessment of Function and the Environment for Rehabilitation-Health Outcome Measurement and Evaluation (known as the SAFER-HOME) is being involved in a validation process by the psychogeriatric team.

　　Chin, T,. Oliver, R., Tamaki, T., Faibish, S., & Sisson, H. (2001). *The Safety Assessment Function and the Evaluation*/SAFER-HOME: unpublished work.

There is evidence of positive change after services. For instance, physical rehabilitation clients demonstrated positive changes in disability and handicap scores. The caregivers involved with psychogeriatric clients had become more competent and had fewer burdens, and the safety concerns of older adult clients had decreased after receiving occupational therapy services.[13]

The client feedback system utilizes a cross-sectional survey. A Client Feedback Questionnaire was developed that included items from agency—developed questions and a standardized questionnaire. The questionnaire was designed to have a sixth to seventh grade reading level. In the year 2000, the agency received feedback from 893 clients. Most clients were satisfied with the occupational therapist's personal skills. Family members had an appreciation for the occupational therapist's suggestions and knowledge. Managers and occupational therapists studied the survey results. Consequently, action plans were developed to address areas that needed improvement (e.g., client respondents stated that they wanted more visits). Therefore, guidelines were established so that occupational therapists could communicate more effectively to clients concerning the length of services and frequency of visits as predetermined by the referrers and the finders.[13]

The Service Outcome System and the Client Feedback System have enhanced the agency's ability to blend practice and evidence. "The blending process has provided useful information for use in clinical practice, quality management, and outcome research."[13, p. 220] The utilization of these systems is an ongoing process as indicated by the authors.

CONCLUSION

Occupational therapy is at the threshold in establishing a body of literature and methods that are based on evidence-effective practice. With this new way of looking at client care, there will be, in all likelihood, a continuing variety of practice settings that will be involved in utilizing evidence-based practice. There is no doubt that with this strong emphasis upon sharing literature, expertise, methods, and research results that clinicians will be enabled to experience greater access to information that can only enhance and improve the quality of care of our clients.

REFERENCES

1. Sackett, D. L., Richardson, W. S., Rosenberg, W. M., & Haynes, B. R. (1997). *Evidence-based medicine: How to practice and teach EBN.* New York: Churchill Livingstone.

2. Law, M. (2000, August 28). Evidence-based practice: What can it mean for me? *OT Practice, 5*(17), 16-18.

3. Taylor, M. C. (1997). What is evidence-based practice? *British Journal of Occupational Therapy, 60*, 470-474.

4. Kielhofner, G. & Henry, A D. (1988). Development and investigation of the Occupational Performance History Interview. *Am J Occup Ther, 42*, 489-498.

5. Law, M., Baptise, S., Carswell, A., McColl, M., Polatajko, H., & Pollock, N. (1998). *Canadian occupational performance measure* (3rd Ed.). Ottawa, Canada: Canadian Association of Occupational Therapists.

6. Mallinson, T., Kielhofner, G., & Mattingly, C. (1996). Metaphor and meaning in a clinical interview. *Am J Occup Ther, 50*, 338-346.

7. McColl, M. A., Paterson, M., Davies, D., Doubt, L., & Law, M. (2000). Validity and community utility of the Canadian Occupational Performance Measure. *Canadian Journal of Occupational Therapy, 67*, 22-30.

8. Abreau, B. C. & Chang Pei-Fen. (2000, October 14). Getting started in evidence-based practice. *OT Practice, 7*(18), CE-1-CE-7.

9. Richardson, W. S., Wilson, M. C., Nishikawa, J., & Hayward, R. S. A. (1995). The well-built clinical question: A key to evidence-based decisions. *ACP Journal Club, 123*(3), A12.

10. Law, M. (2002). *Evidence-based rehabilitation: A guide to practice.* Thorofare, NJ: SLACK Incorporated.

11. Toto, P. E. (2001, December 4). Moving toward evidence-based practice. *Gerontology Special Interest Section Quarterly 4*(24), 4.

12. Guralnik, J. M., Ferrucci, L., Simonsick, E. M., Salive, M., & Wallace, R. B. (1995). Lower extremity function in persons over the age of 70 years as a predictor of subsequent disability. *N Engl J Med, 332*, 556-561. The full text of this article can be accessed online at www.nejm.org.

13. Chiu, T. & Tickle-Degnen, L. (2002, March/April). Learning from evidence: Service outcomes and client satisfaction with occupational therapy home-based services. *Am J Occup Ther, 56*(2), 217-220.

SUGGESTED READING

Holm, M. B. (2001, July 2). The 2000 Eleanor Clarke Slagle Lecture: Our Mandate for the New Millennium: Evidence-Based Practice. *OT Practice, 6*(12), CE-1-CE-16.

The majority of the above text was originally published in the 2000 archival issues of *American Journal of Occupational Therapy* as noted below.

Holm, M. B. (2000). Our mandate for the new millennium: Evidence-based practice, 2000 Eleanor Clarke Slagle lecture. *Am J Occup Ther, 54,* 575-585.

Law, M. & Baum, C. (1998). Evidence-based occupational therapy. *Canadian Journal of Occupational Therapy, 65,* 131-135.

Sackett, D. L., Straus, S. E., Richardson, W. S., Rosenberg, W. M., & Haynes, R. B. (2000). *Evidence-based medicine: How to practice and teach evidence-based medicine* (2nd Ed.). New York: Churchill Livingstone.

THE OCCUPATIONAL THERAPY PRACTICE FRAMEWORK: DOMAIN AND PROCESS—A SUMMARY

APPENDIX

T

In May 2002 the Representative Assembly adopted *The Occupational Therapy Practice Framework: Domain and Process*. The document replaces *The Uniform Terminology for Occupational Therapy—Third Edition* (known as UT-III).

Mary Jane Youngstrom, MS, OTR, FAOTA (Chairperson of the Commission or Practice, 1997-2002) provides a very thoughtful introduction to the Framework in her article, "Introduction to The Occupational Therapy Practice Framework: Domain and Process" that appeared in *OT Practice* on September 16, 2002. This author highly recommends that therapists and assistants carefully read its well-organized and comprehensive contents.

The UT-III provided a generic outline of occupational therapy domain and was designed to create common terminology for the profession's use in a succinct manner. The Framework, a broader document than UT-III, also provides a generic outline of the profession's domain. However, it goes beyond by describing the domain and outlines process.

The process explains how occupational therapy services occur within this domain. The process is built upon the structure of the domain, on the basis of suggestions by the profession's membership. Terminology that is used by the World Health Organization's International Classification on Functioning, Disability, and Health (ICF-2001), was carefully reviewed and selectively incorporated into this newly revised document.[1]

DOMAIN AND OCCUPATION

In her book, *Occupational Therapy: Configuration of a Profession*, Ann Mosey describes domain as an area of human experience where members of a profession offer assistance to other persons.[2]

Occupation can be broadly described as participation in daily life activities. The Framework utilizes the following definition for occupation:

"Activities… of everyday life are named, organized, and given value and meaning by individuals and a culture. Occupation is everything people do to occupy themselves, including looking after themselves... enjoying life... and contributing to the social and economic fabric of their communities."[3]

As Youngstrom states, "Occupations are seen as central to a person's sense of identity as well as to his or her competence and health. The individual's experience of engaging in meaningful occupations is the core area of human experience that is the profession's focus and the basis of our domain."[1, p. CE-2]

The following represents various areas of occupations that are currently considered by occupational therapists and occupational therapy assistants to be an integral part of our profession's domain. These areas are:[1]

- ✧ *Performance in areas of occupation* (activities of daily living, which are also referred to as basic activities of daily living or personal activities of daily living, instrumental activities of daily living, education, work, play, leisure, and social participation)
- ✧ *Performance skills* (motor skills, process skills, and communication/interaction skills)
- ✧ *Activity demands* (objects used and their properties, space demands, social demands, sequencing and timing, required actions, required body functions, and required body structures)
- ✧ *Performance patterns* (habits, routines, and roles)
- ✧ *Context* (cultural, physical, social, personal, spiritual, temporal, and virtual)
- ✧ *Client factors* (body functions and body structures)

The phrase, "engagement in occupation to support participation in context or contexts," is at the top of these areas of occupations that were just described. The basic areas and their parts are more discrete aspects of the domain.[1] "The word *engagement* describes the profession's holistic understanding and supports the profession's belief in valuing individual choice."[1, p. CE-3] Youngstrom further describes interventions, "Interventions are ultimately connected to facilitating the person's ability to participate in meaningful roles and routines."[1, p. CE-3]

OCCUPATIONAL THERAPY PROCESS

Occupational therapy process consists of three broad areas: evaluation, intervention, and outcome. "The process is dynamic and interactive and embedded within a context that influences the client and the process of service delivery. A client-centered approach is used throughout the process."[1, p. CE-5] "What is evaluated, how problems are framed for the intervention, the types of intervention used, and the targeted outcomes all center on the clients' occupations."[1, p. CE-5]

It is during the evaluation process that the therapist determines and evaluates the clients' occupational needs, problems, risks, and concerns. Issues or problems are identified in terms of the client's occupational performance risks (problems). When engaged in intervention, the focus is upon facilitating performance and the occupations that are of interest or needed by the client. To facilitate an improvement in performance, specifically selected occupations and activities are utilized. "Targeted outcomes are directed at facilitating the client's engagement in occupation to support participation in everyday life situations—an end objective that reinforces the focus of the evaluation and intervention phases."[1, p. CE-5]

During the evaluation process, the initial step is the occupational profile (occupational history, the client's needs, concerns, and problems about engaging in occupations are identified). The client's needs for seeking therapy services are identified, and the client's priorities are clarified.[1] The second phase of the evaluation continues its focus on engaging occupations. However, the focus shifts to analyzing the client's actual occupational performance. Clinical reasoning is used throughout. The basis for the evaluation is gathering information and identifying what hinders and what supports performance. It is this basis that leads to the development of the intervention plan.[1]

Intervention involves three substeps (planning, implementation, and review). It is in the intervention plan that the therapist determines goals, selects approaches, chooses mechanisms for service delivery, identifies outcome measures, thinks about discharge needs, and makes recommendations as they are needed. The client's concerns and priorities are always considered during intervention planning. This is a collaborative process between the client and the practitioner. It is during the intervention implementation that the assistant or therapist may use a variety of interventions (and monitor the response of the client). There are five different interventional approaches (create/promote, establish/restore, maintain, prevent, and modify), and there are four types of interventions (therapeutic use of self; therapeutic use of activities and occupations [purposeful activity, occupation-based activity, and preparatory methods]; education processes; and consultation).[1]

Outcomes may be defined as "dimensions of health toward which interventions are directed."[1, p. CE-7] "Outcome measures are selected early in the intervention process and should be congruent with the client's goals and sensitive to changes that will occur. Measuring and using outcome data occurs throughout the intervention process, and targeted outcomes are revised depending on client priorities and progress."[1, p. CE-7]

This Framework is essential to therapists and assistants in assisting them to help individuals engage in occupations and in supporting participation in the occupations.[1]

REFERENCES

1. Youngstrom, M. J. (2002, September 16). Introduction to The Occupational Therapy Practice Framework: Domain and Process. *OT Practice, 7,* CE-1–CE-8.

2. Mosey, A. C. (1981). *Occupational therapy: Configuration of a profession.* New York: Raven.

3. Law, M., Polatajko, H., Baptiste, S., & Townsend, E. (1997). Core concepts of occupational therapy. In E. Townsend (Ed.), *Enabling occupation: An occupational therapy perspective* (p. 32). Ottawa, Ontario: Canadian Association of Occupational Therapists.

INDEX

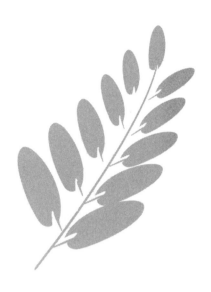

Build Your Library

Along with this title, we publish numerous products on a variety of topics. We are sure that you will find the titles below to be an essential addition to your library. Order your copies today or contact us for a copy of our latest catalog for additional product information.

ELDER CARE IN OCCUPATIONAL THERAPY, SECOND EDITION

Sandra Cutler Lewis, MFA, OTR/L

528 pp., Hard Cover, 2003, ISBN 1-55642-527-9, Order #35279, $39.95

Elder Care in Occupational Therapy has been extensively revised into a new and completely updated second edition. This pragmatic text presents up-to-date information in a user-friendly format that seamlessly flows from one subject to the next. From wellness to hospice, this edition offers a broad yet detailed discussion of occupational therapy practice that is devoted to older adults.

EVIDENCE-BASED REHABILITATION: A GUIDE TO PRACTICE

Mary Law, PhD, OT(C)

384 pp., Soft Cover, 2002, ISBN 1-55642-453-1, Order #44531, $36.95

Evidence-Based Rehabilitation: A Guide to Practice is designed as an entry-level book on evidence-based practice in rehabilitation. Specifically written for rehabilitation practitioners, this exceptional text is not designed to teach students how to do research, but rather how to become critical consumers of research, therefore developing skills to ensure that their rehabilitation practice is based on the best evidence that is available.

VISION, PERCEPTION, AND COGNITION: A MANUAL FOR THE EVALUATION AND TREATMENT OF THE NEUROLOGICALLY IMPAIRED ADULT, THIRD EDITION

Barbara Zoltan, MA, OTR

232 pp., Soft Cover, 1996, ISBN 1-55642-265-2, Order #32652, $29.95

This extraordinary book is an indispensable reference for outlining the theoretical basis for visual, perceptual, and cognitive deficits, as well as specific procedures for the evaluation and treatment of these deficits.

Contact Us

SLACK Incorporated, Professional Book Division
6900 Grove Road, Thorofare, NJ 08086
1-800-257-8290/1-856-848-1000, Fax: 1-856-853-5991
orders@slackinc.com or www.slackbooks.com

ORDER FORM

QUANTITY	TITLE	ORDER #	PRICE
	Elder Care in Occupational Therapy, Second Edition	35279	$39.95
	Evidence-Based Rehabilitation: A Guide to Practice	44531	$36.95
	Vision, Perception, and Cognition, Third Edition	32652	$29.95
		Subtotal	$
		Applicable state and local tax will be added to your purchase	$
		Handling	$4.50
		Total	$

Name: _____

Address: _____

City: _____ State: _____ Zip: _____

Phone: _____ Fax: _____

Email: _____

• Check enclosed (Payable to SLACK Incorporated)_____

• Charge my: ____ [Amex] ____ VISA ____ MasterCard

Account #: _____

Exp. date: _____ Signature: _____

NOTE: *Prices are subject to change without notice.*
Shipping charges will apply.
Shipping and handling charges are non-returnable.

CODE: 328